1998
YEAR BOOK OF
ONCOLOGY®

Statement of Purpose

The YEAR BOOK Service

The YEAR BOOK series was devised in 1901 by practicing health professionals who observed that the literature of medicine and related disciplines had become so voluminous that no one individual could read and place in perspective every potential advance in a major specialty. In the final decade of the 20th century, this recognition is more acutely true than it was in 1901.

More than merely a series of books, YEAR BOOK volumes are the tangible results of a unique service designed to accomplish the following:

- to *survey* a wide range of journals of proven value
- to *select* from those journals papers representing significant advances and statements of important clinical principles
- to provide *abstracts* of those articles that are readable, convenient summaries of their key points
- to provide *commentary* about those articles to place them in perspective

These publications grow out of a unique process that calls on the talents of outstanding authorities in clinical and fundamental disciplines, trained literature specialists, and professional writers, all supported by the resources of Mosby, the world's preeminent publisher for the health professions.

The Literature Base

Mosby and its editors survey approximately 500 journals published worldwide, covering the full range of the health professions. On an annual basis, the publisher examines usage patterns and polls its expert authorities to add new journals to the literature base and to delete journals that are no longer useful as potential YEAR BOOK sources.

The Literature Survey

The publisher's team of literature specialists, all of whom are trained and experienced health professionals, examines every original, peer-reviewed article in each journal issue. More than 250,000 articles per year are scanned systematically, including title, text, illustrations, tables, and references. Each scan is compared, article by article, to the search strategies that the publisher has developed in consultation with the 270 outside experts who form the pool of YEAR BOOK editors. A given article may be reviewed by any number of editors, from one to a dozen or more, regardless of the discipline for which the paper was originally published. In turn, each editor who receives the article reviews it to determine whether the article should be included in the YEAR BOOK. This decision is based on the article's inherent quality, its probable usefulness to readers of that YEAR BOOK, and the editor's goal to represent a balanced picture of a given field in each volume of the YEAR BOOK. In addition, the editor indicates when to include figures and tables from the article to help the YEAR BOOK reader better understand the information.

Of the quarter million articles scanned each year, only 5% are selected for detailed analysis within the YEAR BOOK series, thereby assuring readers of the high value of every selection.

The Abstract

The publisher's abstracting staff is headed by a seasoned medical professional and includes individuals with training in the life sciences, medicine, and other areas, plus extensive experience in writing for the health professions and related industries. Each selected article is assigned to a specific writer on this abstracting staff. The abstracter, guided in many cases by notations supplied by the expert editor, writes a structured, condensed summary designed so that the reader can rapidly acquire the essential information contained in the article.

The Commentary

The YEAR BOOK editorial boards, sometimes assisted by guest commentators, write comments that place each article in perspective for the reader. This provides the reader with the equivalent of a personal consultation with a leading international authority—an opportunity to better understand the value of the article and to benefit from the authority's thought processes in assessing the article.

Additional Editorial Features

The editorial boards of each YEAR BOOK organize the abstracts and comments to provide a logical and satisfying sequence of information. To enhance the organization, editors also provide introductions to sections or individual chapters, comments linking a number of abstracts, citations to additional literature, and other features.

The published YEAR BOOK contains enhanced bibliographic citations for each selected article, including extended listings of multiple authors and identification of author affiliations. Each YEAR BOOK contains a Table of Contents specific to that year's volume. From year to year, the Table of Contents for a given YEAR BOOK will vary depending on developments within the field.

Every YEAR BOOK contains a list of the journals from which papers have been selected. This list represents a subset of approximately 500 journals surveyed by the publisher and occasionally reflects a particularly pertinent article from a journal that is not surveyed on a routine basis.

Finally, each volume contains a comprehensive subject index and an index to authors of each selected paper.

The 1998 Year Book Series

Year Book of Allergy, Asthma, and Clinical Immunology: Drs. Rosenwasser, Borish, Boguniewicz, Nelson, Routes, and Spahn

Year Book of Anesthesiology and Pain Management®: Drs. Tinker, Abram, Chestnut, Roizen, Rothenberg, and Wood

Year Book of Cardiology®: Drs. Schlant, Collins, Gersh, Graham, Kaplan, and Waldo

Year Book of Chiropractic®: Dr. Lawrence

Year Book of Critical Care Medicine®: Drs. Parrillo, Balk, Calvin, Franklin, and Shapiro

Year Book of Dentistry®: Drs. Meskin, Berry, Jeffcoat, Leinfelder, Roser, Summitt, and Zakariasen

Year Book of Dermatologic Surgery®: Drs. Greenway, Barrett, Papadopoulos, and Whitaker

Year Book of Dermatology and Dermatologic Surgery: Drs. Thiers and Lang

Year Book of Diagnostic Radiology®: Drs. Osborn, Groskin, Dalinka, Maynard, Pentecost, Rebner, Ros, Smirniotopoulos, and Young

Year Book of Drug Therapy®: Drs. Lasagna and Weintraub

Year Book of Emergency Medicine®: Drs. Wagner, Dronen, Davidson, King, Niemann, and Roberts

Year Book of Endocrinology®: Drs. Bagdade, Braverman, Horton, Kannan, Landsberg, Molitch, Morley, Nathan, Odell, Poehlman, Rogol, and Ryan

Year Book of Family Practice®: Drs. Berg, Bowman, Davidson, Dexter, and Scherger

Year Book of Gastroenterology®: Drs. Aliperti and Fleshman

Year Book of Geriatrics and Gerontology®: Drs. Burton, Beck, Ostwald, Rabins, Reuben, Roth, Shapiro, and Whitehouse

Year Book of Hand Surgery®: Drs. Amadio and Hentz

Year Book of Hematology®: Drs. Spivak, Bell, Ness, Quesenberry, Wiernik, and Horowitz

Year Book of Infectious Diseases: Drs. Keusch, Barza, Bennish, Poutsiaka, Skolnik, and Snydman

Year Book of Medicine®: Drs. Cline, Frishman, Jett, Klahr, Malawista, Mandell, McCallum, and Utiger

Year Book of Neonatal and Perinatal Medicine®: Drs. Fanaroff, Maisels, and Stevenson

Year Book of Nephrology, Hypertension, and Mineral Metabolism: Drs. Schwab, Bennett, Emmett, Hostetter, Kumar, and Toto

Year Book of Neurology and Neurosurgery®: Drs. Bradley and Gibbs

Year Book of Nuclear Medicine®: Drs. Gottschalk, Blaufox, Neumann, Strauss, and Zubal

Year Book of Obstetrics, Gynecology, and Women's Health: Drs. Mishell, Herbst, and Kirschbaum

Year Book of Occupational and Environmental Medicine®: Drs. Emmett, Frank, Gochfeld, and Hessl

Year Book of Oncology®: Drs. Ozols, Eisenberg, Glatstein, Loehrer, and Tallman

Year Book of Ophthalmology®: Drs. Wilson, Augsburger, Cohen, Eagle, Grossman, Laibson, Maguire, Nelson, Penne, Rapuano, Sergott, Spaeth, Tipperman, Ms. Gosfield, and Ms. Salmon

Year Book of Orthopedics®: Drs. Morrey, Beauchamp, Currier, Tolo, Trigg, and Swiontkowski

Year Book of Otolaryngology–Head and Neck Surgery®: Drs. Paparella and Holt

Year Book of Pathology and Laboratory Medicine®: Drs. Raab, Cohen, Olson, Sirgi, and Stanley

Year Book of Pediatrics®: Dr. Stockman

Year Book of Plastic, Reconstructive, and Aesthetic Surgery®: Drs. Miller, Bartlett, Garner, McKinney, Ruberg, Salisbury, and Smith

Year Book of Psychiatry and Applied Mental Health®: Drs. Talbott, Ballenger, Frances, Lydiard, Meltzer, Schowalter, and Tasman

Year Book of Pulmonary Disease®: Drs. Jett, Maurer, Ryu, Strollo, and Wenzel

Year Book of Rheumatology®: Drs. Panush, Hadler, LeRoy, Liang, Reichlin, Simon, and Weinblatt

Year Book of Sports Medicine®: Drs. Shephard, Drinkwater, Eichner, Torg, Alexander, and Mr. George

Year Book of Surgery®: Drs. Copeland, Bland, Deitch, Eberlein, Howard, Luce, Seeger, Souba, and Sugarbaker

Year Book of Thoracic and Cardiovascular Surgery®: Drs. Ginsberg, Wechsler, and Williams

Year Book of Urology®: Drs. Andriole and Coplen

Year Book of Vascular Surgery®: Dr. Porter

1998 The Year Book of ONCOLOGY®

Editor-in-Chief
Robert F. Ozols, M.D., Ph.D.
Senior Vice President of Medical Services, Fox Chase Cancer Center, Philadelphia, Pennsylvania

Mosby

St. Louis Baltimore Boston Carlsbad Naples New York Philadelphia Portland London
Madrid Mexico City Singapore Sydney Tokyo Toronto Wiesbaden

Mosby
Dedicated to Publishing Excellence

A Times Mirror Company

Associate Publisher: Gretchen C. Murphy
Developmental Editor: Jacquelyn M. Leonard
Production Editor: Pat Costigan
Project Supervisor, Production: Joy Moore
Production Assistant: Karie House
Manager, Literature Services: Idelle L. Winer
Illustrations and Permissions Specialist: Steve Ramay

1998 EDITION

Printed in the United States of America
Composition by Reed Technology and Information Services, Inc.
Printing/binding by Maple-Vail

Editorial Office:
Mosby, Inc.
11830 Westline Industrial Drive
St. Louis, MO 63146
Customer Service: customer.support@mosby.com
www.mosby.com/Mosby/CustomerSupport/index.html

International Standard Serial Number: 1040-1741
International Standard Book Number: 0-8151-9710-1

Associate Editors

Burton L. Eisenberg, M.D.
Professor of Surgery, Temple University School of Medicine; Chairman, Department of Surgery, Fox Chase Cancer Center, Philadelphia, Pennsylvania

Eli Glatstein, M.D.
Professor of Radiation Oncology, Hospital of University of Pennsylvania, Philadelphia, Pennsylvania

Patrick J. Loehrer, Sr., M.D.
Professor of Medicine, Section of Hematology/Oncology, Indiana University Medical Center, Indianapolis, Indiana

Martin S. Tallman, M.D.
Assistant Professor, Division of Hematology/Oncology, Northwestern University Medical School; Director, Clinical Leukemia Research Program of Robert H. Lurie Cancer Center of Northwestern University, Chicago, Illinois

Table of Contents

Journals Represented xiii
1. Cancer Etiology and Epidemiology 1
2. Cancer Biology, Markers, and Diagnosis 13
3. Breast Cancer 61
4. Gynecologic Malignancies 85
5. Prostate Cancer 103
6. Genitourinary Cancer 115
7. Gastrointestinal Cancer 139
8. Adult Leukemia 197
9. Adult Lymphoma 207
10. Pediatric Solid Tumors 225
11. Brain Tumors 227
12. Lung Cancer 231
13. Head and Neck Cancer 243
14. Skin Cancer 255
15. Sarcomas 261
16. Bone Marrow Transplantation and Stem Cell Support 279
17. Basic Radiation Therapy and Radiation Biology 291
18. Pharmacology 307
19. Novel Therapy 321
20. Complications of Therapy 333
21. Supportive Care 345
Subject Index. 357
Author Index 387

Journals Represented

Mosby and its editors survey approximately 500 journals for its abstract and commentary publications. From these journals, the Editors select the articles to be abstracted. Journals represented in this YEAR BOOK are listed below.

American Journal of Human Genetics
American Journal of Pathology
American Journal of Public Health
American Journal of Surgery
American Surgeon
Annals of Internal Medicine
Annals of Oncology
Annals of Surgery
Annals of Surgical Oncology
Annals of Thoracic Surgery
Archives of Otolaryngology-Head and Neck Surgery
Archives of Surgery
Blood
Bone Marrow Transplantation
British Journal of Cancer
British Journal of Surgery
British Journal of Urology
British Medical Journal
Canadian Journal of Surgery
Cancer
Cancer Research
Chest
Clinical Cancer Research
Clinical Infectious Diseases
Diseases of the Colon and Rectum
European Journal of Cancer
Experimental Hematology
Gynecologic Oncology
Head and Neck
Human Pathology
International Journal of Radiation, Oncology, Biology, and Physics
Journal of Clinical Investigation
Journal of Clinical Oncology
Journal of Cutaneous Pathology
Journal of Nuclear Medicine
Journal of Surgical Oncology
Journal of Thoracic and Cardiovascular Surgery
Journal of Urology
Journal of the American College of Surgeons
Journal of the American Medical Association
Journal of the National Cancer Institute
Lancet
Leukemia
New England Journal of Medicine
Proceedings of the National Academy of Sciences
Radiology
Radiotherapy and Oncology

Southern Medical Journal
Surgery
Thorax
Western Journal of Medicine
World Journal of Surgery

Standard Abbreviations

The following terms are abbreviated in this edition: acquired immunodeficiency syndrome (AIDS), cardiopulmonary resuscitation (CPR), central nervous system (CNS), cerebrospinal fluid (CSF), computed tomography (CT), deoxyribonucleic acid (DNA), electrocardiography (ECG), health maintenance organization (HMO), human immunodeficiency virus (HIV), intensive care unit (ICU), intramuscular (IM), intravenous (IV), magnetic resonance (MR) imaging (MRI), and ribonucleic acid (RNA).

Note

The Year Book of Oncology is a literature survey service providing abstracts of articles published in the professional literature. Every effort is made to assure the accuracy of the information presented in these pages. Neither the editors nor the publisher of the Year Book of Oncology can be responsible for errors in the original materials. The editors' comments are their own opinions. Mention of specific products within this publication does not constitute endorsement.

To facilitate the use of the Year Book of Oncology as a reference tool, all illustrations and tables included in this publication are now identified as they appear in the original article. This change is meant to help the reader recognize that any illustration or table appearing in the Year Book of Oncology may be only one of many in the original article. For this reason, figure and table numbers will often appear to be out of sequence within the Year Book of Oncology.

1 Cancer Etiology and Epidemiology

Cancer Undefeated
Bailar JC III, Gornik HL (Univ of Chicago)
N Engl J Med 336:1569–1674, 1997 1–1

Introduction.—Even with intensive clinical and basic science research, cancer continues to be a major cause of morbidity and mortality. Because of advances in diagnostic techniques, the reported incidence of cancer is not a reliable indicator of trends in incidence over time. Age-adjusted mortality is a more useful measure of progress in the fight against cancer. Trends in age-adjusted mortality were analyzed to assess the progress made against cancer from the 1970s to the 1990s.

Methods.—The analysis used National Center for Health Statistics data on all cancer deaths and on deaths from cancer at specific sites from 1970 through 1994. Data on cancer deaths also were broken down by age, race, and sex. Age-specific mortality rates were calculated and adjusted to the 1990 age distribution of the U.S. population.

Results.—Age-adjusted cancer mortality increased from 189.6 per 100,000 population in 1970 to 200.9 per 100,000 in 1994. Age-adjusted all-cancer mortality decreased steadily for several decades, then reached a plateau before decreasing 1% from 1991 to 1994. Groups achieving the greatest reduction in cancer mortality were African-American men and individuals younger than 55 years old. In recent years, white men age 55 years or older have had a reduction in mortality. These trends include changes in mortality from specific types of cancer, including stomach, cervical, and uterine cancer and leukemia; reductions in cigarette smoking, achieved decades ago; and improvements in cancer screening. For childhood cancers, mortality rates have dropped by about 50% since the 1970s, and they continue to drop.

Conclusions.—Recent years have seen some small reductions in cancer mortality, largely because of changes in cancer incidence or early detection. New cancer treatments have had little impact on mortality. These trends suggest that a focus on prevention, with an attendant shift in the focus and funding of research, is the best approach to reducing cancer mortality.

► In 1986, Drs. Bailar and Smith published a treatise titled "Progress Against Cancer?" in which they wrote, "Some 35 years of intense effort focused largely on improving treatment must be judged a qualified failure." Over a decade later, Dr. Bailar (now with Dr. Gornik) revisits the progress we have made. The recent trends in age-adjusted cancer mortality finally appear to be declining. This improvement is particularly noted for those men and women younger than age 55 years (decrease of 25%) and those with leukemia, colorectal cancer, and childhood malignancies. Like a schoolteacher using a fingernail instead of a piece of chalk on a blackboard, these authors remind us that for older patients, cancer-related mortality is increased by 15% to 20%. They also caution us against a unilateral approach to cancer research by stating, "The present optimism about new therapeutic approaches rooted in molecular medicine may turn out to be justified, but the arguments are similar in tone and rhetoric to those of decades past about chemotherapy, tumor virology, immunology and other approaches."

This paper, like the previous one, is provocative in reminding us of the work yet to be done on this disease.

P.J. Loehrer, Sr., M.D.

The Relationship Between Patient Income and Physician Discussion of Health Risk Behaviors

Taira DA, Gelb Safran D, Seto TB, et al (New England Med Ctr, Boston; Tufts Univ, Boston; Beth Israel Deaconess Med Ctr, Boston)

JAMA 278:1412–1417, 1997 1–2

Introduction.—To address the steep annual cost of health risk behaviors upon society, the U.S. Preventive Services Task Force recommended universal risk assessment of patients' alcohol and cigarette consumption, diet, exercise, stress, seat belt, and safe sex practices and discussions of these health risk behaviors with patients, when indicated. It has been found that the prevalence of physician assessment and discussion of health risk behaviors is low despite the physicians believing that health risk behaviors are important risk factors. The relationship between patient income, unhealthy behaviors, the likelihood of physician discussion of these behaviors, and the receptiveness of patients to their physician's advice was examined.

Methods.—A patient-completed mail survey was used to obtain data from 6,549 participants who were all employed. Differences in the prevalence of health risk behaviors, physician discussion of these behaviors, and patient receptiveness to discussions in relation to patient income were discerned with trend tests.

Results.—Physician discussion of health risk behaviors fell far short of the universal risk assessment recommended by the U.S. Preventive Services

Task Force, and unhealthy behaviors were common among all income groups. High-income patients were less likely to be obese and smoke and were more likely to wear seat belts and exercise than low-income patients. However, higher-income patients had increases in stress and alcohol consumption, whereas the proportion of heavy drinkers did not vary significantly. Diet and exercise were more likely to be discussed between physicians and high-income patients than between low-income patients and physicians. However, physicians were more likely to discuss smoking with low-income patients than with high-income patients. Low-income patients were more likely to report attempting to change their behavior based on physician advice among physicians with whom discussions occurred.

Conclusion.—If the U.S. Preventive Services Task Force recommendations are to be fulfilled, physician counseling of patients regarding health risk behaviors should be greatly improved. Alcohol consumption, safe sex, and seatbelt use are the areas where improvement is especially needed. Low-income patients should be identified and counseled on diet and exercise while high-income patients need to be identified and counseled on smoking.

▶ Physicians have a significantly positive impact on health risk behaviors of patients. Despite recognizing numerous risk factors for many diseases, physicians have been inconsistent in their role as patient counselors. This trial suggests that patients, in the group that needs the advice the most (i.e., the lower socioeconomic population), do worse. There are many reasons for this, including coexistent medical problems (which are often multiple and severe), communication problems, costs, time constraints, and the lack of perceived benefit by the physicians. This study reminds health care providers of our responsibilities to effect positive change.

P.J. Loehrer, Sr., M.D.

Molecular Damage in the Bronchial Epithelium of Current and Former Smokers

Wistuba II, Lam S, Behrens C, et al (Univ of Texas, Dallas; British Columbia Cancer Agency, Vancouver; Johns Hopkins Univ School of Hygiene and Public Health, Baltimore, Md; et al)

J Natl Cancer Inst 89:1366–1373, 1997 1–3

Background.—Lung cancers attributed to smoking have been associated with multiple genetic changes and the presence of preneoplastic bronchial lesions. The status of specific chromosomal loci in histologically normal and abnormal bronchial biopsy specimens from current smokers, former smokers, and nonsmokers was determined.

Methods.—Research subjects included 18 current smokers, 24 former smokers, and 21 nonsmokers. Multiple bronchial biopsy specimens were obtained by fluorescence bronchoscopy. Eight chromosomal regions were examined using 15 polymorphic microsatellite DNA markers.

Findings.—Eighty-six percent of the patients with histories of smoking had loss of heterozygosity (LOH) in 1 or more biopsy specimens. Twenty-four percent of this group showed LOH in all biopsy specimens. About half of the histologically normal specimens obtained from smokers showed LOH. However, the frequency of LOH and the severity of the histologic change did not correspond until the carcinoma in situ stage. Loss of heterozygosity on chromosomes 3p and 9p was more common than on chromosomes 5q, 17p, and 13q. Sixty-four percent of the smokers showed microsatellite changes. There were no genetic changes in nonsmokers.

Conclusions.—Genetic changes similar to those detected in lung cancers are apparent in the nonmalignant bronchial epithelium of current and former smokers. These changes may persist for many years after quitting smoking.

► It seems to me that the most important genetic information with respect to cancer that has been delineated in the last 15 years is that cancer represents a cascade of mutations, not just 1 simple mutation. There are multiple events that take place in the evolution of what we call a cancer, and this group of investigators studying lung cancer is largely responsible, along with a few other laboratories, for shedding light on this problem.

In this study, they look at the status of specific chromosomal changes in normal and abnormal bronchial biopsy specimens from current and former smokers, as well as specimens from nonsmokers. The investigators report LOH and microsatellite alterations in both current and former smokers but no statistically significant difference between the 2. Loss of heterozygosity was seen in 86% of patients who had histories of smoking. About half of the histologically normal specimens from smokers showed LOH, but the frequency of LOH and the severity of the histologic changes did not correspond until the point at which carcinoma in situ was able to be detected. A set of biopsy specimens from smokers that exhibited either normal or preneoplastic changes showed an LOH at multiple chromosomal sites, which is an observation frequently made in carcinoma in situ and in invasive cancer. No genetic alterations were detected in nonsmokers. The important point is that once genetic changes actually occurred and mutations became incorporated into the cells' constitutional makeup, those genetic changes persisted for many, many years after the cessation of smoking.

I believe that this work on the evolution of mutations in high-risk smokers will serve to be the basis of a new approach to lung cancer in the next century. I think we will be able to screen for high-risk patients, obtain cells via bronchoscopy, analyze these cells for mutations such as p53, and others, and, at some propitious level of change, treat these patients on an interventional, preventive basis by means of photodynamic therapy or retinoids.

E. Glatstein, M.D.

The Accumulated Evidence on Lung Cancer and Enviromental Tobacco Smoke

Hackshaw AK, Law MR, Wald NJ (St Bartholomew's and Royal London School of Medicine and Dentistry)

BMJ 315:980–988, 1997 1–4

Introduction.—Exposure to environmental tobacco smoke can be measured in nonsmokers via increased urinary and blood concentrations of tobacco-specific carcinogens. The risk of lung cancer in lifelong nonsmokers exposed to environmental tobacco smoke was evaluated.

Methods.—A MEDLINE search was performed to identify epidemiologic trials on the risk of lung cancer in nonsmokers who did and did not live with a smoker. Thirty-seven trials were identified (4,626 patients). The risk estimate in this cohort was compared with that from linear extrapolation of the risk in smokers using 7 investigations of biochemical markers of tobacco smoke intake. Urine or saliva concentrations of cotinine and nicotine were used to estimate the risk of lung cancer in nonsmokers exposed to environmental tobacco smoke by extrapolating from the risk in smokers. The relative risk of lung cancer was estimated in lifelong nonsmokers according to whether their spouses currently smoked or had never smoked.

Results.—Pooled data from 37 investigations revealed an excess risk of lung cancer of 24% in nonsmokers who lived with a smoker. After adjusting for the effect of bias and dietary confounding, the adjusted excess risk was 26%. There was a significant dose-response association between the risk of lung cancer and both the number of cigarettes smoked by the spouse and the duration of exposure. The indirect and direct estimates of excess risk were similar: 19% and 26%, respectively.

Conclusion.—Females who have never smoked have an estimated 24% higher risk of lung cancer if they live with a smoker. There is a dose-response correlation between a nonsmoker's risk of lung cancer and the number of cigarettes smoked and years of exposure to environmental tobacco smoke.

▶ It has been a decade since the first evidence of a relationship between environmental (or second-hand) smoke and lung cancer has emerged. Although some smoking advocates have discounted the impact of environmental smoke, the analysis of 37 studies involving over 4,000 patients shows that an excess lung cancer risk among nonsmokers is clearly evident and that there is a dose-response relationship. This paper provides an excellent review of accumulated evidence regarding environmental smoke collected thus far.

P.J. Loehrer, Sr., M.D.

The National Cancer Data Base Report on Malignant Epithelial Ovarian Carcinoma in African-American Women

Parham G, Phillips JL, Hicks ML, et al (Univ of Arkansas, Little Rock; American College of Surgeons, Chicago; Henry Ford Hosp, Detroit; et al)

Cancer 80:816–826, 1997 1–5

Introduction.—Several studies have shown that there is not a universal access to excellent medical care in the United States. For example, blacks have more leg amputations than whites, and these differences can persist even after adjustments are made for income and variations in clinical characteristics. The fifth cause of cancer death affecting black women is ovarian carcinoma. Outcomes of gynecologic cancers affecting black women were compared with those of white women.

Methods.—Black women and non-Hispanic white women who received a diagnosis of invasive epithelial tumors of the ovary were compared. The white women were classified as "White–same facility" or "White–other facility." The white women from the same facility classification were those

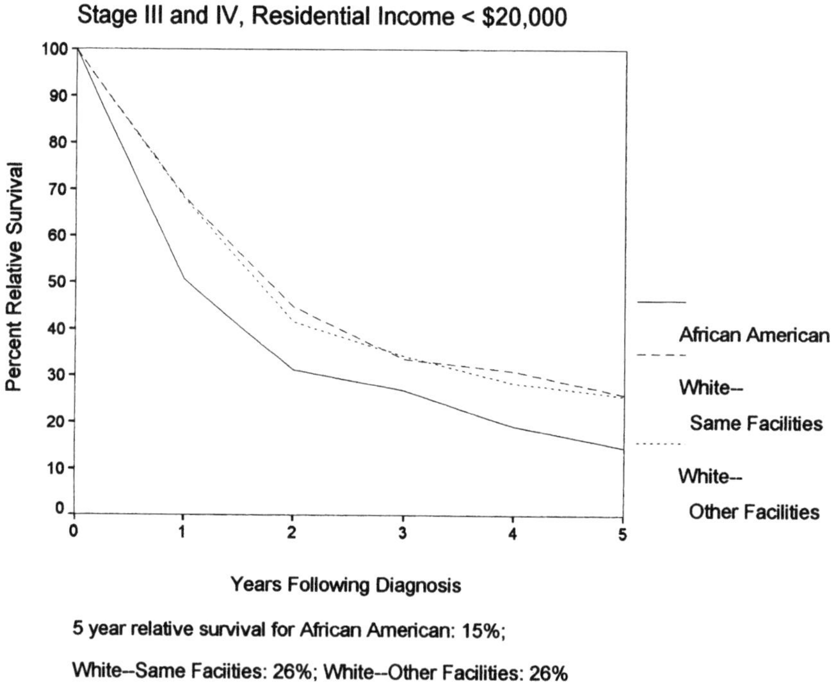

FIGURE 3, C.—Relative survival by income, stage, and racial groups in patients with invasive malignant epithelial ovarian carcinoma diagnosed 1985–1988. Patients had stage III and IV disease, and residential income of less than $20,000. Five-year relative survival for African Americans, 15%; White–same facilities, 26%; White–other facilities, 26%. Source: National Cancer Data Base. (Courtesy of Parham G, Phillips JL, Hicks ML, et al: The National Cancer Data Base report on malignant epithelial ovarian carcinoma in African-American women. *Cancer* 80:816–826. Copyright 1997, American Cancer Society. Reprinted by permission of Wiley-Liss, Inc., a subsidiary of John Wiley & Sons, Inc.)

who were in the same hospital as a substantial number of black women, and those classified in another facility were white women who were treated in hospitals that had a very few number of black women treated. A history of prior cancer was not evident in any of the women.

Results.—Black women with advanced invasive epithelial ovarian cancer were more often treated with chemotherapy only and less often treated with surgery and chemotherapy. White women were twice as likely to receive appropriate treatment than their black counterparts. Regardless of income, black women had poorer survival rates than white women from the same or different hospitals (Fig 3, C). Black women had stage IV disease diagnosed more often among the staged patients when compared with both groups of white women.

Conclusions.—Less aggressive treatment was given to black women with advanced epithelial ovarian carcinoma, and they had a poorer prognosis when compared with white women.

▶ This study raises many disturbing questions regarding the treatment of ovarian cancer in African-American women. Why are these women frequently not treated with aggressive surgery and combination chemotherapy? It is apparent that African-American women frequently wait too long to seek medical attention for symptoms associated with ovarian cancer progression. But advanced disease at presentation is not likely to account for the substandard therapy that these women receive. It is imperative that behavioral studies be performed to determine the roles of education, physician mistrust, misrepresentation of outcomes, physician bias, and economic incentives in the decision-making process, which leads unnecessarily to inferior survival for African-American women afflicted with ovarian cancer.

R.F. Ozols, M.D., Ph.D.

Over-the-Counter Analgesics and Risk of Ovarian Cancer

Cramer DW, Harlow BL, Titus-Ernstoff L, et al (Harvard Med School, Boston; Dartmouth-Hitchcock Med Ctr, Lebanon, NH)

Lancet 351:104–107, 1998 1–6

Background.—Evidence suggests that aspirin and other nonsteroidal anti-inflammatory drugs (NSAIDs) decrease the risk for colorectal cancer. The effect of over-the-counter analgesics on the risk of ovarian cancer was tested.

Methods.—In a case-control study, over-the-counter analgesic use among 563 women with epithelial ovarian cancer was compared with that of 523 women from the general population. Over-the-counter analgesic use was determined in interviews.

Findings.—After adjustment for age; study center; education; religion; parity; oral contraceptive use; and menstrual, arthritis, or headache pain, aspirin use was associated with an 0.75 odds ratio for ovarian cancer risk; other odds ratios were ibuprofen, 1.03; and paracetamol, 0.52. Compared with no use, the lower risk associated with paracetamol was more apparent for daily use (0.39), for more than 10 years of use (0.4), and for more than 20 tablet-years (0.45).

Conclusion.—Paracetamol use was significantly inversely associated with ovarian cancer risk. Aspirin use was modestly, but nonsignificantly, inversely related to ovarian cancer risk. Ovarian cancer risk was not associated with ibuprofen use.

▶ This is the first report of a possible protective effect of acetaminophen use upon the risk of ovarian cancer. A major problem of this study is that there is no strong biological rationale as to how acetaminophen could possibly decrease the risk of ovarian cancer. Furthermore, there are possible medical risks associated with long-term and excessive use of acetaminophen. Without further confirmatory studies and a biological hypothesis as to the mechanism of a protective effect, it is way too early to recommend acetaminophen as a chemopreventive agent for ovarian cancer.

R.F. Ozols, M.D., Ph.D.

Survival of *BRCA1* Breast and Ovarian Cancer Patients: A Population-based Study From Southern Sweden

Jóhansson OT, Ranstam J, Borg A, et al (Univ Hosp, Lund, Sweden)

J Clin Oncol 16:397–404, 1998 1–7

Introduction.—For developing breast cancer, a positive family history of breast cancer is a well-known risk factor. How family history of breast cancer influences survival of breast cancer patients is still not clear. Mutations in the gene *BRCA1* confer a high risk for development of breast and ovarian cancer, but whether carriers of *BRCA1* have a better or worse survival than other breast or ovarian cancer patients is still not known. Survival of breast and ovarian cancer patients belonging to families carrying *BRCA1* germline mutations was compared with survival of a population-based comparison group.

Methods.—Survival in a population-based group with 28,281 invasive breast cancers and 7,011 ovarian cancers diagnosed over 37 years was compared with survival in 71 patients with *BRCA1*-associated cancer (33 breast cancer, 7 breast and ovarian cancer, and 31 ovarian cancer) from 21 families with *BRCA1* germline mutations (Fig 1).

Results.—On direct comparison no apparent survival advantage was found for patients with *BRCA1*-associated breast cancers. Survival was equal to or worse than that in the comparison group after adjustment for age and calendar year of diagnosis. Survival appeared equal or worse in comparison with survival in an age- and stage-matched control group. An initial survival advantage was noted that disappeared over time for *BRCA1*-associated ovarian cancers. Multivariant analyses cannot adequately be analyzed because of this time dependency. Survival appeared

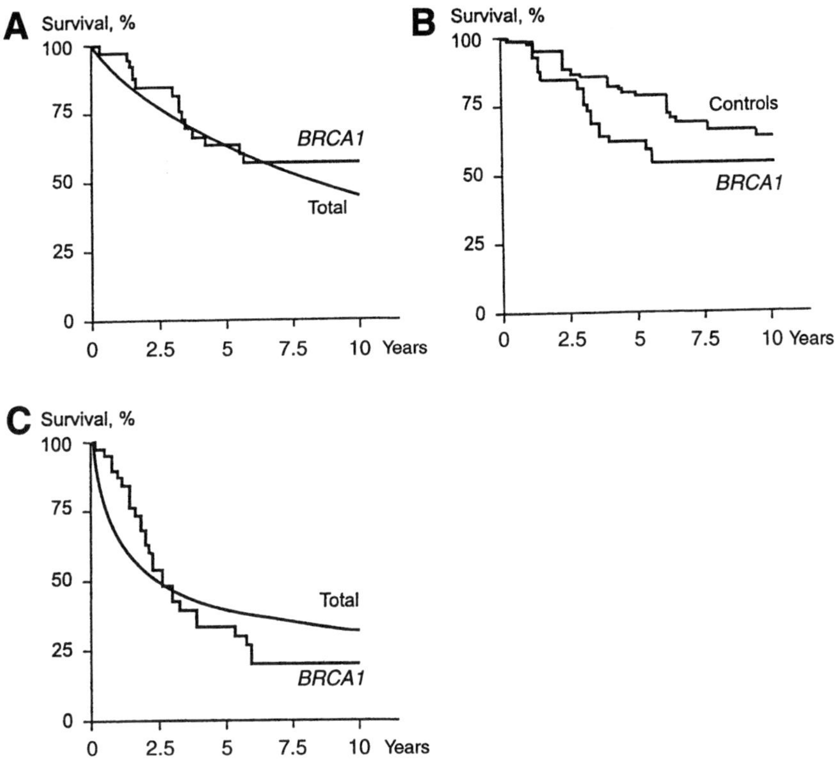

FIGURE 1.—A, overall survival of *BRCA1* breast cancer cases diagnosed from 1958 to 1995 (n = 40) vs. survival of all other breast cancer patients (n = 28,281) diagnosed in south Sweden from 1958 to 1995. B, overall survival of *BRCA1* breast cancer cases diagnosed from 1958 to 1995 (n = 40) and a comparative group (n = 112) of age- and stage-matched breast cancer cases. C, overall survival of *BRCA1* ovarian cancer cases diagnosed from 1958 to 1995 (n = 38) vs. survival of all other ovarian cancer patients (n = 7,011) diagnosed in south Sweden from 1958 to 1995. (Courtesy of Jóhannsson OT, Ranstam J, Borg A, et al: Survival of *BRCA1* breast and ovarian cancer patients: A population-based study from Southern Sweden. *J Clin Oncol* 16:397–404, 1998.)

equal or worse when compared with that in the age- and stage-matched control group.

Conclusion.—For carriers of a *BRCA1* mutation, survival may be similar or worse than that in patients with ovarian or breast cancer in general, according to the adverse histopathologic features found in *BRCA1* tumors. Families that carry a *BRCA1* mutation must be under surveillance.

▶ Germline mutations in *BRCA1* increase the risk for both breast and ovarian cancer. The lifetime risk for development of ovarian cancer for *BRCA1* carriers is estimated to be 16% to 40%. The impact of a mutated *BRCA1* gene on the natural history of ovarian cancer and breast cancer compared with the sporadic forms of these diseases remains controversial. Rubin et al.[1] reported an improved survival for women with ovarian cancer if they were carriers of the mutated *BRCA1* gene. This population-based study from Sweden suggests that, if anything, the prognosis for women with breast and ovarian cancer who are carriers of the mutated gene is worse than for these diseases in general. The results indicate the need to develop effective prevention strategies in these women.

R.F. Ozols, M.D., Ph.D.

Reference

1. Rubin S, Benjamin I, Behbakht K, et al: Clinical and pathological features of ovarian cancer in women with germ-line mutations of *BRCA1*. *N Engl J Med* 335:1413–1416, 1996.

Prospective Seroepidemiologic Study of Human Papillomavirus Infection as a Risk Factor for Invasive Cervical Cancer

Dillner J, Lehtinen M, Björge T, et al (Karolinska Inst, Stockholm; Natl Public Health Inst at Helsinki; Inst for Epidemiological Cancer Research, Oslo, Norway; et al)

J Natl Cancer Inst 89:1293–1299, 1997 1–8

Objective.—Human papillomavirus (HPV) infection, infection with other sexually transmitted diseases such as *Chlamydia trachomatis*, and cigarette smoking are risk factors for invasive cervical cancer. The individual contributions of each of these risks have not been established. The HPV-associated risk for invasive cervical cancer was assessed in a prospective study.

Methods.—Blood samples were obtained from 700,000 residents of Finland, Norway, and Sweden. Women were followed for 5 years, and the 182 women with a diagnosis of invasive cervical cancer were age-matched with 538 controls in a nested case-control study. *Chlamydia trachomatis,* HPV, and serum serology were determined at enrollment. Relative risks for cervical cancer were estimated using conditional regression analysis.

Results.—Infection with HPV was associated with an increased risk of cervical cancer (relative risk [RR] = 2.4). Neither smoking nor *C. trachomatis* infection increased the risk significantly. Infection with HPV16 increased the relative risk of squamous cell carcinoma in the low sexually transmitted disease prevalence cohort (RR = 11.8). Infection with HPV18 increased the relative risk of adenocarcinoma in all cohorts (RR = 3.4).

Conclusion.—Infection with HPV16 increased the relative risk of squamous cell carcinoma in the low sexually transmitted disease prevalence cohort (RR = 11.8). Infection with HPV18 increased the relative risk of adenocarcinoma in all cohorts (RR = 3.4). Smoking and *C. trachomatis* infection did not increase those risks.

▶ This definitive study clearly presents the importance of known risk factors for invasive cervical cancer. Antibodies against HPV were associated with a marked increased risk of cervical cancer. Seropositivity for HPV16 was associated primarily with an increased risk of squamous cell carcinoma, whereas HPV18 seropositivity was associated with risk of cervical adenocarcinomas. This association was most evident in populations with a low prevalence of sexually transmitted diseases (STDs). In populations with a high risk of STDs, it appears that a saturation level of exposure among control subjects is reached, resulting in HPV exposure no longer being the major measurable risk factor for cervical cancer. This does not obviate the causal role of HPV in cervical cancer in patients with a high prevalence of STDs.

R.F. Ozols, M.D., Ph.D.

2 Cancer Biology, Markers, and Diagnosis

Decline in Telomerase Activity as a Measure of Tumor Cell Killing by Antineoplastic Agents in Vitro

Faraoni I, Turriziani M, Masci G, et al (Univ of Rome; Istituto Dermopatico dell'Immacolata, Rome; Univ of Texas Southwestern Med Ctr, Dallas)

Clin Cancer Res 3:579–585, 1997 2–1

Background.—Telomerase is a ribonucleoprotein DNA polymerase that adds an enzyme to the ends of chromosomes in dividing cells to ensure stability and prevent aging. In terminally differentiated cells, telomerase activity is sparse or absent, whereas most tumor cells express telomerase activity. It is therefore believed that telomerase activity may be useful as a marker for neoplastic cell survival. This possibility was examined in telomerase-positive human tumor cells treated by antineoplastic agents in vitro.

Methods.—Human cell lines from T-cell leukemia (Jurkat), histiocytosis (U937), breast adenocarcinoma (MCF-7) and its subline that is resistant to doxorubicin (MCF-7/DOXO), and normal endometrial cells were used. Cells were exposed in vitro to the antitumor drugs *cis*-diamminedichloroplatinum(II)(CDDP), doxorubicin, and temozolomide (TEMO). Telomerase activity was assessed by the telomerase repeat amplification protocol (TRAP).

Findings.—In the Jurkat cell line, both CDDP and doxorubicin (at concentrations inhibiting cell growth by 50%) inhibited telomerase activity by 24 hours of treatment (73% and 63% inhibition, respectively). In the U937 cell line, TEMO had a similar effect on telomerase activity (41% inhibition at 48 hours, 90% inhibition at 72 hours). Doxorubicin treatment of the MCF-7 cell line showed 94% and 98% inhibition of telomerase activity at 48 and 72 hours. Treatment of cell lines by a drug to which those cell lines are resistant (e.g., treatment of MCF-7/DOXO by doxorubicin) did not affect telomerase activity.

Conclusions.—As the antineoplastic drugs killed tumor cells, telomerase activity decreased substantially. The TRAP assay needs only 15 tumor cells for analysis, and even fine-needle aspiration can supply this amount. Thus, the monitoring of telomerase activity may prove useful for assessing cell chemosensitivity to particular antineoplastic agents.

▶ This is another paper on telomerase and its almost ubiquitous association with cancer. This Italian study indicates that successful destruction of tumor cells by drugs is associated with a significant decline in detectable telomerase activity. The study suggests that resistance of cancer cells to various chemotherapeutic agents might be able to be monitored simply by following telomerase activity. This could prove to be a useful chemosensitivity assay, but it obviously requires considerable additional investigation.

E. Glatstein, M.D.

▶ It has recently been demonstrated that telomerase expression is strongly correlated with cell immortalization and the malignant phenotype. It is expressed in continuously dividing cells and helps maintain chromosomal stability. In the absence of telomerase activity, repetitive sequences are not added to the ends of chromosomes during cell division and this shortening leads to an inhibition of cell proliferation. Telomerase activity is increased in the majority of tumor tissues and is not expressed in terminally differentiating cells of most organs. This study describes a novel test to measure telomerase activity after treatment with antineoplastic agents. The findings support a larger study to determine whether an in vitro chemosensitivity assay based on detection of telomerase activity may be used to identify active agents for individual patients.

R.F. Ozols, M.D., Ph.D.

Telomerase Activity in Ordinary Meningiomas Predicts Poor Outcome
Langford LA, Piatyszek MA, Ruishu XU, et al (Univ of Texas, Houston; Univ of Texas, Dallas; Geron Corp, Menlo Park, Calif)
Hum Pathol 28:416–420, 1997 2–2

Introduction.—Telomerase is an enzyme that stabilizes the length of telomeres, long stretches of repetitive DNA sequences that prevent the chromosome ends from being recognized as broken DNA molecules in need of repair. Nearly all types of cancer are associated with telomerase reactivation, which may be essential for unlimited cell proliferation. It can be difficult to tell whether meningiomas are malignant or not, because there are no histologic or karyotypic abnormalities that are clearly associated with aggressive clinical behavior. Telomerase activity was compared with clinical behavior in ordinary meningiomas.

Methods.—The study included 52 patients undergoing surgery for meningioma. Each tumor was evaluated for telomerase activity using the telomeric repeat amplification protocol, a highly sensitive assay. Neo-

TABLE 1.—Clinical Data and Telomerase Activity for 52 Tumor Samples From 52 Patients

Tumor	No.	No. of Telomerase-Positive Biopsies (%)	No. of Telomerase-Negative Biopsies (%)	Age Range at Time of Surgery (yr)	Mean Age at Time of Surgery (yr)	Male-Female Ratio
Ordinary meningioma	30	5 (17)	25 (83)	11–80	53	8:22
Atypical meningioma	13	12 (92)	1 (8)	36–79	59	8:5
Malignant meningioma	9	9 (100)	0	30–75	60	4:5
Total	52	26 (50)	26 (50)	11–80	57	20:32

Note: Some patients had multiple biopsy samples evaluated (data not shown); in these cases, telomerase assay results were similar.
(Courtesy of Langford LA, Piatyszek MA, Ruishu XU, et al: Telomerase activity in ordinary meningiomas predicts poor outcome. *Human Pathol* 28:416–420, 1997.)

plasms with and without detectable telomerase activity were identified, and the patients in these 2 groups were compared for freedom from recurrence.

Results.—Half of the tumors had detectable telomerase activity (Table 1). Twenty-two tumors were classified as malignant or atypical; all but 1 of these had detectable telomerase activity. Most patients with these tumors had a poor outcome. The remaining 30 tumors were ordinary, i.e., morphologically benign meningiomas. Seventeen percent of these tumors had detectable telomerase activity. Three of 5 patients with telomerase-positive ordinary meningiomas had rapid tumor regrowth after gross total resection, whereas the other 2 patients had other primary cancers. The presence of telomerase activity in an ordinary meningioma was highly significantly correlated with poor prognosis.

Conclusions.—Assessment of telomerase activity may be relevant in benign meningiomas. The finding of telomerase positivity suggests that the apparently benign tumors may have a population of immortal cells. Studies of telomerase activity may be useful in identifying benign meningiomas that are likely to recur after complete surgical resection. The findings open the way to new treatments aimed at blocking telomerase.

▶ Telomerase is an enzyme that stabilizes the length of the telomere during cell division. It appears to be increased in activity with almost every kind of cancer that is imaginable. Indeed, it may actually prove to be necessary for unlimited cell proliferation, although at present that is not clear. This is a provocative study from Texas that looked at 52 cases of meningiomas of which half had detectable telomerase activity. Of the 22 neoplasms that were thought to be malignant or atypical, 21 had detectable telomerase and patients with those tumors in general did poorly. Of the 30 patients whose tumors were thought to be morphologically benign, 5 had tumors that also showed detectable telomerase activity. Three of those patients had rapid regrowth of tumor and the other 2 patients had other primary malignancies.

It is certainly conceivable that telomerase acticivity may be a valuable test in selecting patients with meningiomas that should receive additional treatment beyond surgery. Only time will tell on this, but these are provocative data that need corroboration.

E. Glatstein, M.D.

Fascin, a Sensitive New Marker for Reed-Sternberg Cells of Hodgkin's Disease: Evidence for a Dendritic or B Cell Derivation?

Pinkus GS, Pinkus JL, Langhoff E, et al (Harvard Med School, Boston; Rutger's Univ, Piscataway, NJ; Univ of California, Los Angeles)

Am J Pathol 150:543–562, 1997 2–3

Introduction.—The origin of the Reed-Sternberg cell, the hallmark of Hodgkin's disease, remains controversial despite the discovery of this disease more than 150 years ago. A localization pattern that appeared

TABLE 3.—Detection of Fascin and Epstein-Barr Virus in Hodgkin's Disease and Selected Non-Hodgkin's Lymphomas

Diagnosis	Number of cases positive/number of cases evaluated EBV positive*	Fascin positive
Hodgkin's disease		
Nodular sclerosis	27/121 (22%)	121/121 (100%)
Mixed cellularity	24/33 (73%)	33/33 (100%)
Lymphocyte depletion	2/2	2/2
Lymphocyte predominance	0/14	0/14
Post-transplant B cell lymphoproliferative disorders	8/8 (100%)	3/8 (38%)
B cell lymphomas in HIV$^+$ patients	8/12 (67%)	3/12† (25%)

*Only cases evaluated for both EBV and fascin were included. Studies for EBV latent membrane protein were performed for Hodgkin's cases. For other lymphomas, EBV detection included studies for EBNA-2, LMP, Southern blot analysis, and/or in situ hybridization for EBV RNA (EBER-1).

†All fascin-positive cases were also EBV-positive and represent 3/8 (38%) of EBV-positive cases.

Abbreviation: EBV, Epstein-Barr virus.

(Courtesy of Pinkus GS, Pinkus JL, Langhoff E, et al: Fascin, a Sensitive New Marker for Reed-Sternberg Cells of Hodgkin's Disease: Evidence for a Dendritic or B Cell Derivation? *Am J Pathol* 150:543–562, 1997. Permission granted: Copyright American Society for Investigative Pathology.)

highly restricted to dendritic cells was demonstrated in human peripheral blood cells with the use of a monoclonal antibody to human fascin, a 55-kd actin-bundling protein initially isolated from HeLa cells. A comprehensive staining profile for fascin in normal and neoplastic lymphoid tissues was defined. To determine whether reactivity for fascin may provide insights into the pathogenesis of Hodgkin's disease, a large series of Hodgkin's disease of various histologic types and a variety of non-Hodgkin's lymphomas were evaluated.

Methods.—There were 187 cases of Hodgkin's disease retrieved, with 132 having nodular sclerosis, 34 having mixed cellularity, 14 with lymphocyte predominance, 2 with lymphocyte depletion, and 5 that were unclassified. These were compared to neoplastic tissues of 14 reactive lymph nodes, 4 thymuses, and 3 spleens. The comparison also included 156 specimens that involved B- or T-cell neoplasms. Fixed tissues were used to perform all the studies.

Results.—Reactivity was highly selective and localized predominantly in dendritic cells in nonneoplastic tissues. This protein was localized to medullary dendritic cells in the thymus. Only dendritic cells were reactive for fascin in the peripheral blood. In the Hodgkin's disease cases, nearly all Reed-Sternberg cells and variants were immunoreactive for fascin. Strong diffuse cytoplasmic staining and frequently assumed dendritic shapes, producing an interdigitating meshwork or syncytial network of cells, were exhibited in the neoplastic cells. L&H variants were nonreactive in all 14 patients with nodular lymphocyte predominance type (Table 3). By contrast, reactivity for fascin was demonstrated in 24 of 156 (15%) other lymphoid neoplasms, and this evaluation included 127 B cells, 27 T cells, and 2 null-cells.

Conclusion.—For detection of certain dendritic cells in normal and neoplastic tissues, fascin represent a highly effective marker. Fascin also is extremely consistent as a marker for Reed-Sternberg cells and variants of Hodgkin's disease, except for L&H types. In difficult cases, fascin may help distinguish between Hodgkin's disease and non-Hodgkin's disease. In the majority of nonlymphocyte predominance cases, the highly selective B-cell marker did not support a B-cell derivation for Reed-Sternberg cells. The Epstein-Barr virus may induce fascin expression, thus in patients with Epstein-Barr virus, the possibility that viral induction of fascin in lymphoid or other cell types must be considered.

▶ Ever since I started working in this field, we have been arguing about the origin of the Reed-Sternberg cell in Hodgkin's disease. This is an interesting paper that talks about fascin, which appears to be a distinct protein seen in a variety of lymphoid tissues. In peripheral blood, only dendritic cells react for fascin, but what was remarkable was that in Hodgkin's disease virtually all the Reed-Sternberg cells or their variants were immunoreactive for this substance. The authors suggest that the derivation of the Reed-Sternberg cell could well be dendritic in origin, particularly the interdigitating reticulum cell in the nodular sclerosing type. On the other hand, they also suggest that the expression of fascin could be induced by the Epstein-Barr virus infection of B cells. This appears to be an important step in answering the question of where the Reed-Sternberg cells originate, although they have not resolved that issue quite yet. The illustrations are impressive, and hopefully this article will be helpful in answering that perplexing question regarding Hodgkin's disease.

E. Glatstein, M.D.

High Levels of Wilms' Tumor Gene (wt1) mRNA in Acute Myeloid Leukemias Are Associated With a Worse Long-term Outcome

Bergmann L, Miething C, Maurer U, et al (JW Goethe Univ, Frankfurt, Germany)

Blood 90:1217–1225, 1997 2–4

Background.—Studies of patients with Wilms' tumor have identified the tumor suppressor gene wt1, which encodes for a zinc finger DNA-binding protein that is a transcription factor with mostly repressing activity on different target genes. Expression of wt1 is frequently found in patients with acute myeloid leukemias, and thus may be a useful marker of minimal residual disease or prognosis. Expression of wt1 mRNA was evaluated as a prognostic indicator and predictor of relapse in patients with AML.

Methods.—Studies were performed in totally bone marrow–derived blasts of 139 patients with AML. One hundred twenty-nine patients were studied at initial diagnosis of AML, and 22 of these were studied again at first relapse. The remaining 10 patients were initially studied at first relapse. Expression of wt1 mRNA was studied in each sample. In 77 patients, wt1 mRNA expression was studied during follow-up. The researchers used a wt1-specific reverse transcription–polymerase chain reaction (RT-PCR), and classified the amplification product as not, weakly, moderately, or strongly amplified. Quantitative analysis of the PCR products was performed in representative cases. Expression of wt1 was correlated with various factors, including age, French-American-British (FAB) subtype, phenotype, karyotype, and long-term survival.

Results.—Seventy-seven percent of samples, at diagnosis and at first relapse, showed detectable wt1 mRNA. This finding was unrelated to age, previous myelodysplastic syndrome, or FAB subtype, although only 40% of M5 leukemias showed wt1 transcripts. Levels of wt1 mRNA were unrelated to treatment response or karyotype-determined prognostic group. Among patients with newly diagnosed AML, 3-year overall survival was 13% for those with high levels of wt1 vs. 38% for those with undetectable or low wt1 levels. For de novo AML, survival was 12% and 43%, respectively. The wt1-related differences in survival were more marked for patients younger than 60 years. All patients who went into complete remission became negative for wt1.

Conclusions.—The Wilm's tumor gene appears to be a significant prognostic indicator in AML, with high wt1 mRNA expression associated with a worse long-term outcome. Performing wt1 analyses on routine bone marrow specimens may provide additional prognostic information, as well as define the quality of remission and provide an early predictor of disease relapse. More research is needed to define the role of wt1 in detecting minimal residual disease or its role in the pathogenesis of acute leukemias.

▶ Because of the considerable interest in determining prognostic factors for patients with newly diagnosed AML, this report demonstrating that expression of the tumor suppressor gene wt1 confirms an unfavorable prognosis is of interest. We are now learning that a variety of prognostic factors can be used to predict prognosis, including white blood cell count at diagnosis, karyotype, the expression of multidrug resistance, and Wilm's tumor gene expression. However, the latter now provides an actual potential mechanism of resistance of leukemia cells.

M.S. Tallman, M.D.

Use of Hematopoetic Cytokines to Accelerate the Recovery of the Immune System in Irradiated Mice

Frasca D, Guidi F, Arbitrio M, et al (Lab of Immunology, Rome)
Exp Hematol 25:1167–1171, 1997 2–5

Background.—These authors have previously shown that interleukin (IL)-3 can induce the differentiation and growth of thymocytes and splenic T and B lymphocytes in mice with radiation-induced damage to the bone marrow (200 to 500 cGy). Subsequent research has indicated that IL-11 has similar effects. In this article, they report on the utility of IL-3 and IL-11 in combination to promote hematopoiesis in mice with radiation-induced bone marrow damage.

Methods.—Four groups of 3- to 6-month-old mice were used. The control group received no irradiation. The other groups each received total body irradiation with 500 cGy. For each of 7 days these animals received 0.1 mL phosphate-buffered saline solution with 0.1% bovine serum albumin. The second group was given 5 μg of human recombinant IL-11 alone on days 1 through 5. Groups 3 through 7 received 5 μg IL-11 in combination with 4–8 μg of murine recombinant IL-3 on days 1 through 5. Four animals in each group were killed on day 7. Thymocyte, splenocyte, and bone marrow cell counts were performed.

Findings.—Irradiation with 500 cGy significantly decreased the thymocyte count and mitotic activity. The injection of IL-11 alone did little to improve these parameters. However, IL-11 in combination with IL-3 significantly increased the thymocyte count and the mitotic response. The best response occurred with an IL-3 dose of 7 μg and the IL-11 dose of 5 μg. This optimal dose returned all thymocyte cell levels to normal by 7 days. Results for splenocyte count and T- and B-lymphocyte mitotic responses were similar, in that IL-11 had no effect on its own, but had a significant effect when combined with IL-3 in doses from 6 to 8 μg. Irradiation of bone marrow cells caused more cells to be in the S phase of the cell cycle and less cells to be in the G_0/G_1 phase. Again, immediate treatment with 5 days of IL-3 and IL-11 restored cell fractions to levels in mice that had not been irradiated.

Conclusions.—In mice, radiation-induced damage to thymus and spleen cells could be reversed by a combination of IL-3 and IL-11. It is suspected that IL-11 acts very early to stimulate hematopoietic progenitor cells, and then IL-3 helps these cycling cells differentiate. This synergistic effect of IL-3 and IL-11 suggests a role for these interleukins in treating patients undergoing radiation therapy to prevent radiation-induced injury to bone marrow.

▶ Perhaps it is because I am a radiation oncologist, but I find this article interesting in that it evaluates two of the newer cytokines (IL-3 and IL-11) in terms of their ability to induce differentiation in growth of a variety of lymphocytes and thymocytes after exposure to radiation therapy. We have known for a long time that radiation therapy is immunosuppressive, and these agents apparently are able to minimize some of those effects, at least in mice. I think it would be of considerable interest to study their effects in patients. Perhaps these cytokines can prevent at least some of the known immunosuppression that is associated with radiation therapy.

E. Glatstein, M.D.

Detection of Mutant K-*ras* DNA in Plasma or Serum of Patients With Colorectal Cancer

Kopreski MS, Benko FA, Kwee C, et al (Pennsylvania College Univ, Hershey)

Br J Cancer 76:1293–1299, 1997 2–6

Background.—The recognition that extracellular DNA circulates in the plasma and serum of patients with colorectal cancer has enabled new approaches to detection and monitoring. A polymerase chain reaction (PCR) assay was used to demonstrate mutant K-*ras* DNA in the plasma or serum of such patients.

Methods.—Thirty-one patients with metastatic or unresected colorectal cancer and 28 healthy volunteers were studied. Plasma or serum was fractionated from blood obtained from both groups, and DNA was extracted by a sodium chloride or gelatin precipitation method. The DNA was then amplified in a 2-stage PCR assay using selective restriction enzyme digestion to enrich for mutation K-*ras* DNA.

Findings.—Mutant K-*ras* DNA was found in the plasma or serum of 39% of the patients. In all cases, the findings were confirmed by sequencing. Such mutations were not present in any of the healthy persons. K-*ras* mutations were identified in plasma or serum regardless of sex, primary tumor location, principal site of metastasis, or proximity of chemotherapy and surgery to blood sampling. Tumor specimens, available from 19 patients, were also assayed for *ras* mutations and compared with blood specimens.

Conclusion.—Mutant K-*ras* DNA is readily detectable by PCR in the plasma or serum of patients with advanced colorectal cancer. Thus, plasma- or serum-based nucleic acid amplification assays may be a valuable way of monitoring and potentially detecting colorectal cancer.

▶ Molecular medicine is already changing traditional beliefs regarding the malignant phenotype in humans. As more sophisticated techniques that can be applied in routine clinical oncology evolve, genetic risk factors, molecular targets for potential therapeutic intervention, and definition of new intracellular diagnostic and prognostic features will become part of patient management.

This paper describes several types of methodologies used for extracting and amplifying tumor DNA (mutated K-*ras*) in the plasma or serum of patients with colon cancer. Techniques of PCR can be used to detect minute quantities of RNA or DNA in either cellular blood fraction, serum, or tumor specimens, and multiplex assays can expand the scope of detection for specific, but less clustered, gene mutations. Application to clinical medicine in terms of early detection of primary or recurrent disease, response to therapy, or actually directing specific therapy await more extensive data accumulation and subsequent clinical trials.

B.L. Eisenberg, M.D.

Relationship Between Lifetime Ovulatory Cycles and Overexpression of Mutant p53 in Epithelial Ovarian Cancer

Schildkraut JM, Bastos E, Berchuck A (Duke Univ, Durham, NC)

J Natl Cancer Inst 89:932–938, 1997 2–7

Background.—The number of ovulatory cycles appears to be related to the development of ovarian epithelial cancer. It has been hypothesized that a greater number of ovulatory cycles increases ovarian cancer risk by inducing DNA damage associated with proliferation during ovarian surface repair after ovulation. The relationship between lifetime number of ovulatory cycles and mutation of the p53 tumor-suppressor gene (TP53) in ovarian tumors was studied.

Methods.—Participants in the Cancer and Steroid Hormone study were included in the case-control study. One hundred ninety-seven case patients with invasive ovarian epithelial cancer and 3,363 control subjects 20- to 54-years-old were included. Overexpression of p53 protein in paraffin-embedded ovarian cancer tissue blocks indicated p53 gene mutation.

Findings.—Women with cancers overexpressing p53 protein had a higher mean number of lifetime ovulatory cycles than those who were p53 negative. Women with p53-positive tumors were more likely to have had moderate or high numbers of ovulatory cycles than those with p53-negative tumors. Women with p53-positive tumors were significantly more likely to have had moderate or high numbers of cycles than control subjects after adjustment for age, menopausal status, and nulliparity.

Conclusion.—A greater number of ovulatory cycles may be related to increased amounts of proliferation-associated DNA damage and an increased risk of p53-positive (but not p53-negative) epithelial ovarian cancer. These findings support the notion that there may be more than one developmental pathway in the pathogenesis of such cancer.

► It has long been known that a woman's risk for ovarian cancer is related directly to the number of ovulatory cycles. Any condition that decreases ovulations, such as pregnancy and oral contraceptive use, decreases a woman's risk. It is also known that ovarian cancer is a heterogeneous disease and numerous molecular alterations have been identified. This interesting study provides some persuasive evidence that there is more than 1 pathway for the pathogenesis of ovarian cancer. Those ovarian cancers that may be associated with increased ovulatory cycles can be characterized by increased mutations of the tumor suppressor gene p53. One of the many functions of the p53 protein is to block division of cells that have sustained DNA damage, permitting DNA repair, or if the damage is irreparable, to initiate apoptotic cell death. In the absence of p53 or in the presence of mutated dysfunctional p53, damaged cells will continue to proliferate, increasing the risk of tumor formation. Studies such as this are important in finding strategies to prevent the development of ovarian cancer. Tumors that are associated with ovulation are targets for agents that could interfere with ovulation. For example, epidemiologic studies have already shown that oral contraceptives significantly decrease lifetime risk for ovarian cancer, particularly in women nulliparous or those with a positive family history. Strategies aimed at prevention of ovarian tumors not associated with ovulation will be dependent on unraveling the pathogenic mechanisms involved.

R.F. Ozols, M.D., Ph.D.

Serum Inhibin and Disease Status in Women With Ovarian Granulosa Cell Tumors

Boggess JF, Soules MR, Goff BA, et al (Univ of Washington, Seattle)
Gynecol Oncol 64:64–69, 1997 2–8

Background.—Normal granulosa cells of the ovary secrete inhibin, an important growth factor within the ovary. Inhibin levels were found to be elevated in women with granulosa cell tumors of the ovary. Thus, are inhibin levels useful as a marker of granulosa cell tumors? Whether monitoring inhibin levels was useful in the treatment and follow-up of these patients was investigated.

Methods.—This retrospective analysis involved 15 patients aged 27–78 years with proved granulosa cell tumors who had undergone a bilateral oophorectomy. All patients provided serum samples for the measurement of inhibin concentrations. Levels of inhibin were analyzed by radioimmunoasssay to determine their correlation with disease status. Patients with no symptoms and no clinical findings of disease were considered to be in remission.

Findings.—Serum inhibin levels ranged from 0 to 7,470 U/L. Four of 15 patients had measurable recurrent disease and elevated inhibin levels; tumor burden and inhibin level showed a strong correlation ($r^2 = 0.96$). Another 4 patients who were in remission but later had a recurrence also had elevated inhibin levels; the increase in inhibin level predated disease recurrence by a median of 11.5 months. The remaining 7 patients were in remission for 9–53 months. In 4 of these patients whose disease was staged, the 2 patients with stage I disease had no measurable inhibin, whereas the 2 patients with metastatic disease (stage IIC and IIIa) had elevated inhibin levels.

Conclusions.—There is a strong relationship between the inhibin level and granulosa cell tumors, with an elevated level indicating disease. Inhibin levels were undetectable in patients who were disease-free. Although more research is needed, monitoring serum inhibin levels could help identify those patients most likely to benefit from adjuvant chemotherapy to reduce the risk of recurrence.

► Granulosa cell tumors of the ovary are uncommon and account for only 2% to 5% of ovarian malignancies. Inhibin is a member of the TGF-β family of growth factors and is secreted by granulosa cells of normal ovarian follicles. On the basis of previous studies that suggested elevated inhibin levels were common in patients with granulosa cell tumors of the ovary, the investigators performed a retrospective analysis to determine whether serum inhibin levels provided clinically useful information in the treatment or follow-up of patients with granulosa cell tumors of the ovary. Although questions remain regarding the sensitivity and specificity of the currently available inhibin assays in patients who have ovarian function, the results of this study do suggest that there is a correlation between inhibin levels and tumor burden. Measurement of inhibin may be useful in detection of early recurrence, as well as for monitoring response to treatment in patients with granulosa cell tumors of the ovary.

R.F. Ozols, M.D., Ph.D.

Risk of Diagnosis of Ovarian Cancer After Raised Serum CA 125 Concentration: A Prospective Cohort Study

Jacobs IJ, Skates S, Davies AP, et al (St Bartholomew's Hosp, London; Harvard Med School, Boston)

BMJ 313:1355–1358, 1996 2–9

Background.—Serum levels of CA 125 are commonly used as markers of ovarian cancer. However, their role as a screening tool is not known. A large group of women were evaluated to determine the relationship between CA 125 levels and the risk for ovarian cancer.

Methods.—Over almost 4 years, 19,464 women 45 years of age or older with ovarian cancer were evaluated by annual incidence screening (n = 9,344) or annual postal questionnaire (n = 10,120) for 3 years. Patients with a CA 125 blood level of 30 U/mL or more were examined by abdominal US and, if results were abnormal, the patient was referred for surgery. The cumulative and relative risks of developing ovarian or fallopian tube cancer (i.e., the index cancers) given a particular CA 125 level were determined.

Findings.—A total of 47,755 screening tests for CA 125 levels were performed. Of those, 1,180 (2.5%, from 767 patients) showed a serum CA 125 level of 30 U/mL or more, with 49 patients having an index cancer. At 1, 3, 5, and 7 years of follow-up, the sensitivity of the CA 125 level to identify these cancers was 75%, 54%, 48%, and 47%, respectively. The overall specificity of the CA 125 level to identify these malignancies was 97%, and its positive predictive value was 3%. The cumulative risk of developing an index cancer was 0.0022, but patients with a CA 125 level less than 30 U/mL were significantly less at risk than those with CA 125 levels of 30 U/mL or more or those with levels greater than 100 U/mL (0.0012 vs. 0.030 vs. 0.149, respectively). Likewise, the relative risk of developing an index cancer increased as the CA 125 level increased (relative risk 1 year after a screening, from 0.13 to 36 to 205 for CA 125 levels less than 30, 30 or more, and greater than 100 U/mL, respectively).

Conclusions.—Less than 3% of all women screened showed elevated CA 125 levels. Nonetheless, as the serum CA 125 level increased, so did the relative and cumulative risks for ovarian or fallopian tube cancer in these postmenopausal women. But, although the serum CA 125 level can certainly indicate risk in women with clinically advanced disease, its role in the diagnosis of such malignancies in their preclinical stages is still undetermined. Thus, whether the serum CA 125 level can be used as a screening tool remains unanswered.

▶ This study clearly defines the increased risk for ovarian cancer associated with an elevated CA 125 level. However, the problem with CA 125 screening is the low positive predictive value, which is defined as a percentage of screen-positive women who actually have ovarian cancer. Most women who have an elevated CA 125 will not have ovarian cancer and the positive predictive value in this study was 3.1%. Consequently, there is an unacceptably high level of false positive test results. The strategy used by the investigators is to follow up a patient with an elevated CA 125 level with an US examination, and if that result is abnormal, then to proceed to surgery. It should be emphasized that although this study demonstrates that a raised serum CA 125 level is associated with a high risk for development of ovarian cancer, it does not establish the efficacy of a screening program for ovarian cancer. There is no randomized study that has yet shown that screening for ovarian cancer using CA 125 levels or transvaginal sonography or both procedures is associated with a decreased mortality from this disease.

R.F. Ozols, M.D., Ph.D.

Contribution of *BRCA1* Mutations to Ovarian Cancer

Stratton JF, Gayther SA, Russell P, et al (WellBeing Ovarian Cancer Research Centre, Cambridge, England; Cancer Research Campaign Human Cancer Genetics Research Group, Cambridge, England; Royal Marsden Hosp, London)

N Engl J Med 336:1125–1130, 1997 2–10

Background.—Mutations in the *BRCA1* gene carry a risk for the inheritance of breast and ovarian cancer in some families. However, its role in these cancers in the general population is not known. The frequency of *BRCA1* mutations in women with ovarian cancer who did not necessarily have a family history of ovarian cancer was examined.

Methods.—Blood samples were drawn for DNA analysis from 374 women with ovarian cancer who were younger than 70 years old. Only 31 patients reported a family history of ovarian cancer. Genomic DNA was extracted by standard methods and the *BRCA1* coding sequence was analyzed by multiplex heteroduplex analysis. Variant patterns underwent sequencing. Results of chromosomal analysis in these patients were compared with those of 380 normal chromosomes in 190 women without ovarian cancer.

Findings.—Six variants of a probable germ-line *BRCA1* mutation were found in 13 women (3%). One patient had an in-frame deletion of GAT near the zinc-finger domain, and the other 12 had truncation mutations.

Of those 12, 9 (75%) had a family history of ovarian cancer or breast cancer or both. Furthermore, all 12 had serous cystadenocarcinomas of the ovary.

Conclusions.—In this general population, 3% of women with ovarian cancer had a *BRCA1* mutation; assuming a testing sensitivity of 70%, then, the true proportion of such mutations in the general population would be 5%. In women with a family history, there was a strong association between *BRCA1* mutation and serous cystadenocarcinoma of the ovary. It is suggested that genetic testing in women with a family history of at least 1 case of breast cancer before age 60 years or 1 case of ovarian cancer in a first- or second-degree relative would detect most *BRCA1* mutations (9 of 13 in this study).

▶ Ovarian cancer is primarily a disease of the elderly population and the median age of diagnosis is approximately 60 years. Hereditary ovarian cancer is characterized by early onset and patients frequently receive the diagnosis premenopausally. *BRCA1* mutations account for a majority of women with a hereditary ovarian cancer syndrome, which is often associated with breast cancer and other tumors as well. In that group of women, there is considerable uncertainty regarding how best to manage and counsel those who are *BRCA1* carriers. This study demonstrates that the vast majority of women with epithelial ovarian cancer are unlikely to harbor mutations in *BRCA1*. Almost 400 women with ovarian cancer who were unselected for family history were examined, and *BRCA1* mutations were found in only 13 women (3%). It has been reported that some genetically isolated populations, such as Ashkenazi Jews, have a higher prevalence of *BRCA1* mutations. Although *BRCA1* mutations perhaps account for the majority of hereditary ovarian cancers, it is possible that other mutations, such as *BRCA2* and genes associated with mismatched repair, for example, may also be associated with increased risk of ovarian cancer.

This study also points out the problems associated with strategies for screening women for *BRCA1* mutations. It is clear that women without a family history of ovarian cancer should not be screened for *BRCA1* mutations. For example, if genetic testing were restricted to women with at least 1 relative with breast cancer diagnosed before the age of 60 or 1 case of ovarian cancer in a first- or second-degree relative (in addition to the index case), a majority of women who have *BRCA1* mutations would have been detected (9 of 13) in this study. As the authors point out, with such a policy only 20% of women with ovarian cancer would be screened.

R.F. Ozols, M.D., Ph.D.

Expression of Angiogenesis-related Genes and Progression of Human Ovarian Carcinomas in Nude Mice
Yoneda J, Kuniyasu H, Crispens MA, et al (Univ of Texas, Houston)
J Natl Cancer Inst 90:447–454, 1998 2–11

Introduction.—Ovarian cancer is the leading cause of death from gynecologic cancer with a mortality rate of about 50%. In the majority of patients, metastasis has occurred within the peritoneum by the time of diagnosis, and lesions can give rise to ascitic tumor cells with survival being inversely associated with tumor size and accumulation of ascites. The growth and spread of neoplasms depends on the formation of angiogenesis, and several angiogenic molecules have been identified in the last decade, including basic fibroblast growth factor. The proliferation of endothelial cells is induced by vascular endothelial growth factor and active neovascularizatoin has been associated with the levels of matrix metalloproteinase-2 and matrix metalloproteinase-9. The relationship between the expression of various angiogenic molecules and the pathologic behavior of 5 different human ovarian cancers growing in nude mice was investigated.

Methods.—Into the peritoneal cavity of female NC4-nu/nu nude mice, 5 different human ovarian carcinomas were injected individually. Immunohistochemical analysis, in situ hybridization of messenger RNA, and Northern blot analysis were used to determine the expression of basic fibroblast growth factor, vascular endothelial growth factor/vascular permeability factor, interleukin-8, and collagenase type IV (Fig 1).

Results.—Solid lesions and ascitic tumors were produced by 3 of the carcinomas, whereas only solid lesions were produced by the remaining 2 carcinomas. Rapidly progressive disease was produced by 2 of the carcinomas, slow disease was produced by 2, and intermediate disease was produced by 1. Expression of vascular endothelial growth factor/vascular permeability factor was directly associated with the formation of ascites, and expression of interleukin-8 was inversely associated with survival. Through the lesions, the number of blood vessels was high in rapidly growing tumors. Most vessels and infiltrating macrophages were located at the periphery in slow-growing tumors.

Conclusion.—The pattern of the disease and its progression are associated with the expression of various genes that regulate angiogenesis in human ovarian carcinomas. New approaches to the treatment of ovarian cancer may be found by targeting specific genes that regulate angiogenesis.

► Specific genes regulate angiogenesis, which is essential for tumor growth and progression. This important study is among the first to examine the expression of various genes that regulate angiogenesis and the pattern of metastases of specific tumors. The authors' experimental model consisted of ovarian cancer cells implanted into nude mice. The carcinomas that produced ascites had increased expression of vascular endothelial growth factor/vascular permeability factor and survival was inversely associated

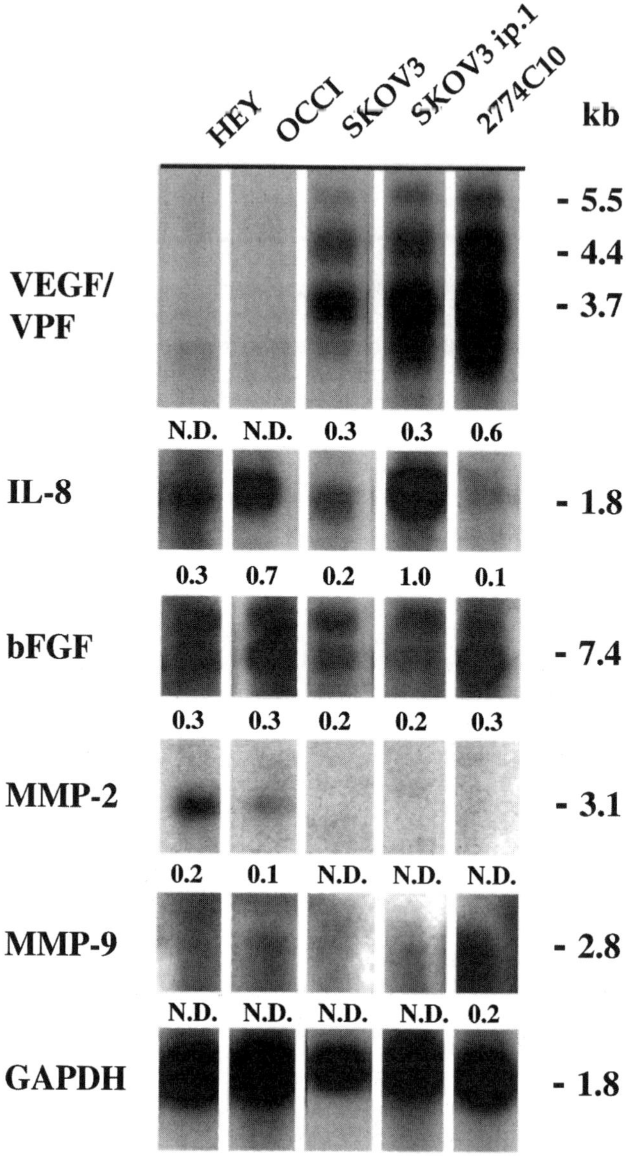

FIGURE 1.—Northern blot analysis for angiogenesis-related genes in 5 human ovarian carcinomas (i.e., HEY-A8 [HEY], OCCI, SKOV3, SKOV3ip.1, and 2774-C10) growing in culture. Polyadenylated messenger RNA (mRNA) (5 μg per lane) was used to detect the specific mRNA transcripts. A rat glucose-6-phosphate dehydrogenase (GAPDH) probe was used as an internal control. For densitometric quantitation, the ratio of the area between the specific transcripts and the 1.3-kilobase (kb) GAPDH transcript was compared and is recorded for each case. *Abbreviations*: *N.D.*, not detected; *VEGF/VPF*, vascular endothelial growth factor/vascular permeability factor; *IL-8*, interleukin 8;*bFGF*, basic fibroblast growth factor; *MMP*, matrix metalloproteinase. (Courtesy of Yoneda J, Kuniyasu H, Crispens MA, et al: Expression of angiogenesis-related genes and progression of human ovarian carcinomas in nude mice. *J Natl Cancer Inst* 90:447–454, 1998, by permission of Oxford University Press.)

with expression of interleukin-8. These results not only point out the importance of angiogenesis inhibition, but also identify specific gene targets.

R.F. Ozols, M.D., Ph.D.

Telomerase Activity in Benign and Malignant Epithelial Ovarian Tumors

Wan M, Li W-Z, Duggan BD, et al (Univ of South California, Los Angeles)

J Natl Cancer Inst 89:437–441, 1997 2–12

Introduction.—Among the most lethal of the gynecologic cancers is the ovarian epithelial tumor; however, not all of these tumors are malignant. Cystadenomas are made up of secretary cells and are considered neoplastic. Tumors of low malignant potential (LMP) also are found in the ovarian epithelial tumor category, and their apparent benign clinical behavior has led some to believe that they should be considered variants of cystadenomas. As a means of better defining the similarities between ovarian LMP tumors and either cystadenomas or carcinomas, the expression of the enzyme telomerase, which is generally expressed in malignant tumor cells, was examined. Telomerase activity was compared in ovarian carcinomas and cystadenomas.

Methods.—There were 64 consecutive ovarian tumors that were subdivided into 27 cystadenomas, 17 LMP tumors, and 20 carcinomas. Without knowledge of the telomerase results, tumor subtyping was conducted. Without knowledge of tumor types, telomerase assays were interpreted. The telomeric repeat amplification protocol assay was used to determine telomerase activity. Fisher's exact test was used to evaluate the differences in the proportions of tumors expressing this enzyme in each subgroup.

Results.—In all 20 carcinomas and in all 17 LMP tumors, telomerase activity was detected. In 19 of the 24 cystadenomas, however, telomerase activity was not detected. There was a statistical significance in the differences of rates of telomerase expression in carcinomas or LMP tumors and in cystadenomas. A variant called papillary cystadenomas accounted for all 5 of the telomerase-positive cystadenomas.

Conclusions.—In spite of their benign clinical course, LMP tumors should be separated from cystadenomas. Papillary cystadenomas should be reclassified as variants of LMP tumors because of the finding of telomerase expression. Expression of telomerase is thought to be essential for continuous growth in adult tumors; thus its lack in ovarian cystadenomas raises questions about the alleged immortality of these tumors.

► Telomeres are specialized structures at the ends of eukaryote chromosomes with characteristic DNA sequences that are vital for DNA replication and cell division. Telomeres become progressively shorter with each cell division and thereby permit cells to undergo only a limited number of divisions. Tumor cells have activated telomerase that restores the length of telomeres and may be critical in sustaining continuous cell division, a characteristic of malignancy. Not only is telomerase a new key target for development of specific inhibitors that may be useful in therapy, but measurement of telomerase activity may also be useful in diagnosis. In addition, it is clear that telomerase activity can be used to unravel mechanisms of molecular carcinogenesis. This study demonstrates that the uncontrolled growth exhibited by ovarian tumors of low malignant potential can be accounted for, in part, by the presence of telomerase expression in these tumors. Telomerase activity may be useful in separating benign and malignant precursors of ovarian tumors.

R.F. Ozols, M.D., Ph.D.

Quantitative Differences in Telomerase Activity Among Malignant, Premalignant, and Benign Ovarian Lesions

Kyo S, Takakura M, Tanaka M, et al (Kanazawa Univ, Japan; Nippon Gene Co Ltd, Toyama, Japan)

Clin Cancer Res 4:399–405, 1998 2–13

Introduction.—Telomerase activity has been found in a variety of malignant tumors, irrespective of tumor type, but little is known about its activity in premalignant and benign lesions. For quantitation of telomerase activity, stretch polymerase chain reaction has recently been developed. In a variety of malignant, premalignant, and benign lesions of the ovary, telomerase activity was quantitatively determined using this new technique.

Methods.—In a variety of ovarian lesions, including 36 ovarian cancers, 5 ovarian low potential malignancy lesions, 10 ovarian cysts, and 12 normal ovaries, telomerase activity was quantitatively determined using a recently developed stretch polymerase chain reaction assay. Normalized to control activity (100 units) in the C33A cell line, telomerase activity was given in relative units.

Results.—In ovarian cancer, telomerase activity was 51±7 units and was significantly higher than in ovarian cysts (10±2 units), ovarian low potential malignancy lesions (7±3 units), and normal ovaries (10±2 units) (Fig 3). Low telomerase activity of less than 30 units was seen in all ovarian low potential malignancy lesions, ovarian cysts, and normal ovaries. The level of telomerase activity did not differ significantly among these. The clinical stage of ovarian cancer and the level of telomerase activity were significantly correlated.

Conclusion.—Telomerase activity in low potential malignancy lesions and ovarian cysts was clearly distinguished from that found in ovarian cancers. In cancer, significant levels of telomerase activation frequently occurred, but in premalignant and benign lesions, it rarely occurred. In the development of cancer, telomerase activation is suggested to be a critical step. In metastatic ovarian tumors, telomerase activity was significantly lower than in primary ovarian tumors, possibly because telomerase activity was diluted by the abundant stromal tissues characteristic of this tumor type.

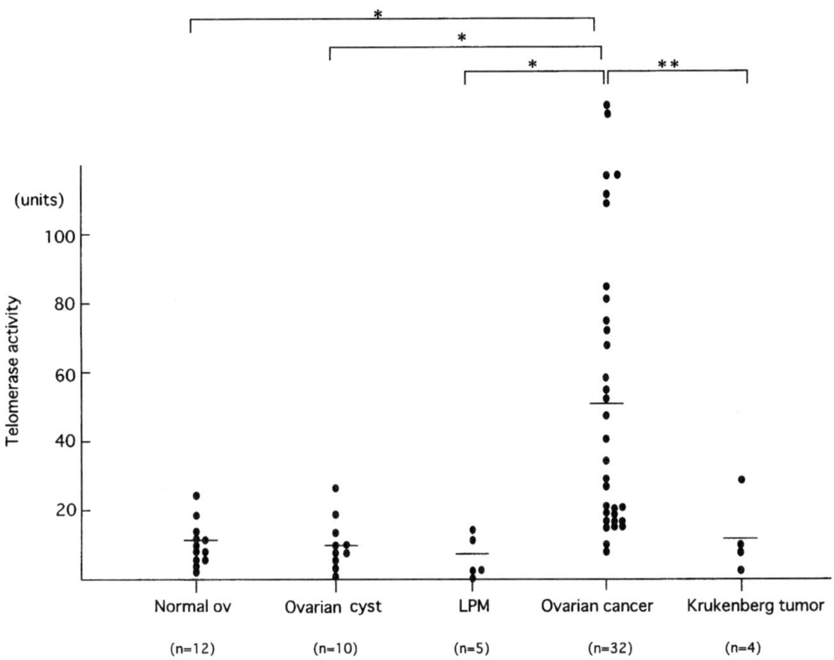

FIGURE 3.—Telomerase activity in ovarian tumors. Levels of the telomerase activities in various ovarian lesions were determined by stretch polymerase chain reaction assay. The activity was normalized to control activity (100 units) in C33A cells and given in relative units. $*P < 0.001$; $**P = 0.007$; $***P = 0.02$. *Abbreviation*: *LPM*, low potential malignancy. (Courtesy of Kyo S, Takakura M, Tanaka M, et al: Quantitative differences in telomerase activity among malignant, premalignant and benign ovarian lesions. *Clin Cancer Res* 4:399–405, 1998.)

▶ Telomeres (distal ends of human chromosomes) are thought to be involved in cellular senescence or conversely in cellular immortality. Telomere length is dependent upon the activity of telomerase. Repression of telomerase activity leads to shortening of telomere repeats and to senescence. Telomerase reactivation stabilizes telomere length and facilitates continual cell replication, which is a hallmark of neoplastic growth. Support for the importance of telomerase activity in ovarian cancer pathogenesis is provided by this study, which measured activity of this enzyme in ovarian cysts, tumors of low malignant potential, and in invasive epithelial tumors. The increased activity of this enzyme in invasive carcinomas thus may have some diagnostic applications. Perhaps more importantly, telomerase inhibition is a potential new therapeutic target.

R.F. Ozols, M.D, Ph.D.

The Costs and Effects of Cervical and Breast Cancer Screening in a Public Hospital Emergency Room

Mandelblatt J, Freeman H, Winczewski D, et al (Mem Sloan Kettering Cancer Ctr, New York; Harlem Hosp Ctr, New York)

Am J Public Health 87:1182–1189, 1997 2–14

Introduction.—Many minority women and women of low socioeconomic status are not exposed to traditional cancer screening programs, tending instead to depend upon the emergency room for their primary care. Reported are costs and effects of implementing a cervical and breast cancer screening program in a public hospital emergency department.

Methods.—The costs and effects of opportunistic emergency department screening for cervical and/or breast cancer were compared with those incurred during routine hospital screening efforts. Life expectancy and costs associated with each strategy were assessed.

Results.—The cost of creating a dedicated cervical cancer screening program was $212,187, or $329 per woman screened. The undiscounted cost-effectiveness results for creating new programs were $4,050 for cervical cancer, $403,203 for breast cancer, and $4,375 for joint cervical and breast cancer per year of life saved. When screening was added to an existing emergency department program, these figures were smaller: $429, $21,324, and $479, respectively, per year. The cost-effectiveness results were impacted by the number of women screened and rates of completion of treatment after an abnormal screening finding.

Conclusion.—Cervical and breast cancer screening in an emergency department setting was relatively expensive for the number of women screened. For this type of program to be cost effective, more intensive recruitment and follow-up strategies are needed.

► For those of us who have worked in a hospital caring for patients of lower socioeconomic status or predominantly minority patients, it is clearly recognized that the emergency department is often relied upon for primary care. To encourage health-seeking behaviors by patients, 2 approaches can be considered: (1) changing the behavior of patients (using a primary care office rather than the emergency department) and (2) using screening tools in the emergency department. Although it would appear that the former approach is clearly more cost effective, successful modulation of patient behavior has been largely ineffective. The cost effectiveness of the second approach is discussed in this paper. The data presented provide a useful background for a discussion of the economic issues of cancer prevention procedures in a public setting.

P.J. Loehrer, Sr., M.D.

Prevalence and Contribution of BRCA1 Mutations in Breast Cancer and Ovarian Cancer: Results From Three U.S. Population-based Case-Control Studies of Ovarian Cancer

Whittemore AS, Gong G, Itnyre J (Stanford Univ, Calif)

Am J Hum Genet 60:496–504, 1997 2–15

Objective.—*BRCA1* mutations increase the risk of both breast and ovarian cancer. Familial cancer risk data from 3 U.S. population-based case-control studies of ovarian cancer were evaluated to provide an estimate of the mutation prevalence and penetrance of *BRCA1* in the general population.

Methods.—The incidence of breast and ovarian cancer was determined in mothers and sisters of 922 women with epithelial invasive (n = 651), borderline (n = 169), or unknown malignant potential (n = 102) ovarian cancer and of 922 control women. Model fitting and goodness of fit testing were used to estimate mutation prevalence and the presence of *BRCA1* in the general population.

Results.—Among the 922 patients with ovarian cancer, there were 55 mothers and 31 sisters with breast cancer and 22 mothers and 6 sisters with ovarian cancer. Among the 922 controls, 42 mothers and 19 sisters had breast cancer and 5 mothers and 2 sisters had ovarian cancer. The prevalence of *BRCA1/BRCA2* mutations in the general population is estimated to be 0.0014 according to the model. The risks of ovarian and breast cancers in carriers is dramatically higher than in noncarriers. The cumulative risk for breast cancer at age 80 is 73.5% for carriers and 6.8% for noncarriers. For ovarian cancer, the respective risks are 27.8% and 1.8%. These estimates for breast and ovarian cancer because of the presence of the *BRCA1* gene are low. Population-based estimates put the proportion of breast and ovarian cancers, by age 80, because of *BRCA1/BRCA2* mutations at 3.0% and 4.4%, respectively. The data are less clear cut in the case of 169 women with borderline ovarian cancers.

Conclusion.—The present study estimates that 3.0% of all U.S. breast cancers and 4.4% of all U.S. ovarian cancers are caused by mutations in the *BRCA1* gene. Larger, population-based, multiethnic studies should be conducted to confirm the frequencies and penetrances of specific mutations.

► This important study pooled family breast cancer data and ovarian cancer data from 3 population-based case-control studies to estimate the frequency and penetrance of mutations conferring increased risk of ovarian cancer and breast cancer. Frequency of *BRCA1* mutation carriers in the general population is low and estimated at 1 in 345 individuals in this present study. The present study also estimates that *BRCA1* mutations account for only 3% of all U.S. breast cancers and for less than 5% of all U.S. ovarian cancers. The estimated risk of ovarian cancer by age 80 years was 27.8% in carriers and 1.8% in noncarriers. These estimates are important for appropriate counseling of women with a strong family history of ovarian cancer who may be considering the merits of undergoing testing for *BRCA1* mutations.

R.F. Ozols, M.D., Ph.D.

Cost-effectiveness of Extending Screening Mammography Guidelines to Include Women 40 to 49 Years of Age

Salzmann P, Kerlikowske K, Phillips K (Univ of California, San Francisco)

Ann Intern Med 127:955–965, 1997 2–16

Introduction.—Screening mammography is universally recommended for females ages 50–69 because of its proven efficacy and reasonable cost-effectiveness. Pooled findings of large, randomized controlled trials indicate there is no mortality reduction in females ages 40–49 after 7 to 9 years of screening. A significant reduction is apparent after 10–14 years of screening. Some analyses suggest screening is less cost-effective in females ages 40–49, compared to older females, but other analyses suggest screening is also cost-effective in younger females. The cost-effectiveness of screening mammography in women of different ages was compared.

Methods.—Results of biennial screening of females ages 50–69 years was compared with that of females with no screening. Screening performed every 18 months from ages 40–49 years, followed by biennial screening from ages 50–69 years, was compared with biennial screening for females ages 50–69 years. Life expectancy, costs, and incremental cost-effectiveness were assessed. The costs of screening mammography examinations, evaluating abnormal mammograms, and treating breast cancer were examined.

Results.—The screening of females ages 50–69 improved life expectancy by 12 days at a cost of $704 per woman, yielding a cost-effectiveness ratio of $21,400 per year of life saved. When screening included females ages 40–49, life expectancy was improved by 2.5 days at a cost of $676 per female. The incremental cost-effectiveness of screening females ages 40–49 years was $105,000 per year of life saved. There was a 75% chance that screening mammography in females ages 50–69 years cost less than $50,000 per year of life saved, compared with a 7% chance in females 40–49 years.

Conclusion.—The cost-effectiveness ratio of screening mammography for females ages 40–49 years was almost 5 times that of the cost-effectiveness of screening for older females. It is recommended that mammogram screening programs focus on the 50- to 69-year age group, for whom the benefits are clear and the costs are acceptable.

▶ In 1997, when the NIH Consensus Panel met to discuss recommendations for screening mammography for women between the ages of 40 and 49, the panel agreed to disagree. The incidence of breast cancer in this population of women is greater than in those women who are younger, but it remains 2–3 times lower than in older women. As a consequence, more women must be screened to find breast cancer in this younger population, and thus the cost per year of lives saved is greater. This is a balanced article which states the facts and figures that can be used on both sides of this issue.

P.J. Loehrer, Sr., M.D.

The Role of Numeracy in Understanding the Benefit of Screening Mammography

Schwartz LM, Woloshin S, Black WC, et al (Veterans Affairs Med Ctr, White River Junction, Vt; Dartmouth Med School, Hanover, NH)

Ann Intern Med 127:966–972, 1997 2–17

Introduction.—The National Institutes of Health Consensus Panel recommended that screening mammography for women aged 40–49 years not be routinely performed, and that the women make their own decisions about the need for screening based on their personal evaluation of risks and benefits. However, it is not known how well the patients understand quantitative information, and whether they can understand and manipulate numbers. It is thought that patients with some facility with basic probability and numerical concepts, known as numeracy, can find quantitative information to be meaningful. Women's comprehension of messages about mammography was studied to learn more about the role of numeracy in communicating information about risk.

Methods.—There were 500 female veterans who were asked to complete one of 4 questionnaires, which differed only in how the same information on average risk reduction with mammography was presented. The questionnaire was completed by 61% of the women who had a median age of 68 years and of which 96% were high school graduates. The total number of correct responses to 3 simple tasks was the score for numeracy (Fig 1). With and without mammography, participants estimated their risk for death from breast cancer. A woman's ability to adjust her perceived risk according to the risk reduction data presented was used to judge accuracy.

Results.—There was poor accuracy in applying risk reduction information and numeracy. For example, one third of the women indicated that 1,000 flips of a fair coin would result in less than 300 heads. Numeracy was strongly related to accuracy, with an accuracy rate of 5.8% for a numeracy score of 0. For a numeracy score of 1, the accuracy rate was 8.9%. For a numeracy score of 2, the accuracy rate was 23.7%. For a numeracy score of 3, the accuracy rate was 40%.

Conclusion.—Numeracy was strongly related to gauging the benefit of mammography accurately, regardless of how information was presented. To communicate quantitative information about risks and benefits, more effective formats are needed.

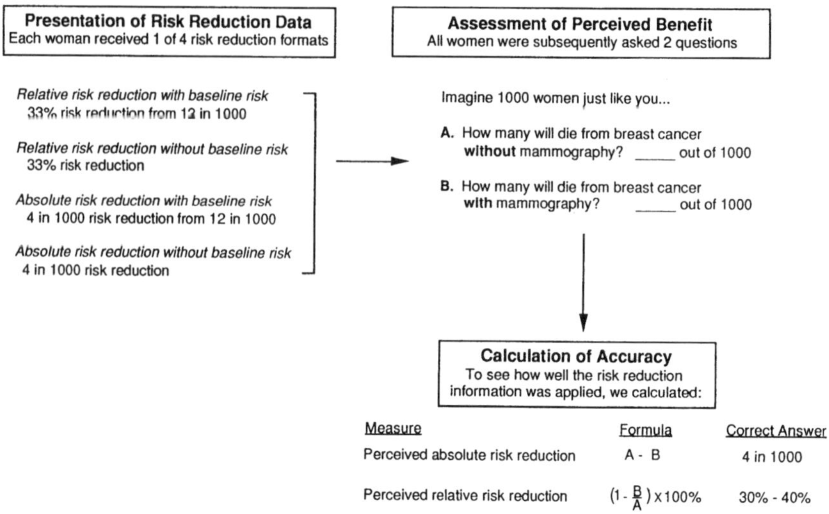

FIGURE 1.—Overview of the task presented to a woman completing the survey and the investigator's measures of her ability to apply risk reduction information accurately. The relation between the measure of accuracy and numeracy was subsequently assessed. (Courtesy of Schwartz LM, Woloshin S, Black WC, et al: The role of numeracy in understanding the benefit of screening mammography. *Ann Intern Med* 127:966–972, 1997.)

► When health care providers talk to patients, it is not only important that they understand what they are trying to communicate, but just as important that the *patients* understand also. This is an interesting article, which addresses how women from New England process information about numbers and statistics. Every day, we attempt to influence patients with facts and figures. The ability to influence "properly" in large part depends upon how we process this information. This study shows that the perceived benefit of mammography varies greatly among differing individuals and emphasizes a need to have alternative forms of communications with our patients.

P.J. Loehrer, Sr., M.D.

Recommendations for Follow-up Care of Individuals With an Inherited Predisposition to Cancer: II. *BRCA1* and *BRCA2*

Burke W, for the Cancer Genetics Studies Consortium (Univ of Washington, Seattle; et al)

JAMA 277:997–1003, 1997 2–18

Introduction.—Mutations in the *BRCA1* and *BRCA2* genes are associated with an inherited predisposition to breast and ovarian cancer. A task force with expertise in medical genetics, oncology, primary care, gastroenterology, and epidemiology was formed by the Cancer Genetics Studies Consortium, which is sponsored by the National Human Genome Research Institute. The recommendations of the task force for the follow-up care of patients with an inherited predisposition to cancer were reported.

Data.—A MEDLINE search was conducted, as well as an evaluation of bibliographies of articles identified by MEDLINE, to find studies examining cancer risk, surveillance, and risk reduction in individuals genetically susceptible to breast and ovarian cancer. Quality of evidence was determined using criteria of the U.S. Prevention Service Task Force.

Provisional Recommendations.—Early screening for breast cancer and ovarian cancer are recommended for individuals with *BRCA1* mutations. For those with *BRCA2* mutations, early screening for breast cancer is recommended. No recommendations are made by the task force for or against prophylactic mastectomy or oophorectomy. These surgeries are an option for mutation carriers, but there is no evidence of benefit. There have been documented case reports of cancer in patients who have undergone prophylactic surgery.

Conclusions.—Counseling regarding these recommendations should consider the uncertainties in risk estimates and in the efficacy of cancer surveillance for genetically susceptible individuals. It must be remembered that these recommendations are based upon potential but unproven benefits. These issues should be jointly evaluated by patients at risk and by their health care providers.

▶ One of the major issues which will need to be addressed during the next decade is the role of genetic testing. As we identify more genetic mutations associated with malignancy and other medical disorders, we must balance the positive predictive value with the potential risks and benefits of such findings. This paper summarizes the recommendations regarding follow-up of patients with *BRCA1* and *BRCA2*. Existing evidence is not sufficient to support or refute prophylactic surgery (mastectomy or bilateral salpingo oophorectomy) to date. This article is a nice reference for both patients and physicians.

P.J. Loehrer, Sr., M.D.

Pathology of Familial Breast Cancer: Differences Between Breast Cancers in Carriers of *BRCA1* or *BRCA2* Mutations and Sporadic Cases

Stratton MR, for the Breast Cancer Linkage Consortium (Haddow Labs, Belmont, Sutton, Surrey, England)

Lancet 349:1505–1510, 1998 2–19

Introduction.—A hereditary predisposition to breast cancer is found in a small proportion of patients with breast cancer, in particular among those who have cancer diagnosed at a young age. The cancer is transmitted as a highly penetrant autosomal dominant trait. A risk of breast cancer has been associated with mutations in *BRCA1* and *BRCA2*, and together they account for about 80% of families with 4 or more instances of breast cancer diagnosed in patients younger than 60 years. In a large collaborative study, the morphological characteristics of breast cancers related to *BRCA1* and *BRCA2* were examined and compared with those of controls who were unselected for a family history of breast cancer.

Methods.—Seven pathologists compared the morphological characteristics of specimens from 440 women with familial breast cancer, of which 188 were carriers of *BRCA1* mutations and 78 were carriers of *BRCA2* mutations, with those of specimens from 547 age-matched controls, unselected for family history.

Results.—The cancers were of a higher overall grade among carriers of *BRCA1* and *BRCA2* mutations when compared to the controls. There were 66% grade 3 cancers among *BRCA1* carriers, 41% grade 3 cancers among *BRCA2* carriers, and 36% among controls. More pleomorphisms, a higher mitotic count, and less tubule formation was seen in *BRCA1*-mutation carriers than among controls, when the 3 grade indices were considered independently, but cancers in *BRCA2*-mutation carriers had less tubule formation but no difference in mitotic count or pleomorphism. Between carriers of *BRCA1* or *BRCA2* mutations and controls, the occurrence of invasive lobular carcinoma and invasive ductal carcinoma was not significantly different. In *BRCA1* carriers (13%), medullary or atypical medullary carcinoma was found more often than in *BRCA2*-mutation carriers (3%) or controls (2%). In *BRCA2*-mutation carriers, tubular carcinoma was less common. Familial cases accounted for the few mucoid carcinomas. Less ductal carcinoma in situ around the invasive lesion was seen among carriers of *BRCA1* mutations than among controls. In familial cancers, lobular carcinoma in situ was less common, but differences were not significant for *BRCA2*-mutations or *BRCA-1* mutation carriers, separately.

Conclusion.—In carriers of *BRCA1* and *BRCA2* mutations, there are differences between breast cancers, and in predisposed women, the histologic features of breast cancers differ from those in sporadic cases. There is a different natural history between breast cancer attributable to *BRCA1* and *BRCA2* mutations or sporadic disease, which may have implications for screening and management.

▶ Genetic testing can provide more information than merely assessing the risk for developing cancer. This article describes morphological differences between the cancers carrying *BRCA1* and *BRCA2* mutations and those of age-matched controls. This information may ultimately lead to a better understanding of the function of these genes. The higher grade of tumor associated with *BRCA1* tumors may suggest alternate treatment strategies for affected patients.

P.J. Loehrer, Sr., M.D.

Histopathologic Validation of the Sentinel Lymph Node Hypothesis for Breast Carcinoma

Turner RR, Ollila DW, Krasne DL, et al (Saint John's Health Ctr, Santa Monica, Calif)

Ann Surg 226:271–278, 1997 2–20

Background.—According to the sentinel lymph node hypothesis, a primary tumor drains to specific (sentinel) lymph node(s). However, does this mean that the sentinel node is the node most likely to be positive for metastatic disease? Whether differences in tumor infiltration exist was determined by comparing the histologic findings in both sentinel and nonsentinel nodes.

Methods.—Research subjects were 103 patients (102 women and 1 man; median age, 55 years) undergoing surgery for invasive breast carcinomas. Intraoperative mapping, sentinel lymph node dissection (SLND), and axillary lymph node dissection (ALND) were performed for all patients. Briefly, for SLND, a dye was injected around the primary tumor. Then, 3–7 minutes later, an incision was made into the axilla, and the lymph channel containing dye was followed until the first staining node(s) was identified. After SLND, levels I and II (and rarely, level III) ALND was performed. Sentinel nodes were examined 3 times, by frozen section analysis, by hematoxylin and eosin (H&E) staining, and by immunohistochemical (IHC) staining. Nonsentinel nodes were also examined 3 times, by H&E staining and by 2 different IHC stainings.

Findings.—The median tumor size was 1.8 cm. Between 1 and 8 (mean, 4) sentinel nodes and between 7 and 37 (mean, 18.9) nonsentinel nodes were examined for each patient. The H&E staining of sentinel nodes indicated metastatic cancer in 33 patients (32%) and no tumors in the remaining 70 patients (68%). However, further IHC staining of the 157 sentinel nodes in these 70 patients identified 10 nodes that did show metastatic disease. Each of these nodes was in a different patient; thus, 10

TABLE 2.—Results of Cytokeratin Immunohistochemical Tests in Nodes That Were Metastasis-free by H&E Examination

	H&E	IHC	IHC Conversion Rate (%)	
Lymph node evaluation				
Tumor in sentinel nodes	0/157	10/157	6.4	
Tumor in nonsentinel nodes only	0/1087	1/1087	0.1	($p < 0.0001$)
Patient evaluation				
Patients with sentinel node metastasis	0/70	10/70	14.3	
Patients with nonsentinel node metastasis only	0/60	1/60	1.7	($p < 0.0001$)

Abbreviations: H&E, hematoxylin and eosin; *IHC*, immunohistochemical tests.

(Courtesy of Turner RR, Ollila DW, Krasne DL, et al: Histopathologic validation of the sentinel lymph node hypothesis for breast carcinoma. *Ann Surg* 226:271–278, 1997.)

TABLE 3.—Final Tumor Status of Sentinel and Nonsentinel Axillary Lymph Nodes

Tumor Status	Number (%) of Patients
All nodes metastasis-free	59 (57.3)
Nodal metastases detected	44 (42.7)
Sentinel node only	25 (24.3)
Sentinel and nonsentinel nodes	18 (17.5)
Nonsentinel nodes only	1 (1.0)
Total	103 (100.0)

(Courtesy of Turner RR, Ollila DW, Krasne DL, et al: Histopathologic validation of the sentinel lymph node hypothesis for breast carcinoma. *Ann Surg* 226:271–278, 1997.)

of 70 patients (14.3%) who had sentinel-node–negative status by H&E staining had sentinel-node–positive disease by IHC staining (Table 2). In total, then, 43 of 103 patients (42%) had sentinel node involvement. In the remaining 60 patients with sentinel-node–negative disease, 1,087 nonsentinel nodes were examined by IHC. In this entire series, only 1 positive node was found (frequency of 0.0009%) (Table 3). Therefore, only 1 of 103 patients had a sentinel node that was negative for disease but a nonsentinel node that was positive for disease.

Conclusions.—Efforts to detect metastatic breast cancer depend on the extent of axillary dissection and the methods of histopathologic examination used. In this study, if H&E and IHC staining both showed the sentinel node to be free of a tumor, then the chance of a nonsentinel node being positive was less than 0.1%. These results confirm the hypothesis that the sentinel node is the most likely node to harbor metastatic disease.

► For the last several years, there has been an interest among surgeons to define the sentinel node for both breast cancer and malignant melanoma. The idea is to use either an isotope or a vital dye to show where the sentinel node is with respect to the primary, and then excise that sentinel node separately and prior to the full dissection. If the sentinel node is negative, the likelihood of finding disease is very low; conversely, the presence of a positive sentinel node is an excellent way to identify those that have other nodes. In this study of breast carcinoma in 103 patients, sentinel node was positive in 33 and negative in 70 patients. If the sentinel node proved to be tumor-free by both histology and immunohistochemical staining, then the probability of other nodes being involved was less than 1%. It would appear the evaluation of the sentinel node was a major improvement in the surgical approach to patients with melanoma and breast cancers.

E. Glatstein, M.D.

Detection of Axillary Lymph Node Metastasis of Breast Carcinoma With Technetium-99m Sestamibi Scintimammography

Tolmos J, Khalkhali I, Vargas H, et al (Univ of California, Los Angeles)
Am Surg 63:850–853, 1997 2–21

Objective.—Whereas nodal metastases predict the presence of systemic disease in patients with breast cancer, axillary dissection without nodal involvement results in unnecessary morbidity. A noninvasive test for axillary metastases is desirable. In vitro studies have shown that technetium-99m sestamibi concentrates in tumor cells. Whether ^{99m}Tc sestamibi scintomammography (SSM) is a reliable technique to predict the presence of axillary metastases was investigated.

Methods.—Scintomammography was performed between June 1992 and December 1995 on 31 women aged 31–67 years with breast cancer. The technique involved acquiring images 5 and 10 minutes after an IV injection of 20 mCi of ^{99m}Tc sestamibi. Planar images were obtained in the lateral prone and in the anterior position with arms raised. Results were interpreted by 2 nuclear medicine physicians blinded to clinical and histologic data. Imaging results were correlated with axillary histologic conclusions.

Results.—Of 11 histologically benign specimens, 9 were SMM benign and 2 were SMM malignant. Of the 20 histologically malignant specimens, 5 were SMM benign and 15 were SMM malignant for a sensitivity of 75%, a specificity of 82%, positive predictive value of 88%, and a negative predictive value of 64%. Interobserver correlation had a κ of 0.49.

Conclusion.—Scintomammography, with a negative predictive value of 64%, is not a reliable method for detecting axillary metastases. The positive predictive value of 88% suggests that improved imaging techniques may improve the reliability of the technique.

► Accurately predicting the presence, location, and extent of metastatic axillary lymph nodes in patients with primary breast cancer would be quite valuable in preoperative staging. Thus far, radiologic evaluation with CT scan and MRI has not provided a highly sensitive means of detecting axillary lymph nodal involvement. The recent advance in lymphatic mapping and sentinel lymph node biopsy, particularly in women with small primary breast cancer, has compared favorably in staging to the gold standard of complete axillary lymphadenectomy. This study from UCLA evaluates technetium-labeled sestamibi scanning of the breast and axilla as an addition to traditional breast cancer imaging techniques. The positive predictive value of 88% for nodal involvement in this series is significant even with a negative predictive value of only 64%. Obviously, refinements in this technique will be important before there is widespread clinical usefulness. However, if a combination of enhanced scanning and sentinel node sampling can accurately identify node positive patients, then the majority of women, especially those with T1 or small T2 breast cancers, would not have to undergo complete staging lymphadenectomy.

B.L. Eisenberg, M.D.

Identification of Clinical Stage A Nonseminomatous Testis Cancer Patients at Extremely Low Risk for Metastatic Disease: A Combined Approach Using Quantitive Immunohistochemical, Histopathologic, and Radiologic Assessment

Leibovitch I, Foster RS, Kopecky KK, et al (Indiana Univ, Indianapolis)

J Clin Oncol 16:261–268, 1998 2–22

Introduction.—Primary nerve-sparing retroperitoneal lymphadenectomy and orchectomy followed by surveillance are the options for managing clinical stage A nonseminomatous germ cell testicular tumors. However, about 70% of all retroperitoneal lymphadenectomies are considered staging procedures and lack therapeutic value. Conversely, 30% of patients may harbor occult metastases, and novel predictors of occult lymph node metastasis have been studied to achieve a more accurate assessment of the risk of occult metastasis. To define the risk of metastasis in low-stage nonseminomatous germ cell tumor patients, quantitative histopathologic evaluation of the primary testicular tumors and proliferative activity by flow cytometry have been found useful. To evaluate the predictive value of a combined staging approach, these 2 independently derived models, which include quantitative radiologic, histopathologic, and immunohistochemical parameters for assessing the risk of occult lymph node metastasis, are used.

Methods.—Orchidectomy specimens and computed tomographic scans were performed on 81 consecutive clinical stage A nonseminomatous germ cell tumor patients, who had primary nerve-sparing retroperitoneal lymph node dissection, and the tests were evaluated blindly in a quantitative fashion. Using previously determined paradigms, these scores were correlated with pathologic stage.

Results.—There were 41 patients who were classified as at low risk for metastasis, using volume of embryonal carcinoma in the orchiectomy specimen, lymph node diameters in the primary landing zones, and MIB-1 staining of the orchiectomy specimen. Pathology stage A disease of retroperitoneal lymph node dissection was seen in 40 of these 41 patients.

Conclusion.—A group of patients at low risk for metastasis can be identified by these parameters, and these patients can be rationally offered surveillance. This model is a 2-arm paradigm that uses stringent and relaxed thresholds according to a histopathologic assessment of the volume of embryonal carcinoma in the primary tumor (Fig 2).

▶ As therapy for advanced germ cell tumor has improved, quite appropriately strategies have also emerged to minimize morbidity for patients with early-stage testicular cancer. One such area of management is in clinical

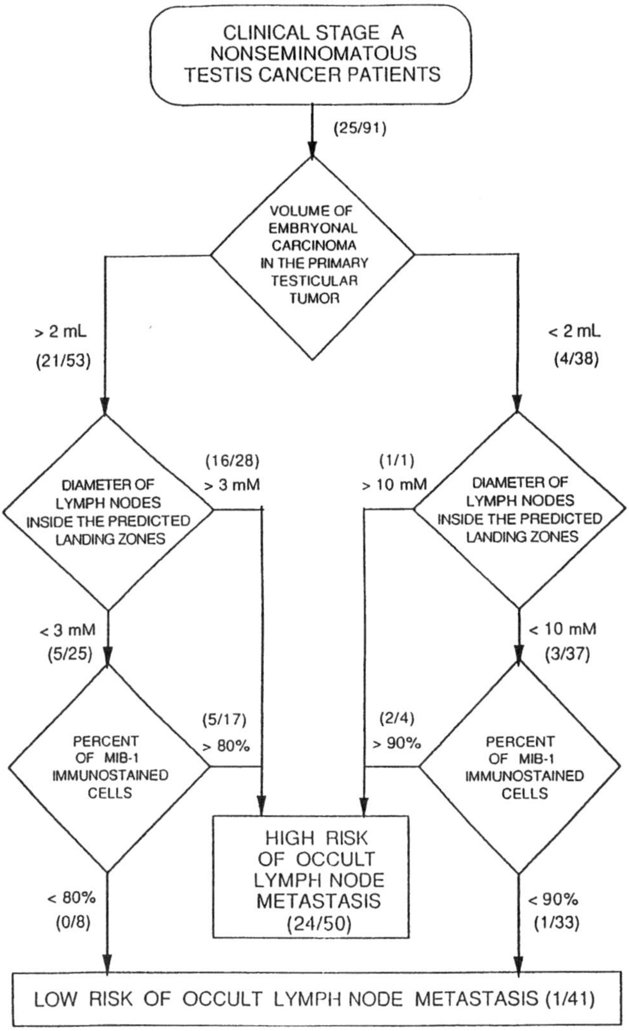

FIGURE 2.—After stratifying for volume of embryonal, different thresholds of lymph node diameters and MIB-1 immunostaining are used. Numbers in parentheses represent pathologic stage B patients and total patients involved. (Courtesy of Leibovitch I, Foster RS, Kopecky KK, et al: Identification of clinical stage A nonseminomatous testis cancer patients at extremely low risk for metastatic disease: A combined approach using quantitative immunohistochemical, histopathologic, and radiologic assessment. *J Clin Oncol* 16:261–268, 1998.)

stage A disease. During most of this century, the primary therapy for clinical stage A testicular cancer has been a retroperitoneal lymph node dissection. This is performed because approximately 30% of patients with a normal abdominal CT scan and serum markers will have involvement of the retroperitoneal lymph nodes. Approximately 70% of patients with involved lymph nodes will be cured with this procedure. Although the morbidity of this procedure has been improved with the use of surgical templates as well as nerve-sparing procedures, it is probably not optimal to perform surgery on all patients with this disease, given that 70% of them will not have nodal involvement. The strategy of management of this disease is divided, but this article defines a population for whom the likelihood of finding positive retroperitoneal lymph nodes is extremely low. These results will need to be validated prospectively to confirm this approach in a multi-institutional setting.

P.J. Loehrer, Sr., M.D.

Androgens Regulate Vascular Endothelial Growth Factor Content in Normal and Malignant Prostatic Tissue

Joseph IBJK, Nelson JB, Denmeade SR, et al (Johns Hopkins Univ, Baltimore, Md)

Clin Cancer Res 3:2507–2511, 1997 2–23

Introduction.—For the expansion of solid tumors beyond 1–3 mm, angiogenesis is a prerequisite. A human and 2 rodent androgen-sensitive prostate cancer sublines were tested to determine whether androgens consistently regulate angiogenesis via control of vascular endothelial growth factor levels. In each of these 3 additional prostate cancer sublines, androgen ablation caused a decrease in the subsequent growth rate. A greater than 60% reduction in tumor vascular endothelial growth factor levels is consistently associated with this growth inhibition. The dose-response ability of androgens to increase vascular endothelial growth factor levels in media of LnCaP cells grown in vitro was tested to evaluate whether androgen regulation of vascular endothelial growth factor is due to a direct effect of androgen on prostatic cells.

Methods.—Male rats were castrated, and the temporal changes in the vascular endothelial growth factor content of ventral prostate tissue were determined, to examine whether androgens regulate vascular endothelial growth factor levels in malignant and normal prostatic tissue. The vascular endothelial growth factor content in expressed prostatic secretion fluid vs. seminal vesicle fluid, obtained from men with prostate cancer, was measured to validate the relevance of these studies to human prostatic disease.

Results.—Within the ventral prostate, vascular endothelial growth factor content decreased to less than 20% 1 week after castration. An eightfold rise in ventral prostate vascular endothelial growth factor content was seen, with subsequent replacement with exogenous androgen to long-term castrated rats, within 1 week. Androgens were found to stimulate vascular endothelial growth factor secretion directly in the LnCaP cells. Elevated levels of vascular endothelial growth factor may contribute to the progression of these prostatic conditions by promoting angiogenesis, as evidenced by the presence of a four–fivefold higher level of vascular endothelial growth factor in prostatic fluid vs. seminal vesicle fluid obtained from benign prostatic hyperplasia and clinically localized prostate cancer patients.

Conclusion.—Stimulation of vascular endothelial growth factor levels is one of the mechanisms for androgen sensitivity for the control of the growth of normal and malignant prostate tissue.

► Since the 1940s, androgens have been recognized as playing a pivotal role in the management of prostate cancer. In addition, androgen production by either orchiectomy or blockade results in atrophy of the prostate epithelium (both malignant and benign). With more sophisticated analysis, we are slowly learning the mechanisms of action of hormonal therapy for this disease. Androgen ablation not only results in apoptosis, but also, as this trial confirms, has the potential role of inhibiting angiogenesis. This article may open the door for alternative treatment strategies for this disease.

P.J. Loehrer, Sr., M.D.

Mitochondrial Genome Damage Associated With Cigarette Smoking
Ballinger SW, Bouder TG, Davis GS, et al (Univ of Vermont, Burlington)
Cancer Res 56:5692–5697, 1996 2–24

Background.—Although the relationship between certain environmental factors and disease has been well documented, the precise mechanisms of cellular injury and disease development remain unclear. Many studies have shown that mitochondral DNA (mtDNA) germline mutations cause a variety of diseases. However, the role of the environment in somatic mtDNA damage, mutation, and human disease is relatively unknown. Mitochondrial genome damage associated with cigarette smoking was explored.

Methods and Findings.—The level of mtDNA damage and deletions were assessed in bronchoalveolar lavage tissues from smokers and nonsmokers. Quantitative, extra-long polymerase chain reaction and a common mtDNA deletion assay were used. Compared with nonsmokers, smokers were found to have 5.6 times the level of mtDNA damage, 2.6 times the damage at a nuclear locus (β-globin gene cluster), and nearly 7 times the level of a 4.9 kb mtDNA deletion (the last being nonsignificant). Both mitochondrial and nuclear genomes showed significantly increased levels of DNA damage in smokers. However, the relative differences were greatest in the mtDNA (Tables 1 and 2).

Conclusions.—Damage to the mtDNA may inhibit oxidative phosphorylation, potentially causing or contributing to chronic lung disease and cancer. Thus, the mtDNA may be a sensitive marker for genetic damage and mutation induced by environmental agents.

► It has not been a good year for the tobacco companies, but I don't care. This is another paper that I think, demonstrates reasonably well the basis for neoplasia secondary to cigarette smoking. In this instance, it appears to be

TABLE 1.—Observed Values, Smokers VS. Nonsmokers

Sample	Age/sex	Pack-years	% deleted	mtDNA Q-XLPCR cpm, mean, SE	β-globin Q-XLPCR cpm, mean, SE	nDNA/mtDNA ratio
Smokers						
1	42/F	45	0.0026	26.54, 22.42	280.95, 90.39	0.052
2	54/F	120	0.031	12.40, 6.50	23.69, 0.74	0.080
3	40/F	20	0.012	2.91, 1.8	4.38, 1.32	0.099
4	43/F	29	0.0002	76.67, 36.03	162.04, 34.94	0.085
5	49/F	30	0.050	8.90, 6.40	289.46, 88.22	0.050
6*	41/F	45	0.001	4.82, 1.98	5.90, 1.63	0.085
Mean, SE	44.83, 2.34	48.17, 14.91	0.016, 0.0083	22.04, 11.45	127.74, 55.28	0.075, 0.0081
Nonsmokers						
7	57/F		0.0015	171.03, 95.99	313.27, 107.78	0.064
8	42/F		0.0006	163.83, 94.95	329.61, 116.42	0.063
9	60/M		0.00056	125.94, 63.84	296.55, 99.69	0.069
10	43/M		0.0034	132.65, 61.61	333.17, 114.44	0.071
11†	40/F		0.00005	65.84, 39.26	302.06, 98.25	0.068
12‡	64/F		0.0077	78.52, 3.22	399.71, 139.16	0.061
Mean, SE	51, 4.29		0.0023, 0.0012	122.97, 17.63	329.06, 127.74	0.066, 0.0016
P values (Independent t-test), Smokers *vs.* nonsmokers	0.23		0.128	0.00072	0.0056	0.291

*Marijuana and cocaine use.
†Formaldehyde exposure.
‡Chlorine exposure.
Abbreviations: F, female; *M*, male; *mtDNA*, mitochondrial DNA; *SE*, standard error.
(Courtesy of Ballinger SW, Bouder TG, Davis GS, et al: Mitochondrial genome damage associated with cigarette smoking. *Cancer Res* 56:5692–5697, 1996.)

TABLE 2.—Mean Values: Smokers Vs. Nonsmokers From Individual Q-XLPCR Experiments

Experiment	cpm Mean	SE	*P* value (independent *t* test)
mtDNA 1			
Smokers	2.05	0.83	0.0097
Nonsmokers	8.62	1.89	
mtDNA 2			
Smokers	25.30	15.01	0.0096
Nonsmokers	201.6	53.09	
mtDNA 3			
Smokers	38.77	20.18	0.00033
Nonsmokers	158.68	9.95	
β-globin 1			
Smokers	91.53	37.97	0.0096
Nonsmokers	216.44	9.35	
β-globin 2			
Smokers	163.95	72.75	0.0044
Nonsmokers	441.69	21.37	

Abbreviations: mtDNA, mitochondrial DNA; *SE,* standard error.
(Courtesy of Ballinger SW, Bouder TG, Davis GS, et al: Mitochondrial genome damage associated with cigarette smoking. *Cancer Res* 56:5692–5697, 1996.)

mtDNA that is damaged by smoking, but I think it is just another indication of what smoking can do. The tragedy of lung cancer is that so much of it is preventable. We live at a time when many people advocate prevention. This is the most preventable cancer we have, and it is our No. 1 problem. How to prevent other cancers is speculative at best, but in another era, someone once wrote a monograph on 6 cases of lung cancer so that posterity would be aware of it!

E. Glatstein, M.D.

Activated Raf-1 Causes Growth Arrest in Human Small Cell Lung Cancer Cells

Ravi RK, Weber E, McMahon M, et al (Johns Hopkins Univ, Baltimore, Md; DNAX Research Inst of Molecular and Cellular Biology, Palo Alto, Calif; Cleveland Clinic Research Inst, Ohio; et al)

J Clin Invest 101:153–159, 1998 2–25

Introduction.—In contrast to the situation with other lung cancers, previous studies have not identified ras mutations in small-cell lung cancer (SCLC). The implication is that activation of the raf-MEK mitogen-activated protein kinases (MAPKs) and other ras-associated signal transduction pathways carries biological consequences distinct from those of other cancers. This study examined the biological effects of raf activation in SCLC cells.

Methods and Findings.—Small cell lung cancer cells were transfected with a gene encoding for a fusion protein. The fusion protein was made up of an oncogenic form of human Raf-1 and the hormone-binding domain of the estrogen receptor (ΔRaf-1:ER), which can be activated by estradiol. Activation of ΔRaf-1:ER led to phosphorylation of MAPK, causing loss of cloning ability in soft agar, suppression of growth capacity, cell accumulation in cell cycle phases G1 and G2, and S-phase depletion. Activation of Raf was associated with induction of the cyclin-dependent kinase (cdk) inhibitor p27^{kip1}, with a decrease cdk2 protein kinase activity. Pretreatment with a MEK inhibitor, PD098059, inhibited all of these effects.

Conclusion.—In SCLC cells, raf can activate signal transduction pathways linked to cell cycle regulatory molecules, thus acting as a growth suppressor gene. The findings show that activation of MAPK by ΔRaf-1:ER leads to cell cycle arrest and that MAPK can activate cdk inhibitors that act to reduce cdk2 activity. Thus, activation of the raf/MEK/MAPK pathway—rather than its inhibition—may be a useful treatment approach in neuroendocrine tumors such as SCLC.

► The ras mutations are reported to be extensive in non–small-cell lung cancer, but they are not seen in SCLC. This study looks at the Raf status in SCLC cells. The authors observed that activation of this pathway caused a dramatic loss in the ability of the cells to clone in soft agar. It suppressed growth capacity, and the cells appeared to pile up in G1 and G2 phases and were depleted from the S phase. These data are taken to demonstrate that the activated Raf-1 stimulates inhibitory pathways of growth that lead to a cell cycle arrest.

The reason this may be important is that these data suggest that this pathway could be a therapeutic target for SCLC and other neuroendocrine tumors. Despite the fact that treatments have improved over the last 15–20 years—at least for limited-stage SCLC—there is still a lot to be desired, and a new strategy could be very helpful. Obviously, this work needs a lot of confirmation, but, if correct, it could represent a whole new approach to what has up to now been frustration in the therapeutic arena.

E. Glatstein, M.D.

Lymph Node Staging in Non–Small Cell Lung Cancer: Evaluation by [^{18}F]FDG Positron Emission Tomography (PET)

Guhlmann A, Storck M, Kotzerke J, et al (Univ of Ulm, Germany)
Thorax 52:438–441, 1997 2–26

Background.—In patients with non–small-cell lung cancer (NSCLC), the presence of lymph node metastases has a major impact on management and prognosis. Disease involving the contralateral mediastinal lymph nodes is considered unresectable. Computed tomography and MRI are of limited aid in staging the mediastinal and nodal metastases of NSCLC. However, positron emission tomography (PET) with 2-[^{18}F]-fluoro-2-deoxy-D-glucose (FDG) is a promising technique for demonstrating not only regional lymph node metastases but also the systemic extent of lung

TABLE 2.—Relationship Between the Nodal Short Axis Diameter and 2-[18F]-Fluoro-2-Deoxy-D-Glucose–Positron Emission Tomography Findings in Patients With Non–Small-Cell Lung Cancer

Nodal short axis diameter (mm)	*N0 PET+*	*PET−*	*N1 PET+*	*PET−*	*N2 PET+*	*PET−*	*N3 PET+*	*PET−*
<5	—	5	—	1	—	—	1	—
5–10	—	4	1	1	5*	—	1	—
11–15	—	1	2	—	4	—	—	—
16–20	—	2	—	—	1	—	2	—
21–25	—	—	—	—	1	—	—	—

Note: Values are number of patients.
*Two patients with N2a nodes were classified as N1 with positron emission tomography; 1 patient with N2 disease was classified as N1 by CT.
Abbreviation: PET, positron emission tomography.
(Reprinted with permission from BMJ Publishing Group from Guhlmann A, Storck M, Kotzerke J, et al: Lymph node staging in non-small cell lung cancer: Evaluation by [18F] FDG positron emission tomography [PET]. *Thorax* 52:438–441, 1997.)

cancer in whole-body scans. The use of FDG-PET for thoracic lymph node staging of patients with NSCLC was investigated.

Methods.—The study included 46 patients undergoing thoracotomy for focal lung tumors. All underwent contrast-enhanced CT and FDG-PET of the chest and mediastinum within 3 weeks before surgery. The tumor proved to be NSCLC in 32 patients. In each case, the diagnosis was made by histopathologic examination of the surgical specimen. Mediastinal lymph node dissection was performed at surgery. The overall accuracy of FDG-PET for preoperative staging was determined, focusing on its ability to differentiate between resectable and unresectable disease.

Results.—Analyzed retrospectively, preoperative FDG-PET had a sensitivity of 80%, specificity of 100%, and accuracy of 87.5% in staging of the thoracic lymph nodes. Computed tomography did not perform as well, with a sensitivity of 50%, a specificity of 75%, and accuracy of 59%. Twelve of 12 patients without lymph node tumor involvement were correctly identified by FDG-PET, as were 3 of 5 patients with N1 disease, 9 of 11 with N2 disease, and 4 of 4 with N3 (unresectable) disease. By comparison, CT identified 9 of 12 patients with N0 disease, 2 of 5 with N1 disease, 6 of 11 with N2 disease, and 2 of 4 with N3 disease (Table 2).

Conclusion.—Noninvasive FDG-PET scanning offers an effective approach to staging of the thoracic lymph nodes in patients with NSCLC. Unlike CT, it can reliably identify patients with conventionally resectable N1/N2 disease and those with unresectable N3 disease. Preoperative staging could be made more accurate by using FDG-PET imaging as an adjunct to CT scanning.

► This German study looked at 46 patients, 32 of whom had NSCLC and 14 of whom had benign processes. The question they asked was whether they could detect nodal disease in the patients who had neoplastic disease. There were no false positives. The FDG-PET methodology proved to be 100% specific in terms of lung cancer, with only 80% sensitivity.

Thus, PET scanning looks to be potentially a good way of assessing the mediastinal nodes by clinical, as opposed to surgical, intervention. The problem is that this is an expensive test, and in today's world, many third party carriers will not pay for it.

E. Glatstein, M.D.

Non-Small Cell Lung Cancer: Nodal Staging With FDG PET versus CT With Correlative Lymph Node Mapping and Sampling

Steinert HC, Hauser M, Allemann F, et al (Univ Hosp, Zürich, Switzerland)
Radiology 202:441–446, 1997 2–27

Background.—Choosing appropriate treatment for cancer depends on accurate tumor staging. Surgical resection is preferred for early stages of bronchogenic carcinoma. Mediastinoscopy can accurately assess mediastinal nodes, though CT and MRI have major limitations in depicting mediastinal lymph node metastases. 2-[fluorine-18]fluoro-2-deoxy-D-glucose (FDG) positron emission tomography (PET) potentially can differentiate lymph nodes from those without metastases. Most studies comparing the accuracy of PET and CT in the staging of mediastinal metastases of lung cancer have used a small sample size or limited numbers of mediastinal lymph nodes, or have had limited surgical correlations. This prospective study compared the accuracy of state-of-the-art partial-body FDG PET and state-of-the-art contrast material-enhanced CT in nodal staging of mediastinal metastases.

Methods.—Both FDG PET and contrast material-enhanced CT were performed in 47 patients with non–small-cell lung cancer: 23 patients had spiral CT and 24 patients had conventional CT. Images were interpreted before surgical staging. A lesion was considered malignant if it had a nodular appearance and intense FDG uptake similar to that of the brain. Nodal stations were localized according to the American Thoracic Society

TABLE 3.—Imaging Findings in 112 Mediastinal Lymph Nodes

Finding	PET	CT
True-positive	25	16
False-positive	1	5
True-negative	83	79
False-negative	3	12
Sensitivity (%)	89	57
Specificity (%)	99	94
Positive predictive value (%)	96	76
Negative predictive value (%)	97	87
Accuracy (%)	97	85

Note: At histopathologic examination, 28 nodes were positive and 84 nodes were negative.

(Courtesy of Steinert HC, Hauser M, Allemann F, et al: Non–small cell lung cancer: Nodal staging with FDG PET versus CT with correlative lymph node mapping and sampling. *Radiology* 202:41–446, 1997. Radiological Society of North America.)

TABLE 4.—N Staging With PET and CT

Staging	N0–N1 (*n* = 34)	N2 (*n* = 7)	N3 (*n* = 6)	All Stages (*n* = 47)
PET				
Correct	33	6	6	45 (96)
Understaged	NA	1	0	1 (2)
Overstaged	1	0	NA	1 (2)
CT				
Correct	30	5	2	37 (79)
Understaged	NA	2	4	6 (13)
Overstaged	4	0	NA	4 (9)

Note: Numbers in parentheses are percentages.
Abbreviation: NA, not applicable.
(Courtesy of Steinert HC, Hauser M, Allemann F, et al: Non–small–cell lung cancer: Nodal staging with FDG PET versus CT with correlative lymph node mapping and sampling. *Radiology* 202:441–446, 1997.)

mapping system. Extensive lymph node sampling of 599 nodes from 191 nodal stations was performed.

Results.—Nodal metastases were confirmed at histopathologic analysis in 29% of patients after mediastinoscopy or thoracotomy. Sensitivity was 89% for PET and 57% for CT for the staging of N2 or N3 disease in mediastinal nodes (Table 3). Specificity was 99% for PET and 94% for CT. The positive predictive value was 96% for PET and 76% for CT. The negative predictive value was 97% for PET and 87% for CT. Accuracy was 96% for PET and 85% for CT. PET was correct in assigning the correct N stage in 96% of cases; CT was correct in 79% of cases (Table 4). Differences between spiral and conventional CT were not significant.

Discussion.—In these study patients, FDG PET was superior to CT in nodal staging of non–small-cell lung cancer. For exact localization of lymph node metastases, emission and transmission-corrected PET scans are needed. It is likely that lesions with FDG activity similar to the FDG activity in the brain are malignant. If these results are confirmed in other studies with larger populations, FDG PET may be considered superior to CT in patients with non–small-cell lung cancer.

▶ This European study of PET scanning and contrast-enhanced CT scans in the staging of lung cancer is an interesting one that suggests that PET is better than CT, with very good sensitivity and specificity. These data appear to suggest that there is a role for the staging of mediastinal nodal disease using PET scanning. The problem is determining who is going to pay for this procedure, as its expense is not inconsequential.

E. Glatstein, M.D.

Advantage of a Residualizing Iodine Radiolabel for Radioimmunotherapy of Xenografts of Human Non–Small-Cell Carcinoma of the Lung

Stein R, Goldenberg DM, Thorpe SR, et al (Garden State Cancer Ctr, Belleville, NJ; Univ of South Carolina, Columbia)

J Nucl Med 38:391–395, 1997 2–28

Background.—The residence time of a radiolabel at the tumor site can be greatly increased through attachment of ^{131}I to monoclonal antibodies (MAbs) through adducts such as dilactitoltyramine (DLT), which remain trapped lyosomally after catabolism of the labeled MAb. Previous research, comparing ^{131}I-DLT with ^{131}I linked to MAb by the conventional chloramine-T methodology, has shown a substantial increase in ^{131}I accretion in a human lung-cancer xenograft model.

Methods.—Biodistribution experiments were conducted to assess the effect of protein dose on the accretion of ^{131}I-DLT-labeled MAb RS11 in tumor and nontumor tissues. In vivo radioimmunotherapy experiments

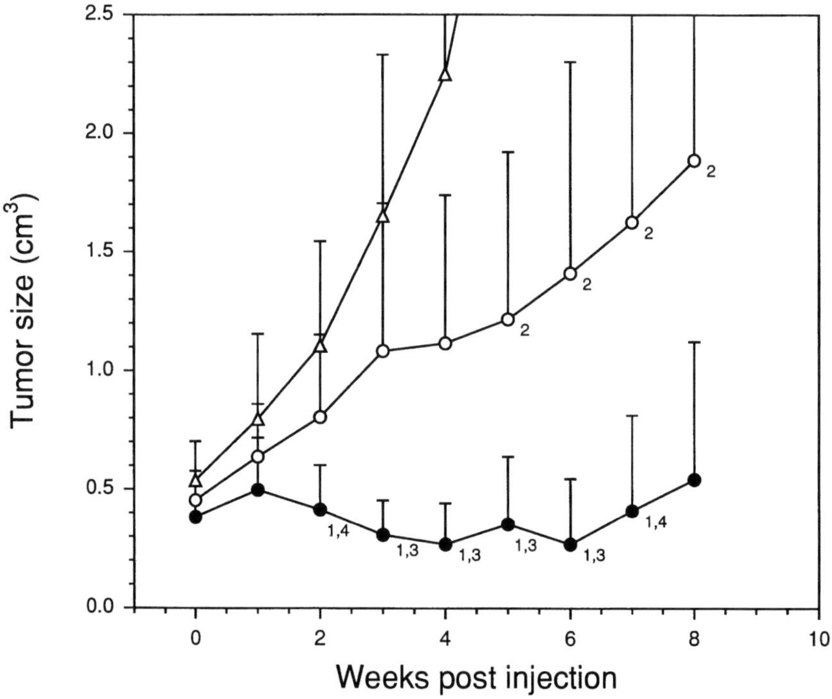

FIGURE 4.—Mean tumor growth. *Points* represent the mean tumor size of the 3 treatment groups. *Error bars* respresent SD and are shown only above the symbol for clarity. *Solid circles* = ^{131}I-labeled DLT-RS11; *open circles* = conventional ^{131}I-labeled RS11; *open triangles* = untreated. $^1P < 0.001$ between treated and untreated groups; $^2P < 0.01$ between treated and untreated groups; $^3P < 0.001$ between the 2 treatment groups; $^4P < 0.01$ between the 2 treatment groups. (Courtesy of Stein R, Goldenberg DM, Thorpe SR, et al: Advantage of a residualizing iodine radiolabel for radioimmunotherapy of xenografts of human non-small-cell carcinoma of the lung. *J Nucl Med* 38:391–395, 1997. Reprinted by permission of the Society of Nuclear Medicine.)

were done to compare the effect of single ^{131}I-DLT-labeled MAb RS11 injections with conventional ^{131}I-labeled RS11 and no treatment.

Findings.—Dosimetry calculations using biodistribution data revealed only small changes in absorbed dose-to-tumor and nontumor tissues with increasing protein dose up to 100 µg. The predicted absorbed dose to tumor ranged from 21,000 to 25,000 cGy/mCi. One 100–µCi dose of ^{131}I-DLT-RS11 resulted in tumor regression. Seven weeks after injection of the radiolabeled MAbs, the tumor volume remained smaller in 73% of the animals given ^{131}I-DLT-labeled RS11 than at the time of MAb injection, compared with 14% in the conventionally labeled ^{131}I-RS11 group and none in the untreated group (Fig 4).

Conclusions.—Residualizing labels such as DLT increase the residence time of radioiodine at the tumor site, thereby enabling an increased dose of radiation to the tumor, while maintaining a lower dose to the dose-limiting organs. Thus this strategy may improve the therapeutic index of radioimmunotherapy.

► Radiolabeled antibodies are still antibodies, i.e., proteins. Because they are proteins, they escape the vasculature suboptimally. The dosimetry will clearly be related to the time that the antibodies are retained on the antigen, which is presumably on the surface or near the surface of the cell. It is interesting that the authors point out that B-cell lymphomas appear to have a lower rate of catabolism of many cell surface–bound MAbs.

These investigators have an innovative approach to trap the iodine inside the cell wall and prolong the exposure of the isotope to its target. I think it will take a lot of work like this to optimize therapeutic radiolabeled antibodies, especially in carcinomas.

E. Glatstein, M.D.

---

bax-Deficiency Promotes Drug Resistance and Oncogenic Transformation by Attenuating p53–dependent Apoptosis

McCurrach ME, Connor TMF, Knudson CM, et al (Cold Spring Harbor Lab, New York; Washington Univ, St Louis)

Proc Natl Acad Sci U S A 94:2345–2349, 1997 2–29

Background.—The p53 protein plays a major role in apoptosis and cell death. However, exactly how p53 is regulated is still unknown. The *bax* promoter may play a role here, in that it has sequence-specific binding sites for *p53* and an excess of p53 increases *bax* expression and triggers apoptosis. The role of *bax* in p53-induced apoptosis was investigated.

Methods.—Mouse embryo fibroblasts (MEFs) were prepared from *p53* and *bax* knock-out mice, such that genotypes were mixed (i.e., some genotypes had no *p53* but did have *bax*, whereas some had neither). The *E1A* oncogene was introduced by gene transfer, to enable the induction of apoptosis based on endogenous p53. The MEFs containing *E1A* were then treated with adriamycin, etoposide, and *cis*-platinum to try to induce p53-dependent apoptosis. Staining was used to confirm apoptotic cell death, and blotting was used to examine gene and protein expression.

Findings.—Drug treatment of MEFs infected with *E1A* that contained *bax* but did not contain *p53* remained viable, but genotypes without *bax* and *p53* had compromised apoptosis. Genotypes with *p53* showed greater (up to six-fold) expression of Bax protein than those without *p53*. Likewise, apoptotic cells without p53 also had no Bax expression. Bax by itself without p53 was not completely successful in inducing apoptosis, although adding the oncogene *E1A* did enhance Bax-induced apoptosis. When cells deficient in *bax* were treated with the oncoproteins Bcl-2 and E1B 19K, p53-dependent apoptosis was suppressed. In the assessment of oncogenic transformation, genotypes with p53 showed less focus formation induced by *E1A* and *ras*. Also, genotypes with p53 and *bax* had no increased effect compared to genotypes containing *bax* without p53.

Conclusions.—Although other substances are also involved, *bax* is an effector of *p53* that helps promote cell death when apoptosis occurs via the *p53* pathway. *bax* is involved in promoting drug resistance and oncogenic transformation, and therefore helps determine p53–dependent chemosensitivity. *bax*-Deficiency was also shown to act in the same genetic pathway as *p53* in effecting oncogenic transformation.

▶ The *p53* mutations are perhaps the most common oncogene mutations in solid tumors. In most studies, *p53* mutations are associated with an inferior prognosis. This study helps define the mechanism responsible for the adverse effects associated with absence of *p53* or *p53* mutations. The p53 protein has been shown to transcriptionally activate *bax*, a *bcl*-2 family member that promotes apoptosis, and p53 appears to coordinate the activities of multiple effectors in the cell. In response to anticancer drugs, p53 promotes apoptosis or cell death. In the absence of p53 or in the presence of a *p53* mutation, exposure to chemotherapeutic agents is not associated with cell death and, consequently, the cell can survive the toxic injury. For these reasons, it is apparent that p53 and its associated pathways become a target for early genetic studies in manipulating the genetic environment of tumors.

R.F. Ozols, M.D., Ph.D.

---

p53-dependent Regulation of *MDR1* Gene Expression Causes Selective Resistance to Chemotherapeutic Agents

Thottassery JV, Zambetti GP, Arimori K, et al (St Jude Children's Research Hosp, Memphis, Tenn; Kumamoto Univ, Japan)

Proc Natl Acad Sci USA 94:11037–11042, 1997 2–30

Introduction.—Previous studies have shown a paradoxic relationship between p53 status and drug sensitivity: when functional p53 is lost, resistance to chemotherapy drugs may be either increased or decreased. This could be related to selective regulation of genes important to the cytotoxic response by p53, specifically, to p53-dependent regulation of multidrug resistance gene (*MDR1*) expression in tumors that normally express this gene. Experiments were performed to see if wild-type p53 regulates the *mdr1* gene.

Methods and Findings.—The experiments used rodent H35 hepatoma cells that express P-glycoprotein (Pgp) and have wild-type p53, into which a transdominant negative (TDN) p53 was introduced. Cells expressing TDN p53 showed greatly increased levels of Pgp and *mdr1a* mRNA. These cells also showed impairment of p53 function, both transactivation and transrepression. Amplification of the *mdr1* gene was not responsible for the enhanced *mdr1a* expression, and the Pgp was functional. Selective insensitivity to Pgp substrates was demonstrated by cytotoxicity assays. Reserpine, a Pgp inhibitor, restored sensitivity to Pgp, which suggested drug retention as the sole basis for loss of drug sensitivity. Further experiments in human LS180 colon carcinoma cells that overexpressed TDN p53 gave similar results.

Conclusions.—Upregulated *MDR1* expression seems to be responsible for p53 inactivation leading to selective resistance to cancer chemotherapy drugs. The results have important ramifications for chemotherapy. The occurrence of p53 mutation in a cancer expressing the *MDR1* gene would be expected to result in a highly multidrug-resistant tumor.

► A deletion or mutation of the p53 tumor suppressor gene is the most frequent alteration in human cancer. This gene is involved in the regulation of a number of cellular functions. Loss of p53 results in decreased susceptibility to apoptotic stimuli, which may account for chemotherapy resistance in some p53–mutated tumors. Paradoxically, p53 mutation is associated with chemosensitivity in other tumors. This study demonstrates that p53-dependent regulation of the *MRD1* gene expression results in selective resistance to chemotherapeutic agents and has obvious potential clinical implications. For example, activating wild-type p53 should make tumors more sensitive to chemotherapy because this could suppress Pgp expression. This phenomenon should predict for synergy between radiation and natural product chemotherapeutic agents, whose intracellular levels are often a function of Pgp expression.

R.F. Ozols, M.D., Ph.D.

Fluorescence Imaging and Spectroscopy of 5-Aminolevulinic Acid Induced Protoporphyrin IX for the Detection of Neoplastic Lesions in the Oral Cavity

Leunig A, Rick K, Stepp H, et al (Univ of Munich, Germany)
Am J Surg 172:674–677, 1996 2–31

Background.—Photodynamic diagnosis with 5-aminolevulinic acid (5-ALA) may be a new alternative for the early detection of oral cancer. The use of 5-ALA has several advantages. This naturally occurring sub-

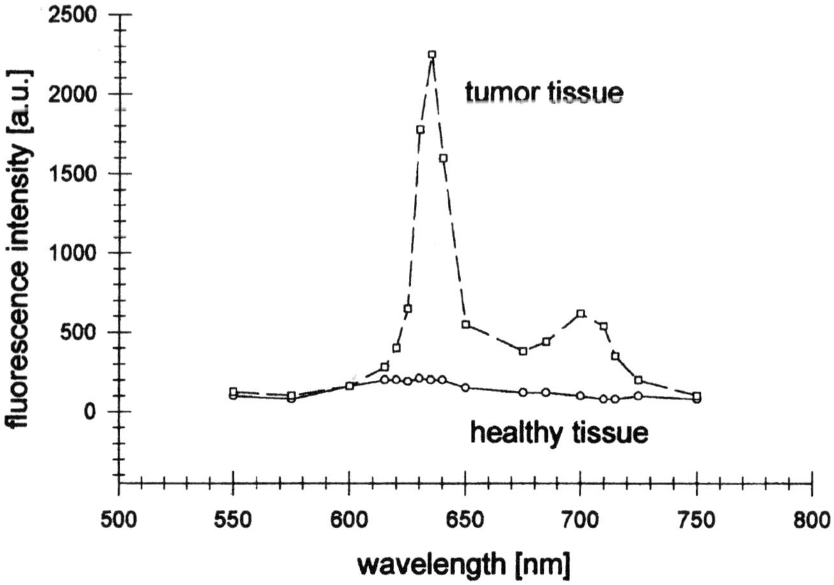

FIGURE 2.—Fluorescence spectra of 5–aminolevulinic acid (5-ALA)–induced protoporphyrin in tumor tissue and the adjacent healthy tissue 1 hour after local application of a 0.4% 5-ALA solution. (Reprinted by permission of the publisher from Leunig A, Rick K, Stepp H, et al: Fluorescence imaging and spectroscopy of 5-aminolevulinic acid induced protoporphyrin IX for the detection of neoplastic lesions in the oral cavity. *Am J Surg* 172:674–677, copyright 1996 by Excerpta Medica Inc.)

stance can be used locally or systemically and metabolizes photosensitizing products rapidly. The efficacy of photodynamic diagnosis after local application of 5-ALA was investigated.

Methods.—In 16 patients with neoplastic lesions of the oral cavity, semiquantitative fluorescence measures were obtained after 5-ALA was applied topically. The time course and type of porphyrin accumulation were assessed in neoplastic and surrounding healthy tissue by analysis of emission spectra of 5-ALA–induced protoporphyrin IX fluorescence.

Findings.—After 5-ALA was applied locally, protoporphyrin IX fluorescence was detected in the oral mucosa in all patients. Protoprophyrin IX accumulated earlier in neoplastic tissue than in surrounding normal tissue. The maximum fluorescence contrast between tumor and host tissue was 10:1, which generally occurred 1–2 hours after application. At that time, the tumor tissue demarcation could be seen with the naked eye (Figs 2 and 4).

Conclusion.—Labeling mucosal lesions of the oral cavity with protoporphyrin IX fluorescence induced by locally applied 5-ALA appears to be a promising diagnostic procedure for neoplastic tumors difficult to see under white light examination. The relevance of this new procedure as a noninvasive, sensitive method for diagnosing oral cancer is under investigation.

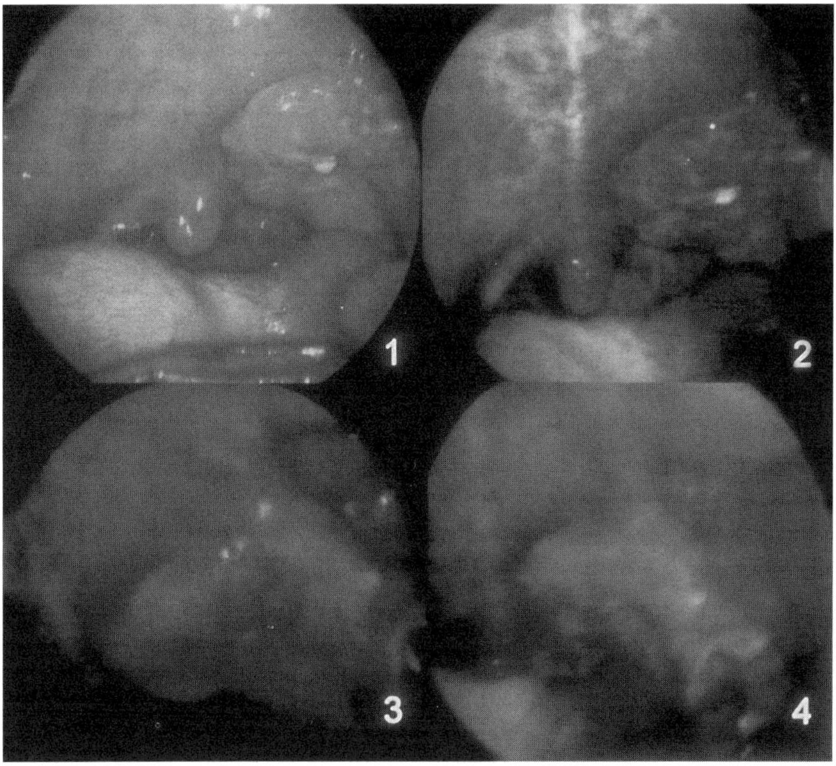

FIGURE 4.—Panel 1 shows the macroscopic findings of a squamous cell carcinoma under white light. **Panel 2** reveals the autofluorescence of this tumor tissue under excitation with blue-violet light before 5-aminolevulinic (5-ALA) application. In contrast to panel 2, an increase of the red fluorescence was observed 1 hour (**panel 3**) and 3 hours (**panel 4**) after topical application of a 0.4% 5-ALA solution. (Reprinted by permission of the publisher from Leunig A, Rick K, Stepp H, et al: Fluorescence imaging and spectroscopy of 5-aminolevulinic acid induced protoporphyrin IX for the detection of neoplastic lesions in the oral cavity. *Am J Surg* 172:674–677, copyright 1996 by Excerpta Medica Inc.)

► 5-Aminolevulinic acid is a phototherapeutic agent, with some additional wrinkles to it. It can be topically applied to cells, and cells gradually metabolize it into a protoporphyrin that can react with laser light and carry out photodynamic therapy. At the same time, it absorbs at other points on the emission spectra. As Figure 4 clearly shows, this can be very helpful in showing the location of cancer in a variety of areas via fluorescence.

Although people are aware of the diagnostic usefulness of these photosensitizing compounds, the technique has been exploited relatively infrequently. I suspect that will change as more people become interested in this form of treatment.

E. Glatstein, M.D.

Identification of Oncofetal Fibronection in Patients With Advanced Epithelial Ovarian Cancer: Detection in Ascitic Fluid and Localization to Primary Sites And Metastatic Implants

Menzin AW, Loret de Mola JR, Bilker WB, et al (Univ of Pennsylvania, Philadelphia)

Cancer 82:152–158, 1998 2–32

Introduction.—Tumor-derived adhesion molecules, such as fibronectin (FN), may play a role in the molecular mechanisms underlying ovarian metastases to the peritoneal cavity. Studies of various types of cancer have shown that oncofetal fibronectin (onfFN) is involved in trophoblast adhesion. The possible association between metastatic ovarian cancer and onfFN production was studied.

Methods.—The study included ascitic fluid samples from 32 patients with epithelial ovarian cancer and from 32 healthy female controls. Samples of primary and metastatic ovarian cancer were available from 14 patients; normal ovarian tissue and small bowel implants of endometriosis were studied for comparison. A nonspecific anti-FN monoclonal antibody, CAF, was used to measure total FN. Specific monoclonal antibodies, FDC-6 and X18A4, were used to identify OnfFN.

Results.—Although both malignant and benign peritoneal fluid specimens showed significant levels of total FN, concentrations were higher in the malignant samples: 172 vs. 76 µg/mL. Concentrations of onfFN were also higher in malignant ascites specimens: 3.4 vs. 0.9 µg/mL with FDC-6 and 5.1 vs. 1.1 µg/mL with X18A4. Immunohistochemical studies of tumor tissue localized FN and onfFN to the stroma around epithelial tumor nests, with more delicate fibrillar staining within the tumor nests. Endometriosis implants showed stromal staining for FN, but not for onfFN.

Conclusion.—Advanced ovarian carcinomas express onfFN, which may play a role in tumor adhesion to peritoneal surfaces. The findings show intense stromal localization of onfFN in primary and metastatic ovarian cancers, as previously shown for other types of carcinomas. The functional significance of onfFN in patients with various malignancies and its possible diagnostic and treatment implications remain to be clarified.

► These investigators looked at FN associated with nonspecific antifibronectal monoclonal antibodies. These antibodies were reacted with ascitic fluids from patients with ovarian cancer and peritoneal fluids from patients without pathology as well as tissue sections of primary and metastatic ovarian implants. Using an enzyme-linked immunosorbant assay, the investigators noted that both malignant and benign peritoneal fluids contained high quantities of FN, although the malignant ascites contained much higher concentrations than did the benign. Their data suggest that onfFN is present in advanced ovarian malignancies. The authors believe that this may play a role in the tumor-associated peritoneal adhesions and other cellular interactions, possibly including peritoneal seeding.

Certainly, the behavior of ovarian cancer features much more reaction with the peritoneal surface than do most other neoplasms, at least on the basis of probability. These results suggest that onfFN may be an important factor in this and may serve as a focal point for new strategy in dealing with ovarian peritoneal seeding.

E. Glatstein, M.D.

3 Breast Cancer

Breast Masses in Women Treated for Childhood Cancer: Incidence and Screening Guidelines

Kaste SC, Hudson MM, Jones DJ, et al (St Jude Children's Research Hosp, Memphis, Tenn; Univ of Tennessee, Memphis)

Cancer 82:784–792, 1998 3–1

Objective.—The risk of breast cancer is increased in children treated for cancer using thoracic radiation therapy. Whether special screening protocols need to be established for specific patient subgroups has not been studied. The incidence of benign and malignant breast lesions was estimated in a group of female patients treated for childhood cancer, and the methods by which the masses were detected were reviewed.

Methods.—Of 1,979 females who were former patients of St Jude's—followed up for an average of 9.9 years—66 received diagnoses of breast abnormalities. Methods of detection, diagnoses of benign or malignant lesion, family history, and treatment history were reviewed.

Results.—There were 53 white women and 13 black women who received a diagnosis of primary malignancy at a median age of 13.8 years. There were 15 patients with primary Hodgkin's disease, 12 with rhabdomyosarcoma, 10 with germ cell tumor, 5 with acute lymphoblastic leukemia, 5 with non-Hodgkin's lymphoma, 4 with osteosarcoma, 3 with acute myelocytic leukemia, 2 with other leukemia, 2 with Wilms' tumor, 2 with carcinoma, CNS in 1, neuroblastoma in 1, soft-tissue sarcoma in 1, and other malignancy in 3. Prior treatment for primary cancer included chemotherapy for 16, chemotherapy plus radiation for 38 (including breast tissue in 22), and radiation therapy in 3 (including breast tissue in 3). One patient with rare cystosarcoma phylloides had surgery alone for her primary cancer. Additional risk factors included hormone replacement therapy in 12 patients, oral contraceptive use in 14, no pregnancy in 62, and first-degree relative with breast cancer in 6. Of 67 breast masses, 26 were malignant and 41 were benign. Masses were detected by self-examination in 32 and by a physician in 28. Fourteen malignant masses were metastatic and 12 were second primary malignancies. Second primary malignancies were detected at a median of 15.1 years (range 4.4–24.9 years) after the primary malignancy. The 25-year incidence of breast cancer in these patients was 20 times higher than for age- and race-matched controls.

TABLE 6.—Breast Screening Guidelines for Childhood Cancer Survivors Treated With Thoracic Radiation Therapy

Time of screening	Type of screening
Starting at puberty	Breast self-examination
Puberty until age 25 yrs	Clinical breast examination once a yr
Ages 25–40 yrs	Clinical breast examination twice a yr
	Baseline mammogram
	Repeat mammogram every 3 yrs until age 40 yrs
Age 40 yrs and older	Clinical breast examination twice a yr
	Mammogram every yr

(Courtesy of Kaste SC, Hudson MM, Jones DJ, et al: Breast masses in women treated for childhood cancer: Incidence and screening guidelines. *Cancer* 82:784–792. Copyright 1998 American Cancer Society. Reprinted by permission of Wiley-Liss, Inc., a subsidiary of John Wiley & Sons, Inc.)

Conclusion.—Female children treated for cancer have a significantly increased risk of breast cancer and should be instructed in the importance of breast self-examinations and should undergo special screening. Screening guidelines are presented in (Table 6).

▶ With an increasing cure rate for neoplasms of childhood, the long-term effects of therapy are increasingly important. This article nicely illustrates the risk of breast cancer in young women who received radiation therapy to the chest wall for prior childhood malignancies. The authors outline proposed screening recommendations beginning at the age of 25 years. Patients and their parents must be informed of the increased risk of secondary cancers after such therapy.

P.J. Loehrer, Sr., M.D.

HER-2 Expression and Response to Tamoxifen in Estrogen Receptor-positive Breast Cancer: A Southwest Oncology Group Study

Elledge RM, Green S, Ciocca D, et al (Univ of Texas Health Science Ctr, San Antonio; Southwest Oncology Group Statistical Ctr, Seattle; Laboratorio de Reproduccion y Lactancia, Mendoza, Argentina; et al)

Clin Cancer Res 4:7–12, 1998 3–2

Objective.—Whereas overexpression of growth factor HER-2 (erbB-2) predicts a worse outcome in patients with breast cancer, its influence on response to tamoxifen therapy is not clear cut.

Methods.—HER-2 expression was measured in a prospective study of 205 ER-positive tumors in patients with metastatic disease who received tamoxifen as initial metastatic therapy. Response to tamoxifen therapy was compared with patient and tumor characteristics, time to treatment failure, and survival. The median follow-up was 9 years. HER-2 content was analyzed immunohistochemically using the monoclonal antibody TAB 250 and scored according to the proportion of positive membrane-stained tumor cells.

Results.—Using a cutoff immunohistochemical score of 2 for HER-2 positivity, 30% of tumors were HER-2 positive. Estrogen receptor levels and bcl-2 expression were significantly lower in patients who were HER-2 positive. HER-2 status was not related to time-to-treatment failure or to tamoxifen response.

Conclusion.—HER-2 expression does not alter response to tamoxifen therapy in estrogen receptor-positive patients with breast cancer.

▶ Overexpression of HER-2/neu in patients with breast cancer is associated with inferior outcome. In certain breast cancer cell lines, this overexpression may result in tamoxifen resistance, presumably secondary to alteration of the growth factor pathway. In the clinic, retrospective analysis has been inconclusive largely because HER-2/neu overexpression is more commonly seen in estrogen receptor-negative tumors. This study evaluated 205 paraffin-embedded tumors and correlated expression with clinical outcome in previously untreated patients with estrogen receptor-positive tumors. No difference with respect to response rate, time to treatment, and overall survival was noted. The impact of HER-2/neu expression upon outcome of therapy appears to be an interaction of this growth factor with cytotoxic chemotherapy rather than hormonal therapy.

P.J. Loehrer, Sr., M.D.

Tamoxifen and Chemotherapy for Lymph Node–negative, Estrogen Receptor–positive Breast Cancer

Fisher B, Dignam J, Wolmark N, et al (Univ of Pittsburgh, Pa; Allegheny Gen Hosp, Pittsburgh, Pa; Michigan State Univ, East Lansing; et al)

J Natl Cancer Inst 89:1673–1682, 1997 3–3

Introduction.—Before 1985, there were insufficient data to advocate a therapy other than surgery for patients with breast cancer and negative nodes. Subsequent findings from 3 National Surgical Adjuvant Breast and Bowel Project (NSABP) trials led to the recommendation that patients with node-negative breast cancer receive systemic therapy. Findings are reported for the B-20 study of the NSABP, conducted to determine whether chemotherapy plus tamoxifen (TAM) would be more beneficial than TAM alone in the treatment of patients with axillary lymph-node–negative, estrogen-receptor (ER)–positive breast cancer.

Methods.—The study enrolled 2,306 patients between October 1988 and March 1993. They were randomly assigned to 1 of 3 treatment groups before surgery: TAM alone (771 patients); methotrexate, fluorouracil, and TAM (MFT, 767 patients); and cyclophosphamide plus MFT (CMFT, 768 patients). Lumpectomies had been performed in about 45% of patients. Approximately two thirds of tumors were 2 cm in size, and about 20% were ER-negative. The average time spent in the study was 77 months. Patients were followed up for disease-free survival rates, distant disease-free survival rates, and overall survival rates.

Results.—Chemotherapy plus TAM yielded significantly better disease-free survival rates than TAM alone (90% for MFT and 89% for CMFT vs. 85% for TAM through 5 years of follow-up). Both distant disease-free survival rates and overall survival rates showed similar trends: distant disease-free survival rates at 5 years were 92% for MFT, 91% for CMFT, and 87% for TAM; 5-year overall survival rates were 97% for MFT, 96% for CMFT, and 94% for TAM. Both combined regimens reduced the risk of ipsilateral breast tumor recurrence after a lumpectomy and the risk of recurrence at other local, regional, and distant sites compared with TAM alone. The risk of treatment failure was reduced with both types of chemotherapy in all subgroups of tumor size, ER status, and patient age. Risk reduction was greatest, however, in patients 49 years or younger.

Conclusion.—Patients with node-negative breast cancer and ER-positive tumors were found to benefit from TAM, but about one third experienced a treatment failure by 10 years. Thus, even patients considered to have a "good" prognosis—regardless of age, lymph node status, tumor size, or ER status—are candidates for chemotherapy.

▶ The NSABP has conducted seminal trials in the treatment of early-stage breast cancer. This trial, which follows in the tradition of simple, well-designed, well-powered trials, demonstrates that chemotherapy plus TAM is superior to TAM alone in patients with lymph-node–negative and ER-positive tumors. Although no subgroup failed to show an advantage with chemotherapy, the benefit was greatest for women 49 years of age or older. The authors ask 2 important questions in their discussion. First, should all patients with ER-positive tumors and negative lymph nodes (including tumors 1 cm or less) be treated with TAM and chemotherapy? Secondly, is the benefit received (5% or less in disease-free survival, progression-free survival, and overall survival rates) adequate to justify the treatment for all patients? The clinician and the patient must decide the answers to these questions. However, for the time being, this trial suggests that all such patients should be at least advised regarding the potential benefit of chemotherapy.

P.J. Loehrer, Sr., M.D.

Effectiveness of Adjuvant Chemotherapy in Combination With Tamoxifen for Node-positive Postmenopausal Breast Cancer Patients

Castiglione-Gertsch M, and the International Breast Cancer Study Group (Harvard Med School, Boston; et al)

J Clin Oncol 15:1385–1394, 1997 3–4

Objective.—For postmenopausal women with lymph node-positive breast cancer, adjuvant tamoxifen therapy can decrease relapse rate and mortality. It is unclear whether adding chemotherapy to tamoxifen offers

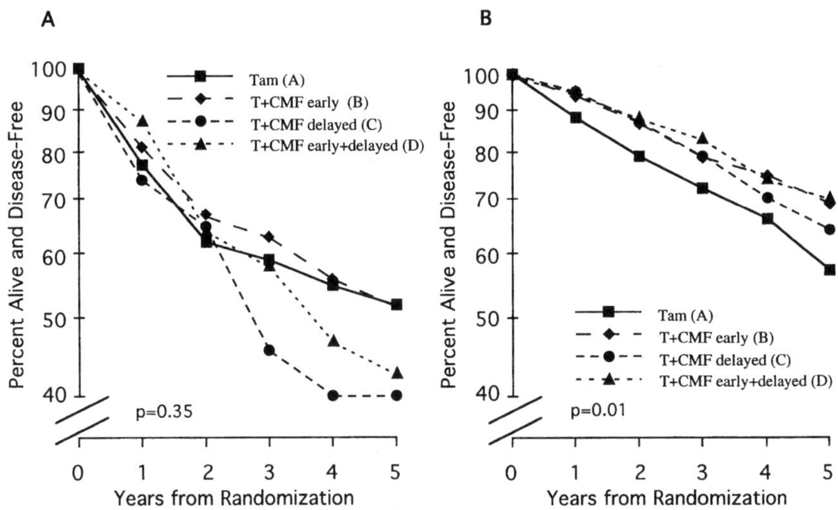

FIGURE 3.—Kaplan-Meier plots of disease-free survival for (**A**) 279 estrogen-receptor (ER)–negative patients and (**B**) 889 ER-positive patients. Numbers of patients at risk at 5 years for each of the treatment groups were: (*A*) 14, (*B*) 23, (*C*) 11, (*D*) 17 for the ER-negative group; and (*A*) 72, (*B*) 77, (*C*) 65, (*D*) 82 for the ER-positive group. *Abbreviations: Tam,* tamifoxen alone; *T + CMF,* tamoxifen plus cyclophosphamide, methotrexate, and fluorouracil. (Courtesy of Castiglione-Gertsch M, and the International Breast Cancer Study Group: Effectiveness of adjuvant chemotherapy in combination with tamoxifen for node-positive postmenopausal breast cancer patients. *J Clin Oncol* 15:1385–1394, 1997.)

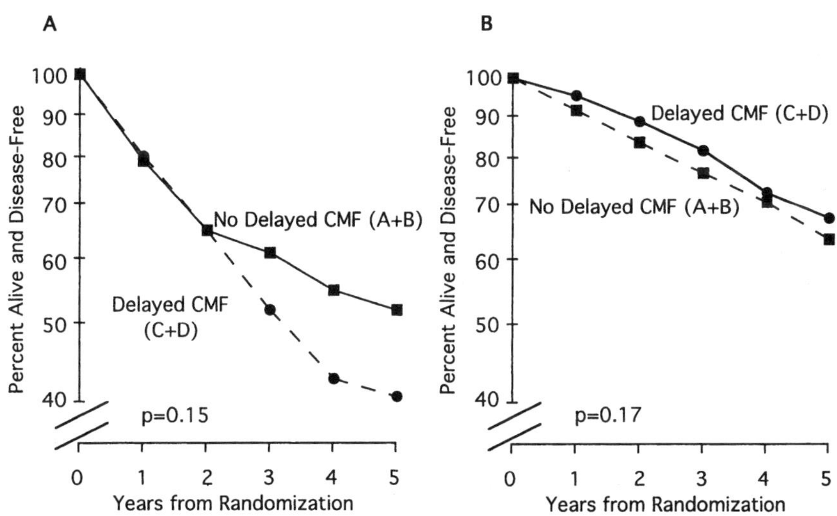

FIGURE 7.—Kaplan-Meier plots of disease-free survival for delayed chemotherapy vs. no delayed chemotherapy for stratified cohort of patients with (**A**) estrogen-receptor (ER)–negative and (**B**) ER-positive primary tumors. Numbers of patients at risk at 5 years for the treatment groups were: delayed, $n = 28$, no delayed, $n = 37$ for ER-negative group; and delayed, $n = 147$, no delayed, $n = 149$ for ER-positive group. *Abbreviation: CMF,* cyclophosphamide, methotrexate, and fluorouracil. (Courtesy of Castiglione-Gertsch M, and the International Breast Cancer Study Group: Effectiveness of adjuvant chemotherapy in combination with tamoxifen for node-positive postmenopausal breast cancer patients. *J Clin Oncol* 15:1385–1394, 1997.)

further benefits. A randomized trial of tamoxifen plus adjuvant chemotherapy for this patient group was conducted.

Methods.—The study included 1,266 postmenopausal women with node-positive breast cancer. They were randomized to receive 5 years of therapy with tamoxifen only; tamoxifen plus early chemotherapy (3 courses of cyclophosphamide, methotrexate, and fluorouracil [CMF] chemotherapy during the first 3 months of treatment); tamoxifen plus delayed chemotherapy (CMF at 9, 12, and 15 months); or tamoxifen plus early and delayed chemotherapy (CMF at 1, 2, 3, 9, 12, and 15 months). The patients were stratified by estrogen-receptor (ER) status. The final analysis included 1,212 patients, with a median follow-up of 60 months.

Results.—Five-year disease-free survival was 64% for patients receiving tamoxifen plus early CMF, compared to 57% for patients not receiving early chemotherapy (hazards ratio [HR] 0.79). However, disease-free survival was unimproved by delayed chemotherapy—61% for patients receiving tamoxifen plus delayed chemotherapy vs. 60% for patients not receiving delayed chemotherapy (HR 0.97) (Fig 3). Chemotherapy—early, delayed, or both—did produce a 22% to 36% reduction in the risk of relapse for patients with ER-positive breast cancer (Fig 7). The risk of relapse was increased slightly but nonsignificantly for patients with ER-negative cancer who received tamoxifen with delayed CMF.

Conclusions.—Adding combination chemotherapy to tamoxifen is beneficial for postmenopausal women with node-positive breast cancer. Three courses of CMF can be given in the first 3 months of long-term tamoxifen therapy. Particularly in patients with ER-negative tumors, tamoxifen should not be started before CMF.

► Adjuvant therapy for patients with node-positive breast cancer is standard treatment. The choice of treatments consist of hormonal therapy, chemotherapy, or both. The optimal schedule or combination has yet to be defined. In patients over the age of 50 with ER-positive tumors, the National Surgical Adjuvant Breast and Bowel Project demonstrated that tamoxifen plus chemotherapy (4 cycles of doxorubicin plus cyclophosphamide) was superior to tamoxifen alone. In contrast, prolonged chemotherapy using a CMF-based regimen with tamoxifen was not superior to tamoxifen alone in a similar patient population. Preclinical data suggest that tamoxifen may adversely modify the side effects of chemotherapy.

Consequently, this paper describes a trial designed to evaluate the role of short-course CMF chemotherapy added to tamoxifen either early in the treatment course, later, or both times. The authors conclude that early chemotherapy did improve the 5-year disease-free survival, compared with hormonal therapy alone. Further, delayed chemotherapy was associated with a trend toward increased relapse in ER-negative patients. This trial supports the preclinical data suggesting the importance of scheduling the tamoxifen in chemotherapy, especially (and perhaps surprisingly) for patients with ER-negative tumors.

P.J. Loehrer, Sr., M.D.

Cyclophosphamide and Fluorouracil Combined With Mitoxantrone Versus Doxorubicin for Breast Cancer: Superiority of Doxorubicin

Stewart DJ, Evans WK, Shepherd FA, et al (Univ of Ottawa, Ont; Toronto Hosp; Toronto-Sunnybrook Regional Cancer Centre; et al)

J Clin Oncol 15:1897–1905, 1997 3–5

Introduction.—Randomized trials in patients with breast cancer which compare single-agent mitoxantrone and single-agent doxorubicin have shown response rates and toxicity to be lower with mitoxantrone. Only 1 trial in breast cancer has shown doxorubicin to have superior survival rates over mitoxantrone as single agents. This article reports a randomized, multicenter trial of combination therapy IV consisting of cyclophosphamide, 500 mg/m^2, plus fluorouracil 500 mg/m^2, combined with either mitoxantrone, 10 mg/m^2, (CNF) or doxorubicin, 50 mg/m^2, (CAF) given every 3 weeks was conducted with 249 patients with advanced breast cancer.

Methods.—Before randomization, patients were stratified according to whether they received earlier adjuvant chemotherapy. Toxicity, response rate, survival time, and quality-of-life were evaluated.

Results.—One-hundred twenty-one patients were randomized to CNF and 128 were randomized to CAF. The response rates for CNF and CAF were 36% (44 patients) and 48% (62 patients), respectively. When only fully assessable patients were included, the response rates were 48% for CNF and 60% for CAF. All except 10 patients had died by last assessment. One and 9 patients receiving CNF and CAF, respectively, were still alive. The median survival for CAF was significantly longer than for CNF (15.2 vs. 10.9 months). The median time to progression was significantly longer for CAF than CNF (5.3 months versus 3.2 months, respectively). When all patients were excluded who failed to meet all eligibility criteria, survival differences were still significant.

Favorable prognostic factors for survival included good performance status; less than 2 organ systems involved by tumor; no lung, liver, or brain involvement; involvement of bone or bone marrow; prior surgery for breast cancer; premenopausal status; 3 or more years from diagnosis to randomization; and treatment with CAF. Significantly more patients treated with CAF than CNF (55% vs. 12%) had grade 3 or greater alopecia. There were no significant differences in any other grade 3 or higher toxicities. Quality of life was similar for both treatment groups.

Conclusion.—Both CAF and CNF are feasible options for patients with advanced breast cancer. Patients in the CAF group had a somewhat higher response rate and survival rate than patients in the CNF group. Alopecia occurred more frequently in the CAF group.

► Few prospective, randomized trials demonstrate significant survival advantages in advanced solid tumors. In the last decade, a number of analogues of active chemotherapeutic agents have been approved, based on comparable activity but with less toxicity. The results of this trial—like carboplatin vs. cisplatin in germ cell tumors—show that the analogue is not quite as effective as a parent compound when examining survival and times to progression. In addition, this trial showed no significant difference in toxicity between the 2 regimens. The trial emphasizes the importance of conducting prospective, randomized trials with solid end points rather than always embracing the newest drug on the block.

P.J. Loehrer, Sr., M.D.

Increased Intensification and Total Dose of Cyclophosphamide in a Doxorubicin–Cyclophosphamide Regimen for the Treatment of Primary Breast Cancer: Findings From National Surgical Adjuvant Breast and Bowel Project B-22

Fisher B, Anderson S, Wickerham DL, et al (Univ of Pittsburgh, Pa; Michigan State Univ, East Lansing; CCOP, Allegheny, Pittsburgh, Pa; et al)

J Clin Oncol 15:1858–1869, 1997 3–6

Background.—The National Surgical Adjuvant Breast and Bowel Project (NSABP) trial B-22 addressed the deficiency of data on the effects of drug doses in patients with breast cancer treated with adjuvant chemotherapy. The effect of different dose intensities and different cumulative doses of a single agent in a multiple-dose regimen was assessed. The 5-year follow-up results are reported.

Methods.—A total of 2,305 women with primary operable breast cancer, positive axillary lymph nodes, and no evidence of metastases were entered into the trial. They were randomly assigned to 1 of 3 groups. Patients in group 1 received 4 courses of standard adjuvant chemotherapy with a doxorubicin–cyclophosphamide (AC) combination; those in group 2 received intensified therapy, that is, the same total dose of cyclophosphamide given in just 2 courses; and those in group 3 received intensified and increased therapy, that is, a double dose of cyclophosphamide given in 4 courses. All patients received the same dose and intensity of doxorubicin. The life-table method was used to assess disease-free survival (DFS) and overall survival rates.

Results.—The 5-year follow-up results showed no significant difference in DFS or overall survival rates among the 3 groups. The DFS rates were 62% in group 1, 60% in group 2, and 64% in group 3. The overall survival rates were 78% in group 1, 77% in group 2, and 77% in group 3. Patterns of survival were similar when analyzed in terms of the number of positive lymph nodes. Patients in groups 2 and 3 experienced more grade 4 toxicity. The observed differences could not be explained by differences in the dose or intensity of cyclophosphamide, by delayed doses, or by the intervals between courses of chemotherapy.

Conclusions.—In patients with node-positive breast cancer, an intensified or increased dose of cyclophosphamide does not improve survival rates. The results are the same whether analyzed by assigned group or by the actual dose received. Intensification and an increased total dose of cyclophosphamide cannot be considered appropriate therapy for women with primary breast cancer.

▶ Since the early 1980s, one of the battle cries regarding chemotherapeutic regimens has been "dose intensity." In retrospective analyses of treatments for breast cancer and other diseases, it appeared that outcome was closely related to the dosage of drugs administered. Whereas it is readily admitted that a threshold dose is important, would further escalation beyond the threshold make a difference?

This trial by the NSABP was a well-designed, adequately powered, prospective randomized trial which evaluated not only dose intensity but cumulative dosage of cyclophosphamide when administered with doxorubicin as adjuvant therapy for women with operable breast cancer and one or more positive lymph nodes. Neither cyclophosphamide dose intensity (mg/m^2/week) or cumulative dose had an impact on outcome when measured as disease-free survival or overall survival.

Whereas other ongoing trials are looking at even more dose-intense regimens, including the use of high-dose chemotherapy with stem cell rescue, it appears that dose escalation of cyclophosphamide, at least, does not appear warranted.

P.J. Loehrer, Sr., M.D.

Breast Conservation After Induction Chemotherapy for Locally Advanced Breast Cancer

Kling KM, Ostrzega N, Schmit P (Olive View-UCLA Med Ctr, Sylmar, Calif)

Am Surg 63:861–864, 1997 3–7

Background.—Neoadjuvant chemotherapy (NC) decreases the size of primary breast cancer in 80% to 90% of patients. One group of patients with locally advanced, operable breast cancer treated with NC was studied prospectively to identify eligibility for breast conservation surgery (BC) and clinical parameters that predict response to chemotherapy.

Methods.—Thirty-two patients with stage IIB and III primary operable breast cancer were assessed between 1991 and 1995. The patients received NC consisting of 3 cycles of 5-fluorouracil, doxorubicin, and cyclophosphamide. Tumor size before chemotherapy was assessed by palpation and mammography. Depending on clinical response, patients were offered BC.

Findings.—The initial mean tumor size was 7 cm, with a range of 4–15 cm. In 53% of the patients, treatment reduced tumor size by more than 50%. Sixty-six percent of the patients were potential BC candidates, with a post-NC pathologic tumor size of less than 4 cm. Sixteen percent of the women had no residual tumor. Thirteen percent underwent BC. Partial response was uncorrelated with patient age, menopausal status, tumor steroid receptor or Her-2/NEU positivity, or initial tumor size.

Conclusion.—The response rate to NC among patients with a clinically negative axilla was 88%. Neoadjuvant chemotherapy can significantly decrease tumor size, enabling subsequent BC treatment.

▶ Early initial studies of multiagent chemotherapy for locally advanced inoperable or inflammatory breast cancer indicated significant local response rates in the order of 50% to 75%. In some reports, pathologic complete response rates were in the 15% to 20% range. This has led to several reports in the literature in the last few years documenting a similar neoadjuvant chemotherapy approach to women with large primary but operable breast cancer with the objective of "downstaging" the primary tumor both in the breast and in the axilla. This paper from a group in California reports on a prospective trial in 32 women with locally advanced breast cancer receiving neoadjuvant chemotherapy followed by mastectomy or, when appropriate, by breast conservation surgery. Although long-term follow-up data are not yet conclusive regarding overall survival or disease-free survival, there is good evidence of adequate response of the primary tumor in the breast.

In this series, partial or greater response occurred in 53% of the patients, and 16% of the patients were pathologically complete responders. It has been my experience with preoperative design protocols that axillary response is quite important in determining prognosis. Those patients who do not experience response in the axillary lymph nodes have a particularly poor prognosis regarding eventual development of systemic disease. More clinical trial data need to be available before any conclusions can be made regarding neoadjuvant chemotherapy in breast cancer; however, good surgical clearance of the axilla is still necessary for prognostic indication and, perhaps, stratification into high-dose density chemotherapy regimens after surgery such as bone marrow transplantation.

B.L. Eisenberg, M.D.

Primary Chemotherapy in Operable Breast Cancer: Eight-Year Experience at the Milan Cancer Institute

Bonadonna G, Valagussa P, Brambilla C, et al (Istituto Nazionale Tumori, Milan, Italy)

J Clin Oncol 16:93–100, 1998 3–8

Introduction.—As part of a multidisciplinary approach for locally advanced inoperable disease, primary chemotherapy for breast cancer has been introduced to achieve prompt tumor response using only a few chemotherapy cycles. Mastectomy was the surgical treatment of choice after drug response. Two consecutive prospective nonrandomized studies were begun in women with large but operable cancers. The 8-year experience achieved in these trials had the aim of decreasing the size of the primary tumor, avoiding mastectomy, and allowing for effective local and distant control.

Methods.—In a 2-year period, 231 women with operable breast cancers measuring 3 cm or more were enrolled. They were tested with 5 different regimens in 7 consecutive groups of 33 patients each. For 3 or 4 cycles, the different drug regimens (cyclophosphamide, methotrexate, and fluorouracil; anthracycline- or mitoxantrone-containing combinations; or doxorubicin alone) were delivered at full dose. In another trial, during a 5-year period 310 women with primary tumors measuring 2.5 cm or more were enrolled. This study involved 3 cycles of single-agent anthracycline delivered as primary chemotherapy. After chemotherapy, the women had breast-sparing surgery in the presence of objective tumor remission. Women at high risk of relapse had additional postoperative chemotherapy, and follow-up was for a median of 65 months.

Results.—The 2 trials had fairly comparable characteristics. Breast-sparing surgery was performed on 85% of women after primary chemotherapy. Surgical specimens failed to show any residual neoplastic cell in 14 patients (3%). The significant variables that influenced the 8-year relapse-free survival were the histologically assessed extent of axillary node involvement and the degree of response to primary chemotherapy. The cumulative risk of local relapse as first event alone was 6.8% in women subjected to a breast-conserving approach.

Conclusion.—In women with tumors of more than 5 cm, primary chemotherapy can be safely administered and can allow breast-sparing surgery in a high fraction of patients (62%). Properly conceived, large randomized studies with more effective and newer drug regimens are warranted to effectively assess the long-term results of this approach.

▶ Dr. Bonadonna and his colleagues at the Istituto Nazionale Tumori in Milan have performed some of the seminal work in the field of breast cancer. Preoperative chemotherapy has long been accepted for locally advanced "inoperable" breast cancer. In addition, in numerous other malignancies such as osteogenic sarcoma, non-small cell lung cancer, head and neck cancer, and others, preoperative chemotherapy or "neoadjuvant" chemotherapy has become commonplace. The use of preoperative chemotherapy in surgically resectable breast cancer has several theoretical and clinical advantages. Preliminary results from the National Surgical Adjuvant Breast Project B-18 randomized trial show no obvious differences in outcome between patients receiving preoperative and patients receiving postoperative chemotherapy. The results of this phase II experience from Milan appear to confirm our suspicions that systemic therapy either before or after local therapy is effective. Prospective randomized trials with longer follow-up, with special attention to quality-of-life issues, will further define the role of preoperative therapy. The potential advantages of downsizing tumors may afford greater options for breast conservation surgery, while not having an adverse effect on survival.

P.J. Loehrer, Sr., M.D.

Adjuvant Radiotherapy and Chemotherapy in Node-positive Premenopausal Women With Breast Cancer

Ragaz J, Jackson SM, Le N, et al (Unit of British Columbia, Vancouver; British Columbia Cancer Agency, Victoria)

N Engl J Med 337:956–962, 1997 3–9

Background.—In women undergoing mastectomies for early breast cancer, postoperative radiotherapy reduces the risk of local relapse. However, radiotherapy after mastectomy has fallen into disuse because of its inability to improve overall survival rates. There is now reason to believe that adding to chemotherapy radiotherapy might improve survival rates. The long-term follow-up of a trial of combined radiotherapy and chemotherapy for breast cancer is reported.

Methods.—Three hundred eighteen premenopausal women with stage I or II breast cancer and positive lymph nodes were enrolled in the trial between 1978 and 1986. After undergoing modified radical mastectomies, the patients were randomly assigned to receive either chemotherapy alone or radiotherapy plus chemotherapy. Chemotherapy consisted of cyclophosphamide, methotrexate, and fluorouracil. Between the 4th and 5th cycles, women in the combined-therapy group received radiotherapy to the chest wall and regional lymph nodes. The median follow-up for survivors was 150 months.

Results.—The recurrence rate was reduced by one third in women receiving chemotherapy plus radiotherapy (relative risk [RR], 0.67; 95% confidence interval [CI], 0.50–0.90). Combined therapy also produced about a 30% reduction in breast cancer mortality (RR, 0.71; 95% CI, 0.51–0.99). Radiotherapy was no more beneficial for women with 4 or more positive lymph nodes than for those with 3 or fewer positive lymph nodes.

Conclusion.—For women undergoing modified radical mastectomies for early, node-positive breast cancer, adding radiotherapy to chemotherapy reduces the risk of local-regional and systemic relapse and reduces breast cancer mortality. Shifting to routine use of radiotherapy for all patients with node-positive breast cancer would be a major change in breast cancer treatment. The results may not apply to patients undergoing breast-conserving surgery followed by breast irradiation.

Postoperative Radiotherapy in High-Risk Premenopausal Women With Breast Cancer Who Receive Adjuvant Chemotherapy

Overgaard M, for the Danish Breast Cancer Cooperative Group 82b Trial (Aarhus Univ Hosp, Denmark; et al)

N Engl J Med 337:949–955, 1997 3–10

Background.—Trial data show that performing radiotherapy after mastectomy reduces the incidence of local-regional recurrence of breast cancer but does not improve survival rates. Most studies of this approach have not used chemotherapy. Postmastectomy radiotherapy in addition to chemotherapy was evaluated for premenopausal women with high-risk breast cancer.

Methods.—The randomized trial included 1,708 women with stage I or II breast cancer treated with mastectomies. All women received adjuvant systemic chemotherapy with cyclophosphamide, methotrexate, and fluorouracil (CMF). One group of patients received 9 cycles of CMF; the other group received 8 cycles of CMF plus chest wall and regional lymph node irradiation. The intended radiation dose to the target volume was 50 Gy in 25 fractions or 48 Gy in 22 fractions. The 2 groups were followed up for a median of 114 months for the study endpoints of local-regional recurrence, distant metastases, disease-free survival rates, and overall survival rates.

Results.—Local-regional recurrence, with or without distant metastases, occurred in 9% of women treated with radiotherapy plus CMF vs. 32% of those treated with CMF alone ($P < 0.001$). The probability of 10-year disease-free survival was 48% for the radiotherapy-plus-CMF group vs. 34% in the CMF-only group ($P < 0.001$). Ten-year overall survival rates were 54% for the former group and 45% for the latter group ($P < 0.001$). On multivariate analysis, postmastectomy irradiation was significantly and independently related to improved disease-free and overall survival rates, regardless of tumor size, number of positive lymph nodes, and histopathologic grade. Data on long-term complications were incomplete, but there was no evidence of a higher death rate among patients with left-side tumors.

Conclusions.—For premenopausal women with high-risk breast cancer, performing radiotherapy in addition to adjuvant chemotherapy after mastectomy reduces the risk of local-regional recurrence and prolongs survival. Both local-regional and systemic disease must be controlled to achieve the best results in breast cancer treatment. Radiotherapy seems to be required for adequate local-regional control in the patient population studied.

► These 2 papers (Abstracts 3–9 and 3–10), published sequentially in the same issue of *The New England Journal of Medicine* support the roles of adjuvant radiotherapy in selective patients after mastectomy for adenocarcinoma of the breast. The combined series involving over 2,000 patients with a median follow-up of 10 to 15 years demonstrated radiotherapy, reduced locoregional recurrence, and prolonged survival. These trials are provocative in light of the fact that overall survival seems to be improved with locoregional radiotherapy.

A few years ago, Cuzick and colleagues[1] performed a meta-analysis including 8 randomized trials and found conflicting results (i.e., survival was inferior for patients with prior radiotherapy). An update suggested that increased cardiac mortality in the radiotherapy group was a major factor in this outcome.[2] Additional studies with long-term follow-up have shown other problems, including sarcomas of the chest wall and postirradiation extremity edema.

Although newer techniques of treatment with the use of electron beam may minimize toxicity, long-term follow-up will continue to evaluate not only mortality but also morbidity. The debate on this issue is far from over.

P.J. Loehrer, Sr., M.D.

References

1. Cuzick J, Stewart H, Peto R, et al: Overview of randomized trials of postoperative adjuvant radiotherapy in breast cancer. *Cancer Treat Rep* 71:15–29, 1987.
2. Cuzick J, Stewart H, Rutgvist L, et al: Cause-specific mortality in long-term survivors of breast cancer who participate in trials of radiotherapy. *J Clin Oncol* 12:447–453, 1994.

Stress and Immune Responses After Surgical Treatment for Regional Breast Cancer

Andersen BL, Farrar WB, Golden-Kreutz D, et al (Ohio State Univ, Columbus)
J Natl Cancer Inst 90:30–36, 1998 3–11

Introduction.—A diagnosis of cancer and cancer treatment are objective, negative events, and severe, acute stress at cancer diagnosis and during recovery is often seen in patients. A range of immune responses may be negatively affected by stress responses. Higher levels of stress may be related to reduced cellular immune responses, such as lowered natural killer cell lysis. The influence of stress on cellular immunity in women with breast cancer, after the diagnosis of breast cancer and during the postsurgical period, was examined.

Methods.—There were 116 patients who were recently treated surgically for invasive breast cancer. Before beginning their adjuvant therapy all women completed a validated questionnaire about the stress of being a cancer patient. A panel of natural killer cell and T-lymphocyte assays was performed on a 60-mL blood sample taken from each patient. To test the contribution of psychological stress to predict immune function, multiple regression models were developed. Variables that might exert short- or long-term effects on these responses were controlled in all regression equations. Other potentially confounding variables were also ruled out.

Results.—Lower natural killer cell lysis was significantly predicted by stress level. Diminished response of natural killer cells to recombinant interferon gamma was significantly predicted by stress level. Decreased proliferative response of peripheral blood lymphocytes to plant lectins and to monoclonal antibody directed against the T-cell receptor was significantly predicted by stress level.

Conclusion.—Cellular immune responses that are relevant to cancer prognosis, such as natural killer cell toxicity and T-cell responses, are inhibited by the physiologic effects of stress. To determine the duration of these effects, their biological and/or behavior mechanisms, and their health consequences, additional longitudinal studies are needed.

▶ Stress has been blamed for many of our ailments, including peptic ulcer disease, hypertension, coronary disease, and cancer. Whereas it seems to be common sense to try to reduce the stress in our lives, the evidence of biological correlative stress in the human body has been evasive. This is a well-conducted study which documents relationships of natural killer cell and T-lymphocyte assays, using validated questionnaires completed by women with breast cancer. The findings are somewhat surprising. Quite appropriately, the authors did not comment upon the impact of stress on survival, but studies in such an area are currently in process.

P.J. Loehrer, Sr., M.D.

Sentinel-node Biopsy to Avoid Axillary Dissection in Breast Cancer With Clinically Negative Lymph-nodes

Veronesi U, Paganelli G, Galimberti V, et al (European Inst of Oncology, Milan, Italy)

Lancet 349:1864–1867, 1997 3–12

Background.—Early diagnosis has resulted in increasing numbers of axillary lymph-node dissections in which nodes are free of disease. This raises questions about the need for the procedure. Whether a single axillary lymph node initially received malignant cells from a breast carcinoma was evaluated, as was the question of whether a disease-free sentinel node reliably predicts disease-free axilla.

Methods.—One hundred sixty-three consecutive patients with operable breast carcinomas were injected with microcolloidal particles of human serum albumin labeled with technetium-99m. The subdermal injection was made close to the tumor site the day before surgery. Scintigraphic images of the axilla and breast were obtained 10 and 30 minutes and 3 hours later. The skin over the site of the radioactive node (sentinel node) was marked. During surgery, the sentinel node was located using a hand-held γ-ray detector probe. This enabled separate removal of the sentinel node through a small axillary incision. After this procedure, a complete axillary lymphadenectomy was performed. The sentinel node was tagged separately from the other nodes, and permanent sections of all nodes removed were prepared for pathologic assessment.

Results.—Sentinel node assessment enabled accurate prediction of axillary lymph-node status in 97.5% of the women in whom the sentinel node was identified. Axillary lymph-node status was predicted accurately in all patients with tumors smaller than 1.5 cm in diameter. In 38% of the patients with metastatic axillary nodes, the only positive node was the sentinel node.

Conclusions.—In most women with breast cancer, lymphoscintigraphy and γ-probe–guided surgery can be used to locate the sentinel node in the axilla. This procedure provides important information about the status of the axillary nodes. Patients without clinical axillary involvement should undergo sentinel-node biopsy routinely, which will spare such women complete axillary dissection when the sentinel node is disease free.

▶ During the past several decades, efforts to minimize surgical morbidity have resulted in an evolution from medical mastectomy to lumpectomy with axillary dissection. Despite this evolution, axillary nodal status remains one of the most important prognostic factors in early-stage disease. Sentinel-node biopsy is a novel technique which was first used to determine nodal drainage patterns in patients with malignancies. This article, by a highly respected group, provides support for sentinel-node biopsy, which ultimately will have further impact on minimizing morbidity in patients with breast cancer.

P.J. Loehrer, Sr., M.D.

Ductal Carcinoma in Situ of the Breast

Fonseca R, Hartmann LC, Petersen IA, et al (Mayo Clinic and Found, Rochester, Minn)

Ann Intern Med 127:1013–1022, 1997 3–13

Background.—The management of ductal carcinoma in situ (DCIS) of the breast is challenging and controversial. The natural history of DCIS and results obtained with various treatments were reviewed.

Methods and Findings.—A computerized MEDLINE search of articles on DCIS published since 1966 was performed. All sources were reviewed critically. There were no randomized trials comparing mastectomy with breast-conserving treatment for patients with DCIS. One large randomized trial demonstrated the efficacy of lumpectomy plus radiotherapy. Although the value of this practice is debated, the presence of comedo necrosis and surgical margin status are often used to predict subsequent recurrence. The risk for in-breast recurrence 5 years after lumpectomy plus radiotherapy is about 8%.

Conclusions.—Lumpectomy followed by radiotherapy appears to be an appropriate treatment for most patients. The effectiveness of lumpectomy alone in selected patients is still debated. The relationship of DCIS to invasive breast cancer will become clearer with more refined molecular analysis.

▶ The YEAR BOOK generally does not include reviews as selected articles. This review on ductal carcinoma in situ of the breast is a notable exception. Although DCIS was once considered uncommon, the rate of the incidence for DCIS (over 23,000 cases per year) is now greater than that of any other histologic type of breast cancer. This is in part secondary to screening mammography. This article provides an excellent summary of the natural history and clinical pathologic findings of this disease.

P.J. Loehrer, Sr., M.D.

Using Autopsy Series to Estimate the Disease "Reservoir" for Ductal Carcinoma In Situ of the Breast: How Much More Breast Cancer Can We Find?

Welch HG, Black WC (Veterans Affairs Med Ctr, White River Junction, Vt; Dartmouth Med School, Hanover, NH; Dartmouth-Hitchcock Med Ctr, Lebanon, NH)

Ann Intern Med 127:1023–1028, 1997 3–14

Background.—The ability to detect early forms of breast cancer will continue to improve. The current study determined how many cases of breast cancer might be found by reviewing autopsy results of women not known to have had breast cancer during life.

Methods and Findings.—Seven autopsy series of such women were identified in a MEDLINE search from 1966 to the present. The prevalence of invasive breast cancer in these studies ranged from 0% to 1.8%, with a median of 1.3%. The prevalence of ductal carcinoma in situ (DCIS) ranged from 0% to 14.7%, with a median of 8.9%. Prevalence was greater among women between 40 and 70 years of age—those likely to have been screened. The mean number of slides examined per breast ranged from 9 to 275. Studies reporting higher levels of scrutiny tended to report more cases of disease.

Conclusions.—A substantial number of DCIS cases go undetected during life. The number of DCIS cases diagnosed depends on how hard pathologists look for the disease and possibly on the threshold for making the diagnosis.

▶ Since 1980, the incidence of DCIS has increased fourfold and now represents nearly half the cases of cancer detected by screening mammography. The natural history of mammography-detected DCIS is unclear, with some but not all patients progressing to invasive breast cancer. This is an interesting article which uses autopsy data to help to define the prevalence of DCIS in the Anglo population. Variability of these numbers depends on the pathologists, the number of samples obtained, and the section depth. If the lower number of estimated probability (5%) is accurate, then as many as 2 million women in the United States may have DCIS. The incidence of invasive cancer is obviously much less than this number. What then should be the threshold for defining DCIS? This problem is reminiscent of the one in prostate specific antigen screening for prostate cancer.

P.J. Loehrer, Sr., M.D.

Overnight Closed Suction Drainage After Axillary Lymphadenectomy for Breast Cancer

Liu CD, McFadden DW (Univ of California, Los Angeles)

Am Surg 63:868–870, 1997 3–15

Background.—The increasing use of breast-conserving surgery has made outpatient surgery, frequently including lymph node dissection, a common treatment option. Seroma formation is the predominant complication after dissection of axillary lymph nodes, occurring in 42% of patients in whom drainage is not used. There is no uniform agreement on drain management after axillary dissection. Placement of drains for excessive durations may increase serum and lymph exudation and predispose the site to retrograde bacterial infection. The efficacy of closed suction drainage for less than 24 hours was evaluated in 50 patients who had undergone axillary lymph node dissection.

Methods.—Fifty women who underwent wide excision of the breast concomitant with level 1 and 2 axillary lymph node dissections, performed by the same surgeon between 1993 and 1996, were included in the study. A 7F closed suction drain was placed inferior to the surgical incision in each patient and was removed within 23 hours of surgery and before discharge. One preoperative and 1-2 postoperative doses of cafazolin were administered to each patient IV. Each woman was re-examined 7–10 days after surgery.

Results.—A mean of 15.5 lymph nodes were sampled from each woman. Nine patients (18%) had evidence of metastasis to the axillary lymph nodes. A seroma formed postoperatively in 1 patient (2%) but had drained spontaneously by the second postoperative day. The remaining 49 patients had no evidence of seroma formation, and no patients experienced wound infections.

Conclusion.—Overnight closed-suction drainage is beneficial to patients receiving breast conservation surgery. The intervention is short term and reduces the risk of seroma formation and infection, as well as the requirement for wound aspiration.

▶ Traditional surgical methods for breast surgery are changing. In most areas of the country, the number of breast conservation cases has increased in frequency and now equals the incidence of mastectomy. Lymphadenectomy remains an important aspect of breast cancer management, providing information with relevance to prognosis and further adjuvant therapy considerations. Surgical management of the axilla can be complicated by the repeated necessity of seroma aspiration and occasional infection from prolonged close suction drain placement. Infection can be a significant problem at times if it delays adjuvant therapy or requires patient hospitalization for antibiotics.

This paper from the University of California demonstrates a small, but favorable, institutional experience with using close suction drainage overnight and then removing the drain, without regard to the extent of drainage, in the morning. In this series of consecutive patients, only 2% had any significant postoperative seroma formation. I believe that this study merits further consideration, perhaps on a larger scale with multiple surgeons participating. If the results are favorable, a quick removal of the suction drain could improve patient comfort and compliance as well as decreasing the incidence of significant surgical problems post lymphadenectomy.

B.L. Eisenberg, M.D.

The Use of Ultrasonography in the Localization of the Lumpectomy Cavity for Interstitial Brachytherapy of the Breast

DeBiose DA, Horwitz EM, Martinez AA, et al (William Beaumont Hosp, Royal Oaks, Mich)

Int J Radiat Oncol Biol Phys 38:755–759, 1997 3–16

Background.—Accurate localization and measurement of the cavity left by breast lumpectomy is required for needle placement in brachytherapy. Frequently, needles must be placed postoperatively, precluding direct observation or the use of surgical clips as methods of determination. Ultrasonography (US) is a promising alternative tool: however, the use of US for identifying the borders of the postlumpectomy cavity has not been well evaluated. The accuracy of US in describing lumpectomy cavity boundaries was evaluated.

Methods.—Borders of breast lumpectomy cavities were identified by US in 38 patients, using a 5.0- or 7.5-MHz linear array transducer, a median of 38 days after tumor excision. The dimensions produced by US were compared with locations estimated by the position of the surgical scar, the presurgical mammography, and the clinical estimate by the physician. Ultrasonography was also used to determine the dimensions of the lumpectomy cavity during needle placement and to verify the accuracy of the placement in 9 patients.

Results.—The dimensions of the lumpectomy cavity were underestimated by clinical examination in 33 patients (87%), and the depth to the chest wall was underestimated by clinical examination in 34 patients (90%), compared with the results of US determination. Ultrasonography was helpful in verifying needle placement in the 9 patients receiving intraoperative US examinations. Needles required repositioning after clinical placement, in 7 of these 9 patients (75%), to provide adequate coverage of the posterior cavity margin localized by US. In 3 patients examined by both US and CT scan, cavity dimensions determined by the 2 modalities were in good agreement as long as the US probe was held normal to the horizontal.

Conclusions.—Accurate identification of the lumpectomy cavity is provided by US, both in estimating target volume for brachytherapy and in verifying needle placement intraoperatively. Ultrasonography is a valuable adjunct method in ensuring precise delivery of irradiation to a specific tissue volume.

► In trying to preserve the breast, there are problems in knowing where the lump was, if it has not been marked by clips at the time of surgery. This paper looks at the value of US of the breast in defining the lumpectomy cavity. Obviously, it is unclear where to put sources for interstitial brachytherapy without identifying the location of where the tumor was. Under anesthesia the exact location can be considerably distorted. These investigators have apparently been very satisfied by using US for localization.

I believe this is a major problem in some of the randomized trials; a lumpectomy by an outside surgeon can make a patient become a real enigma if no clips were placed in the breast to enable radiation oncologists to know where the tumor bed really was.

E. Glatstein, M.D.

Lumpectomy and Radiation Therapy for the Treatment of Intraductal Breast Cancer: Findings From National Surgical Adjuvant Breast and Bowel Project B-17

Fisher B, Dignam J, Wolmark N, et al (Allegheny Univ, Pittsburgh, Pa)

J Clin Oncol 16:441–452, 1998 3–17

Introduction.—Since 1985, the standard treatment for women with intraductal carcinoma-in-situ has been lumpectomy with radiation, but an updated clinical trial had not been conducted. After 8 years, a study was conducted to follow up this information and to evaluate the worth of radiation therapy after lumpectomy.

Methods.—There were 818 women with localized intraductal carcinoma-in-situ who were randomly assigned either to lumpectomy plus radiation at 50 Gy or to lumpectomy. So that resected specimen margins were histologically tumor-free, tissue was removed. There was a mean follow-up time of 90 months, with a range of 67–130 months. Central clinical, mammographic, and pathologic assessments were used to determine size and method of tumor detection. Determinations were also made of estimates of event-free survival and survival, relative risk for event-specific end points, average annual rates of occurrence for specific events, and cumulative probability of specific events composing event-free survival.

Results.—After 5–8 years of follow-up, the benefit of lumpectomy plus radiation was virtually unchanged and was due to a reduction in invasive and noninvasive ipsilateral breast tumors. In both treatment groups, the incidence of locoregional and distant events remained similar (Fig 2). Breast cancer was only infrequently related to deaths. The incidence of invasive ipsilateral breast tumor was decreased from 13.4% to 3.9%, and the incidence of noninvasive ipsilateral breast tumor was decreased from 13.4% to 8.2% in both treatment groups.

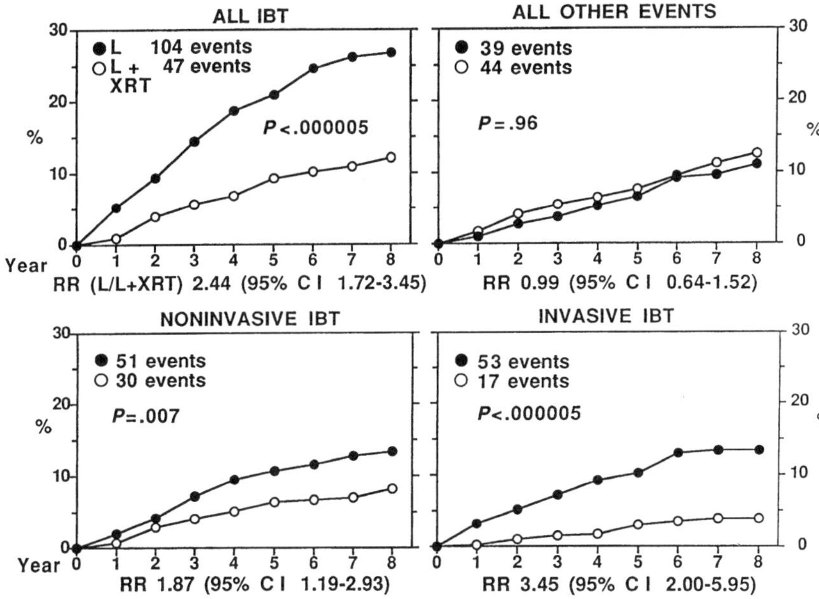

FIGURE 2.—Cumulative incidence of all ipsilateral breast tumors, of noninvasive and invasive intraductal breast tumors, and of all other first events in women treated by lumpectomy or lumpectomy plus radiation. P values are comparisons of average annual rates of failure. (Courtesy of Fisher B, Dignam J, Wolmark N, et al: Lumpectomy and radiation therapy for the treatment of intraductal breast cancer: Findings from National Surgical Adjuvant Breast and Bowel Project B-17. *J Clin Oncol* 16:441–452, 1998.)

Conclusion.—For women with localized, mammographically detected intraductal carcinoma-in-situ, lumpectomy plus radiation is more beneficial than lumpectomy alone, as was evidenced by 8 years of follow-up. Patients in all groups benefited from radiation when evaluated according to the mammographic characteristics of their intraductal carcinoma-in-situ.

▶ Routine mammogram screening has resulted in an increasing number of patients who are diagnosed with clinically undetectable intraductal carcinoma in situ (DCIS). Most of the data about DCIS were previously extrapolated from patients who had invasive tumors and concurrent foci of DCIS. The National Surgical Adjuvant Breast and Bowel Project initiated this prospective randomized trial in 1985 to determine whether radiation therapy is mandated for patients with completely resected DCIS following lumpectomy. The preliminary results of this trial have been previously published. However, it continues to show that lumpectomy plus radiation therapy is superior to lumpectomy alone for patients with localized DCIS detected by mammography. These investigators have yet to define a subset of patients with DCIS who need not be treated with radiation therapy. Nonetheless it is clear that patients need not undergo mastectomy (if all of the lesion is resected) and can be managed quite appropriately with lumpectomy plus radiation therapy.

P.J. Loehrer, Sr., M.D.

Sentinel Lymphadenectomy in Breast Cancer

Giuliano AE, Jones RC, Brennan M, et al (Saint John's Health Ctr, Santa Monica, Calif)

J Clin Oncol 15:2345–2350, 1997 3–18

Background.—There is ongoing debate over the value of routine axillary lymphadenectomy (ALND) for patients with potentially curable breast cancer. The authors have been performing intraoperative lymphatic mapping and sentinel lymphadenectomy (SLND) in breast cancer patients for about 5 years. Their experience suggests that SLND plus immunohistochemical examination can increase detection of axillary metastases. The results of this "mature" SLND technique are reported.

Methods.—The experience included 107 consecutive patients undergoing surgery for potentially curable breast carcinoma. The patients' mean age was 57 years. The typical patient was a postmenopausal woman with a palpable primary tumor undergoing a breast-conserving operation. After SLND, a standard ALND was performed through the same incision. The sentinel nodes underwent intraoperative examination by frozen section. After surgery, the specimens were studied by hematoxylin and eosin staining, as well as by immunohistochemical staining with antibody to cytokeratin. Histologic but not immunohistochemical examination was performed in the nonsentinel nodes.

Results.—One hundred of the 107 patients had an identified sentinel node. The sentinel node showed metastatic involvement in 42 patients, 28 of whom had no other involved axillary nodes. The average number of nodes examined per patient was 1.8 sentinel nodes and 20.2 nonsentinel nodes. Six of the 7 patients with no identified sentinel nodes had no axillary tumor involvement. In this subgroup, axillary status was 100% predicted by SLND. Primary tumor size was related to sentinel lymph node status.

Conclusions.—Sentinel lymphadenectomy, with examination by frozen section and immunohistochemistry, is a minimally invasive, accurate predictor of axillary status in patients with operable breast cancer. The authors are conducting studies to see if it is possible to avoid routine ALND for patients with negative sentinel nodes. Most women with primary breast cancer probably do not need routine ALND.

► This group from the John Wayne Cancer Institute at Saint John's Health Center previously reported their early experience with the clinical use of selective lymphadenectomy, based on the establishment of a sentinel lymph node, in breast cancer patients. This article now includes additional clinical material indicating an improved learning curve, and the results suggest that in selected patients sentinel lymph node mapping and node removal may obviate the need for more complete lymphadenectomy, if the sentinel nodes are indeed negative by both routine hematoxylin and eosin staining and by immunostaining. One must be cautious, however, because clinical trials have not yet matured in number and time interval to prove that sentinel lymph node removal is all that is necessary to stage the axilla. Clearly this technique, employing both blue dye and a radiolabeled tracer, requires a steep learning curve and necessitates consistent individual experience before application to routine practice. Obviously if, after careful scrutiny, matured clinical trials prove the value of sentinel lymph node mapping in breast cancer, then the majority of women with early clinical stage breast cancer would benefit by avoiding the morbidity associated with standard lymph node dissection.

B.L. Eisenberg, M.D.

Axillary Lymph Node Dissection: Is it Required in T1a Breast Cancer?
Chontos AJ, Maher DP, Ratzer ER, et al (St Joseph Hosp, Denver; Kaiser Permanente, Denver)
J Am Coll Surg 184:493–498, 1997 3–19

Background.—Recently, much work has questioned the necessity for dissection of the axillary lymph node for tumors that are 5 mm in diameter or smaller (T1a). Even so, axillary lymph node dissection is still practiced today. This study investigated the necessity for this practice.

Method.—Records of 2,242 breast cancers treated from 1987 to 1994 were reviewed, and primary breast cancer size was noted to find the corresponding incidence of metastases of the axillary lymph nodes. Seventy-four T1a cancers were located. Of these patients, 66 had lymph node dissection performed.

Results.—Of the 66 patients, 3 had corresponding lymph node metastases (4.5%). The records of other institutions were examined as a basis for comparison, and researchers found little difference between their calculated percentage of metastases and that found in other institutions (P greater than 0.10). The authors accounted for a marked difference between their results and those of SEER (Surveillance, Epidemiology, and End Results) by considering the SEER results flawed in that they do not have histologic confirmation of the status of the lymph nodes.

Conclusion.—The data presented in this study suggest that routine dissections of the axillary lymph nodes should not be performed.

► The single most important predictor of disease recurrence is the status of the axillary lymph nodes. Despite advances in defining the molecular basis for breast cancer and associated prognostic implications, most adjuvant treatment trials rely on accurate information relative to axillary lymph node status. In the last several years, there has been increased controversy regarding the necessity of routine axillary lymph node dissection in all women with infiltrating ductal breast cancer. Newer techniques, such as lymphatic mapping and excision of sentinel lymph nodes, may prove to be so sensitive as to render this controversy mute. Certainly, the size of the breast cancer is the significant predictor of the incidence of occult axillary lymph node metastases. However, even small breast cancers—particularly those with infiltrating cancers of less than 1 cm (T1a and T1b) have a diminished, but clinically relevant, incidence of nodal disease.

This article reports a retrospective, single institutional experience with 74 patients with T1a cancers and reveals a 4.5% occult axillary nodal metastasis rate. This concurs with other reports of patients with T1a and T1b cancers with incidences from 3% to approximately 8%. Clearly, the issue here is whether the patient with breast cancer, particularly the premenopausal patient, with node-positive disease will have a change in treatment paradigm by the addition of this risk factor. In all probability, this additional pathologic staging would be meaningful in assessing long-term outcome. Despite the potential cost benefit of eliminating the necessity for lymphatic dissection in all patients with early T1 lesions, it is important to note that this decision may be better made on an individual basis. Axillary lymph node dissection is still the treatment standard.

B.L. Eisenberg, M.D.

4 Gynecologic Malignancies

Patterns of Care for Women With Ovarian Cancer in the United States
Muñoz KA, Harlan LC, Trimble EL (Natl Cancer Inst, NIH, Bethesda, Md)
J Clin Oncol 15:3408–3415, 1997 4–1

Objective.—Ovarian cancer is the fifth most common cancer in women in the United States and carries a 21% 5-year survival for late-stage disease. Survival is influenced by age, histologic grade and type, stage of disease, and tumor rupture. A National Cancer Institute (NIC) study determined the extent to which recommended staging and treatment are being provided to patients with ovarian cancer.

Methods.—Of a sample of 785 women from the NIC Surveillance, Epidemiology, and End Results (SEER) program with diagnosed ovarian cancer in 1991, 399 (50.9%) had presumptive stages I and II disease, 143 (18.2%) had stage III disease, and 242 (30.9%) had stage IV disease. Treatment patterns were determined.

Results.—The average age at diagnosis was 58 years, 87% of patients were white and 5% were black, and 87% had a comorbidity score of 0. Surgery was performed in 54% of women with stages I and II disease, 90% of women with stage III disease, and 64% of women with stage IV disease. Surgery alone in patients with stages I and II, stage III, and stage IV disease was performed in 58%, 11%, and 13%, respectively. Carboplatin-cisplatin chemotherapy plus surgery were provided to 32%, 75%, and 56% of patients, respectively. Nine percent of patients with stage I disease, 14% of those with stage II, 71% of those with stage III, and 53% of those with stage IV disease received the recommended treatment according to stage at diagnosis. Lymph adenectomy was not performed in 66% of patients with stages I and II disease, 57% with stage III, and 83% with stage IV disease. Women with stages I and II, III, and IV disease had extensive surgery in 54%, 90%, and 64% of cases. Younger women were significantly more likely to have surgery than older women. Older women, women with higher comorbidity scores, and women of race other than white were significantly less likely to receive the recommended staging and treatment.

Conclusion.—Women with early stage disease and older women are not receiving the recommended staging and treatment for ovarian cancer. The significant clinical benefits of aggressive treatment of ovarian cancer should be stressed to patients and physicians.

▶ Ovarian cancer is a disease of the elderly population. The importance of accurate surgical staging, cytoreduction, and combination chemotherapy with paclitaxel plus a platinum compound (usually carboplatin) has been widely disseminated in the medical literature and incorporated into clinical guidelines for practice. Yet, it is clear that elderly women are frequently not treated in an appropriate manner. It is a self-fulfilling prophecy to deny elderly women with ovarian cancer effective therapy because they are "too old," "too sick," or because the therapy "does not work." But it appears that this is exactly what is happening in management of elderly patients with ovarian cancer. Our patients and physicians must be educated to the significant clinical benefits that can be derived from aggressive treatment of ovarian cancer. It needs to be emphasized that elderly women with good physiologic function can tolerate not only the surgery, but also current chemotherapy that is tailored to account for differences in physiologic parameters, such as renal function.

R.F. Ozols, M.D., Ph.D.

Enhancing Adherence Following Abnormal Pap Smears Among Low-Income Minority Women: A Preventive Telephone Counseling Strategy

Miller SM, Siejak KK, Schroeder CM, et al (Fox Chase Cancer Ctr, Philadelphia; Georgetown Univ, Washington, DC; Allegheny Univ, Philadelphia; et al)

J Natl Cancer Inst 89:703–708, 1997 4–2

Background.—The incidence of precancerous cervical conditions has been increasing recently. However, prompt initial and long-term follow-up care decreases unnecessary morbidity and mortality. The value of a brief phone counseling intervention among low-income, inner-city women with an abnormal Papanicolaou (Pap) smear result was investigated.

Methods.—The counseling stressed the importance of having an initial and 6-month repeat follow-up diagnostic procedure. In a randomized trial, 192 women received telephone counseling and 203 did not preliminary to an appointment for a repeat colposcopy 6 months after the abnormal Pap smear result. Another 216 women received a telephone appointment confirmation/reminder call only, and 217 received standard care.

Findings.—Logistic regression analysis showed that telephone counseling resulted in significantly greater adherence rates to the initial colposcopy visit compared with telephone confirmation alone. Standard care resulted in significantly lower adherence rates than did telephone confirmation of the appointment. The patients who had received telephone counseling before their initial visit were significantly more likely to keep their 6-month follow-up appointment than those who had received telephone confirmation only. The standard care group had adherence rates similar to those of the phone confirmation group. Lower rates of adherence were associated with forgotten appointments and scheduling conflicts.

Conclusion.—Telephone counseling appears to be an effective strategy for improving initial and long-term compliance with follow-up cervical diagnostic procedures among a traditionally underserved population. More intensive, targeted counseling interventions may be needed for patients with positive Pap smear results and a particular profile of psychological barriers.

▶ Cervical cancer is both a preventable and a highly treatable disease. Widespread screening with the Pap smear has led to a marked decrease in mortality from cervical cancer in the Western world. In contrast, in underdeveloped countries, cervical cancer remains the number 1 cause of mortality from a gynecologic malignancy. However, even in the United States there remains an excessively high number of deaths from cervical cancer. Many of these deaths are in the underserved population.

This important study shows that telephone counseling may be an effective strategy for enhancing initial and long-term adherence to recommendations for monitoring and therapy after an abnormal Pap smear result. In the past, high-risk individuals have frequently not adhered to recommended diagnostic regimens. Although this study demonstrates that behavior modification can be achieved with telephone counseling, more intensive and specific counseling interventions may be required for that subset of women for whom follow-up telephone calls did not lead to adherence to recommended follow-up procedures after an abnormal Pap smear result.

R.F. Ozols, M.D., Ph.D.

The Relationship of Local and Distant Failure From Endometrial Cancer: Defining a Clinical Paradigm

Corn BW, Lanciano RM, D'Agostino R Jr, et al (Thomas Jefferson Univ, Philadelphia; Fox Chase Cancer Ctr, Philadelphia; Bowman Gray School of Medicine, Winston-Salem, NC)

Gynecol Oncol 66:411–416, 1997 4–3

Objective.—Whereas multivariate analysis showed that poor histologic differentiation, deep myometrial invasion, and older age were risk factors for distant failure for endometrial cancer, the model did not characterize the relationship between local and distant failure. With a recently developed statistical method, the relationship of local and distant failure was assessed in women with pathologically staged endometrial cancer treated by hysterectomy followed by adjuvant chemotherapy.

Methods.—Of the 394 patients (70% older than 60 years) with International Federation of Gynecology and Obstetrics (FIGO) stages I-III endometrial cancer, 200 were treated with a median external beam dose of 45 Gy, 166 also received vaginal brachytherapy of median dose 30 Gy, and

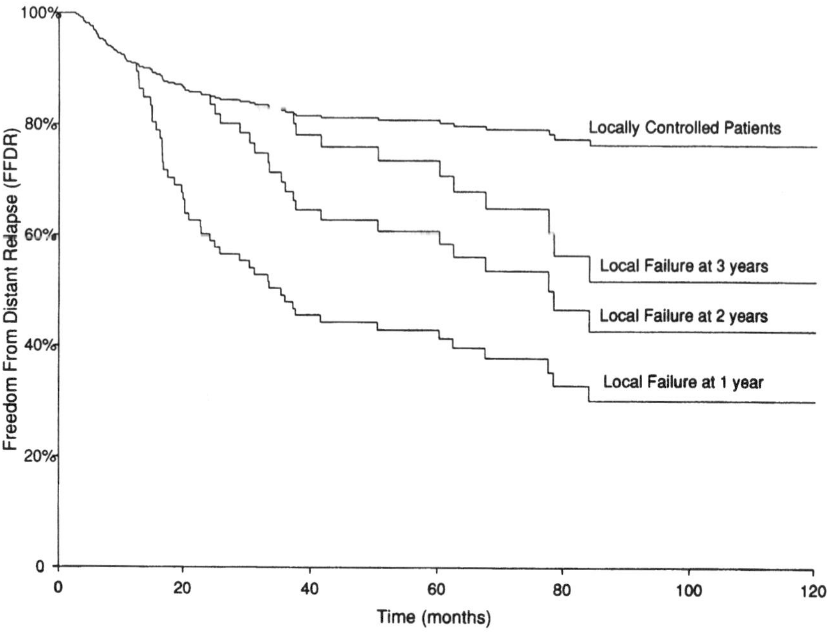

FIGURE 1.—Predicted freedom from distant relapse as a function of local disease status, given at different local failure times. (Courtesy of Corn BW, Lanciano RM, D'Agostino R Jr, et al: The relationship of local and distant failure from endometrial cancer: Defining a clinical paradigm. *Gynecol Oncol* 66:411–416, 1997.)

28 received vaginal brachytherapy only. Patients were followed up for a median of 62 months. Time-to-outcome distributions were estimated using the Kaplan-Meier method and compared using the Mantel-Cox log-rank test.

Results.—Five-year actuarial rate of local failure was 9% and the rate of distant failure was 20%. Univariate analysis showed that high pathologic stage and aggressive histopathologic findings were significantly associated with local failure. In addition to stage and histopathologic findings, poor differentiation was also significantly associated with distant failure. The rate of distant failure was higher among those who had local failure. Distant failure occurred sooner in patients who had local failure than in those with distant failure but not local failure (Fig 1). Women with local failure had 4 times the risk of distant failure as those who did not have local failure. Freedom from distant relapse at 5 years was related to local tumor control, well to moderate differentiation, and low pathologic stages. Local tumor control, younger age, well to moderate differentiation, and early pathologic stage were significantly related to improved 5-year survival.

Conclusion.—There is a significant relationship between local and distant failure in patients with endometrial cancer treated by hysterectomy followed by irradiation. Optimization of local control is important for prolonging survival.

▶ Local failure in endometrial cancer is an unfortunate event not only for the immediate clinical problem in the pelvis, but also because of the increased risk of distant metastases and ultimate death. Whether metastatic disease is a result of the local failure or the local failure is merely a high-risk marker has not been established. Two nationwide trials in progress may help resolve this issue. The Radiation Therapy Oncology Group (RTOG), upon completion of a phase II trial, plans to randomize moderate-risk patients with endometrial cancer to pelvic radiation vs. chemotherapy combined with pelvic radiation. The Gynecologic Oncology Group (GOG), on the other hand, is randomizing a similar group of patients with endometrial cancer to pelvic radiation or chemotherapy. Such studies may help establish the reason why local failure has such a poor prognostic implication for distant metastases in endometrial cancer.

R.F. Ozols, M.D., Ph.D.

Randomized Trial of Cisplatin Versus Cisplatin Plus Mitolactol Versus Cisplatin Plus Ifosfamide in Advanced Squamous Carcinoma of the Cervix: A Gynecologic Oncology Group Study

Omura GA, Blessing JA, Vaccarello L, et al (Univ of Alabama, Birmingham; Roswell Park Cancer Inst, Buffalo, NY; Ohio State Univ, Columbus; et al)

J Clin Oncol 15:165–171, 1997 4–4

Background.—To date, the most active single agents against squamous carcinoma of the cervix identified by the Gynecologic Oncology Group are cisplatin, mitolactol, and ifosfamide. Combinations of cisplatin plus ifosfamide and cisplatin plus mitolactol were compared prospectively with cisplatin alone.

Methods and Findings.—Four hundred thirty-eight patients were randomly assigned to receive cisplatin, 50 mg/m^2; the same dose of cisplatin plus mitolactol, 180 mg/m^2 (both given orally on days 2–6); or cisplatin plus ifosfamide (CIFX), 5 g/m^2, as a 24-hour infusion plus mesna, 6 g/m^2, during and for 12 hours after the ifosfamide infusion. This last regimen was given every 3 weeks for up to 6 courses. Compared with cisplatin alone, CIFX had a significantly greater response rate and a longer progression-free survival time. Response rates were 31.1% and 17.8%, respectively, and median times to progression or death were 4.6 and 3.2 months, respectively. Cisplatin plus mitolactol was not significantly better than cisplatin alone on these measures. Survival was correlated with initial performance score and age. Overall survival did not differ between cisplatin and either of the combinations. Leukopenia, renal toxicity, peripheral neurotoxicity, and CNS toxicity were more common with CIFX.

Conclusion.—Compared with cisplatin alone, CIFX improved response rate and progression-free survival duration in patients with advanced cervical cancer. However, CIFX was associated with greater toxicity and no improvement in survival.

▶ Cisplatin has been the cornerstone of therapy for metastatic or recurrent cervical cancer. Other agents, such as mitolactol and ifosfamide, have also had efficacy. Unfortunately, when these drugs are combined with cisplatin, they lead to increased toxicity. However, they are associated with a higher response rate and a longer progression-free survival without any significant impact upon overall survival. Recommendations are difficult for the clinician in such a situation as there clearly is benefit from having a high response rate and a longer time to relapse. Whether the added toxicity would be clinically beneficial would require more formal quality-of-life analysis. What is obvious, however, is that neither cisplatin or any combination currently studied is very useful for the treatment of patients with metastatic or recurrent ovarian cancer and that new, more active agents are desperately needed.

R.F. Ozols, M.D., Ph.D.

Analysis of the Cost-Effectiveness of Paclitaxel as Alternative Combination Therapy for Advanced Ovarian Cancer

McGuire W, Neugut AL, Arikian S, et al (Ctr for Health Outcomes and Economics, East Brunswick, NJ; Emory Univ, Atlanta, Ga; Columbia Univ, New York)

J Clin Oncol 15:640–645, 1997 4–5

Introduction.—A recent phase III trial suggested that the combination of paclitaxel and cisplatin is more effective in the treatment of advanced ovarian cancer than the standard regimen of cyclophosphamide plus cisplatin. The paclitaxel-cisplatin combination appears to be the new standard of care; however, further data on survival and quality of life are needed. This study compared the cost-effectiveness of paclitaxel-cisplatin with that of cyclophosphamide-cisplatin for patients with advanced ovarian cancer.

Methods.—The pharmacoeconomic analysis used resource utilization data from the phase III trial. The health care resources included in the study model were drug acquisition, physician visits, laboratory and test procedures, inpatient and outpatient treatment, management of adverse reactions, and follow-up costs. The effects of paclitaxel in increasing mean and median survival time were assessed. Kaplan-Meier estimates of the cumulative proportion of surviving patients were used.

Findings.—Including the costs of concomitant medications, the total drug acquisition costs for 6 cycles of treatment were $10,615 for paclitaxel-cisplatin vs. $3,221 for cyclophosphamide-cisplatin. Inpatient costs were identical, but outpatient costs were higher with paclitaxel-cisplatin. The cost of adverse event management was also higher with paclitaxel-cisplatin, particularly for neutropenic fever. Because they survived longer, patients given paclitaxel-cisplatin had somewhat higher follow-up costs.

Total costs for outpatient treatment were $27,320 for paclitaxel-cisplatin vs. $17,964 for cyclophosphamide-cisplatin. Costs per year of life gained were higher with paclitaxel-cisplatin: $19,820 higher for inpatient treatment and $21,222 higher for outpatient treatment.

Conclusions.—The new paclitaxel-cisplatin regimen for advanced ovarian cancer has a higher cost per year of life gained than does standard cyclophosphamide-cisplatin therapy. This additional cost is acceptable, given the substantial benefit achieved. Paclitaxel-cisplatin continues to be a cost-effective alternative on sensitivity analysis. A follow-up pharmacoeconomic analysis of the same phase III trial is planned.

▶ In the era of managed care, economic models will be increasingly important in determining medical resource utilization. A previous randomized trial by the Gynecologic Oncology Group demonstrated that paclitaxel plus cisplatin was clinically superior to cyclophosphamide plus cisplatin. This economic study demonstrates that paclitaxel-based therapy costs approximately $20,000 more per year of life gained, compared with treatment with cisplatin plus cyclophosphamide. It needs to be pointed out that this increase in cost is favorable to previous trials in which the costs per year of life gained ranged from $40,000 to $75,000, and have been considered by health care economists and ethicists to be acceptable.

R.F. Ozols, M.D., Ph.D.

Topetecan Versus Paclitaxel for the Treatment of Recurrent Epithelial Ovarian Cancer

ten Bokkel Huinink W, Gore M, Carmichael J, et al (The Netherlands Cancer Inst, Amsterdam; Weston Park Hosp, Sheffield, England; North Middlesex Hosp, London; et al)

J Clin Oncol 15:2183–2193, 1997 4–6

Background.—Despite platinum-based chemotherapy, most patients with advanced ovarian cancer will eventually experience a relapse and die of their disease. Based on recent studies, the combination of a platinum agent and paclitaxel is becoming the new treatment of choice for recurrent ovarian cancer. However, new agents with new mechanisms of action are needed. The semisynthetic topoisomerase I inhibitor, topotecan, has confirmed activity in patients with progressive ovarian cancer. Topotecan and paclitaxel were compared for use in patients with progressive advanced epithelial ovarian cancer in a phase III trial.

Methods.—The open-label, randomized trial included 226 patients with stage III/IV epithelial ovarian carcinoma that had progressed despite first-line therapy with platinum-based chemotherapy. All had at least 1 lesion that could be measured bidimensionally using imaging studies or physical examination. They were assigned to treatment with either topotecan, 1.5 mg/m^2, given as a 30-minute infusion daily for 5 days every 21 days; or paclitaxel, 175 mg/m^2, given in a 3-hour infusion every 21 days. The 2 treatments were compared for efficacy and toxicity.

Results.—Response rate was 20.5% with topotecan vs. 13.2% with paclitaxel. Thirty percent of patients in the topotecan group and 33% of those in the paclitaxel group had disease stabilization for at least 8 weeks. The median duration of response was 32 weeks with topotecan and 20 weeks with paclitaxel. Median time to progression was 23 and 14 weeks, and median survival was 61 and 43 weeks, respectively. For "resistant" patients who did not respond to previous platinum-based chemotherapy or had progression within 6 months of an initial response, the response rate was 13.3% with topotecan vs. 6.7% with paclitaxel. For "sensitive" patients who had disease progression more than 6 months after an initial response, the response rate was 28.8% with topotecan vs. 20.0% with paclitaxel. Seventy-nine percent of patients treated with topotecan had neutropenia, compared with 23% of those receiving paclitaxel. However, this complication was transient in both groups. Both agents caused usually mild nonhematologic toxic effects.

Conclusions.—In women with advanced ovarian cancer that has progressed despite platinum-based chemotherapy, topotecan is at least as efficacious as paclitaxel. Topotecan is associated with a higher response rate and a longer time to progression. Topotecan offers a new mechanism of action and acceptable toxic effects; it is active even in patients with evidence of platinum resistance and progression on paclitaxel. Studies are currently being conducted to evaluate the role of topotecan in first-line therapy for ovarian cancer.

▶ This study demonstrates that topotecan is an active agent in the treatment of recurrent ovarian cancer. The strengths of the study lie in the randomized nature of the trial and in the independent radiologic review of the responders. However, in the United States, most patients are treated with paclitaxel plus a platinum compound as part of their initial chemotherapy regimen for advanced ovarian cancer. Therefore, the results of this trial, in which initial treatment was a platinum compound plus cyclophosphamide before randomization to either paclitaxel or topotecan as initial second-line therapy, are of interest only in establishing the activity of topotecan.

There clearly is no "drug of choice" for the second-line treatment of recurrent ovarian cancer. There are numerous other agents that have similar activity to topotecan in this clinical situation, including gemcitabine, encapsulated doxorubicin, vinorelbine, and oral etoposide. This latter agent may be of particular relevance to the treatment of recurrent epithelial ovarian cancer in the United States. In a large Gynecologic Oncology Group study, oral etoposide was shown to be an active agent in patients who had progressed on prior treatment with paclitaxel plus a platinum compound.[1] The ultimate utility of topotecan in the treatment of patients with ovarian cancer will primarily rest in its ability to be combined with other active agents to develop more effective initial chemotherapy regimens.

Second-line therapy is primarily palliative. Although the clinical benefits of palliation should not be underestimated, prolongation of survival can primarily be achieved by developing new combination chemotherapy regimens that include novel agents, such as topotecan combined with what currently appears to be the best available combination, which includes paclitaxel plus a platinum compound.

R.F. Ozols, M.D., Ph.D.

Reference

1. Rose PG, Blessing JA, Mayer AR, et al: Prolonged oral etoposide as second-line therapy for platinum-resistant and platinum-sensitive ovarian carcinoma: A Gynecologic Oncology Group Study. *J Clin Oncol* 16:405–410, 1998.

Topotecan in Platinum- and Paclitaxel-resistant Ovarian Cancer

Swisher EM, Mutch DG, Rader JS, et al (Washington Univ, St Louis)
Gynecol Oncol 66:480–486, 1997 4–7

Objective.—Whereas first-line therapy with cisplatin and paclitaxel improves progression-free and overall survival in patients with ovarian cancer, most patients eventually become resistant to platinum and a subset becomes resistant to paclitaxel also. Novel chemotherapeutic agents are needed. The efficacy and toxicity of a 5-day infusion of topotecan in patients with resistant ovarian cancer were evaluated.

Methods.—Twenty patients in a phase I-II study and 16 additional patients treated after protocol closure were given a starting dose of topotecan, 1.25 mg/m²/day, for 30 minutes for 5 days for resistant or recurrent

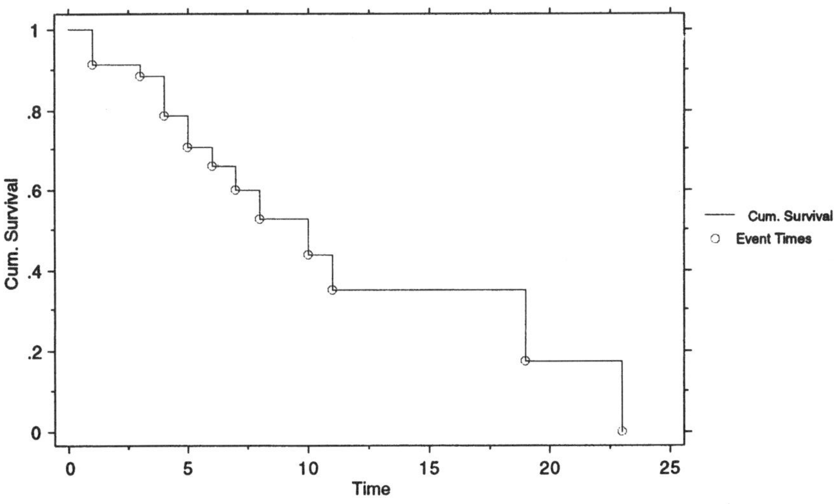

FIGURE 2.—Kaplan-Meier survival curve in months for all 36 patients treated with topotecan. (Courtesy of Swisher EM, Mutch DG, Rader JS, et al: Topotecan in platinum- and paclitaxel-resistant ovarian cancer. *Gynecol Oncol* 66:480–486, 1997.)

ovarian cancer. Response was evaluated in 28 patients receiving more than 1 course of therapy. Toxicity was evaluated in all patients.

Results.—Average age at treatment was 59.5 years (range, 42–74 years). Of the 8 patients receiving only 1 course, 6 died before the second course, 1 received intracavitary radiation treatments, and 1 had severe hematologic toxicity and was changed to another agent. Surgical stage III disease was diagnosed in 29 patients. Toxicity manifested itself as myelosuppression, and most patients had grade 3 or 4 neutropenia and/or thrombocytopenia and grade 3 or 4 anemia. Gastrointestinal effects were minimal. Fatigue was common. There were no complete responses and 4 (14.3%) partial responses among those who were resistant to paclitaxel and platinum. Median survival was 6 months (Fig 2). Half of the patients were able to tolerate subsequent doses of topotecan that were the same or larger than the starting dose.

Conclusion.—Topotecan is effective in some patients with resistance to platinum and paclitaxel. Additional studies in less heavily pretreated patients with other combinations of chemotherapeutic agents are warranted.

► Topotecan is the most recently approved drug for the treatment of refractory ovarian cancer. In the initial studies, topotecan was compared to paclitaxel in patients who had received prior treatment with cyclophosphamide together with a platinum compound. In this recent study, topotecan was examined in patients who were resistant to platinum and paclitaxel. This study demonstrates very modest activity for this agent with considerable toxicity. The overall response rate was 14%. Of the 4 responding patients, 1 was deemed a partial responder only on the basis of a 50% decrease in the serum CA-125 level. Toxicity was significant with 92% of the patients experiencing grade 3 or 4 neutropenia and 67% experiencing grade 3 or 4 thrombocytopenia. This study demonstrates that topotecan is an active agent in this highly refractory group of patients. However, it is also apparent that there are other agents which appear to have similar activity, such as oral VP-16, gemcitabine, encapsulated doxorubicin, and navelbine as well. The fact that topotecan was active in patients with resistance to platinum and paclitaxel provides further impetus for studies in which this agent is evaluated together with paclitaxel and a platinum compound in previously untreated patients with advanced disease. It is apparent, however, that myelosuppression will be a major limiting factor in the development of such combination chemotherapy regimens.

R.F. Ozols, M.D., Ph.D.

Phase II Trial of Oral Altretamine for Relapsed Ovarian Carcinoma: Evaluation of Defining Response by Serum CA125

Rustin GJS, Nelstrop AE, Crawford M, et al (Mount Vernon Hosp, Middlesex, England; Airedale Gen Hosp, Keighley, England; Univ College of London; et al)

J Clin Oncol 15:172–176, 1997 4–8

Background.—More than 60% of patients with advanced ovarian cancer have a relapse within 3 years. In many patients, second-line therapy is successful, but for those who do not respond, other chemotherapeutic agents are needed. Altretamine was examined for its utility as salvage treatment of ovarian cancer in patients with a disease-free interval of 6 months or more.

Methods.—Oral altretamine was used after an initial (n = 55) or a second rescue (n = 11) course of chemotherapy for 66 patients who had been in remission for 6 or more months. Previous regimens had included cisplatin or carboplatin. An increase in the CA 125 level to 50% or more of normal levels or evident disease was used as an indicator of relapse. European Organization for Research and Treatment of Cancer (EORTC) criteria or a decrease in the serum CA 125 level of 50% or 75% over 3 measurements were used to define a response to therapy. Patients underwent from 1 to 12 (median, 5.5) courses of altretamine, 260 mg/m^2 daily in divided doses for 14 days per month.

Findings.—By any criteria (EORTC or CA 125 level), 46% of the patients (26 of 66) showed a response. Responses occurred in 40% of patients evaluated by EORTC criteria and in 39% of patients evaluated by the CA 125 level. Response improved as the disease-free interval increased, from a 35% response rate for a disease-free interval of 6–12 months to a 67% response rate for those with a disease-free interval greater than 24 months. From 5 to 12 months (median, 8 months) passed from the start of altretamine to notable disease progression in the responders; nonresponders had from less than 1 to 20 months (median, 5 months) before the disease progressed. The duration of survival from the start of altretamine dosing varied between less than 1 and 39 months (median, 16 months). The major reported side effects were nausea, vomiting, and fatigue, which were severe enough to cause 10 patients to drop out after 2 courses. Nighttime administration of domperidone, dexamethasone, and chlorpromazine helped control toxicity in most patients. As the study progressed, careful patient selection and the use of antiemetics reduced the incidence of severe nausea and vomiting.

Conclusions.—Oral altretamine was effective in patients undergoing salvage therapy for ovarian cancer who had a disease-free interval of 6 or more months. Success rates improved as the disease-free interval lengthened. Side effects were generally manageable, particularly when antiemetics were given at night. Also, CA 125 levels were as useful as the EORTC criteria in defining a response to altretamine.

▶ Altretamine, previously known as hexamethylmelamine, has been used in the treatment of ovarian cancer for more than 2 decades. This study demonstrates, once again, that it is an active agent in previously treated patients with ovarian cancer. However, most of the patients in this study were not treated with prior paclitaxel-based chemotherapy. In addition, eligible patients were required to have entered a clinical complete remission and to have a disease-free interval greater than 6 months. These 2 factors may account for the high response rate observed in this study. Clinical trials evaluating altretamine in taxol- and platinum-refractory patients are currently in progress by the Gynecologic Oncology Group. This study did, however, have some important implications with regard to evaluating responses based upon the decline in serum CA125 levels. If responses can be assessed solely on the basis of serum CA125 levels, then the need for more expensive CT scanning will be obviated. Furthermore, if serum CA125 levels can be used as a surrogate marker for response, it may be easier to define the activity of new agents, and thereby facilitate approval of their use by regulatory agencies, such as the FDA.

R.F. Ozols, M.D., Ph.D.

Phase II Study of Liposomal Doxorubicin in Refractory Ovarian Cancer: Antitumor Activity and Toxicity Modification by Liposomal Encapsulation

Muggia FM, Hainsworth JD, Jeffers S, et al (Univ of Southern California–Norris Comprehensive Cancer Ctr, Los Angeles; Sequus Pharmaceuticals, Menlo Park, Calif; Sarah Cannon Cancer Ctr, Nashville, Tenn)
J Clin Oncol 15:987–993, 1997 4–9

Background.—Despite initial treatment with cisplatin and paclitaxel, most women with epithelial ovarian cancer will eventually experience a relapse requiring additional treatment. Many forms of salvage therapy have been tried, but have been poorly tolerated and rarely resulted in long remissions. Liposomal doxorubicin has better activity against ovarian cancer xenografts than free doxorubicin does. In a phase I trial, liposomal doxorubicin demonstrated antitumor activity in patients with treatment-refractory ovarian cancer. Liposomal doxorubicin was studied for use in patients with platinum- and paclitaxel-refractory ovarian cancer.

Methods.—The phase II trial included 35 consecutive patients at 2 institutions; the same protocol was followed at both centers. In all patients, disease had progressed after treatment with cisplatin or carboplatin plus paclitaxel, or at least 1 platinum-based and 1 paclitaxel-based regimen. All patients were started on a regimen of IV liposomal doxorubicin, 50 mg/m^2 every 3 weeks. If grade 3 or 4 toxic effects developed, the dose was reduced to 40 mg/m^2. If grade 1 or 2 toxic effects lasted longer than

3 weeks, the interval between treatments was increased to 4 or 5 weeks. The patients were monitored closely and evaluated for response.

Results.—Nine patients responded, including 1 complete and 8 partial responses. Seven of the 9 responses were confirmed with CT. The patients had a median survival of 11 months, and median progression-free survival of 6 months. Grade 3 or 4 nonhematologic toxic effects consisting of either hand-foot syndrome or stomatitis, developed in 13 patients. However, with the described dose modifications, the treatment was well tolerated. There were no problems with drug-related nausea, hair loss, extravasation necrosis, or decreased ejection fraction.

Conclusions.—In this phase II trial, liposomal doxorubicin had antitumor activity against ovarian cancer that had failed to respond to treatment with platinum and paclitaxel. The treatment can produce durable responses in patients with this difficult-to-treat disease. Toxicity is minimal. The results warrant further study of liposomal doxorubicin in combination with other drugs in patients with less refractory ovarian cancer.

► Anthracyclines have had limited activity in the second-line treatment of recurrent ovarian cancer. Liposomal doxorubicin may provide a significant advantage over "naked" doxorubicin in platinum- and paclitaxel-refractory ovarian cancer. Not only was the response rate (26%) encouraging in this trial, the median progression-free survival (5.7 months) and the overall survival (median, 11 months) were also of interest. Furthermore, liposomal doxorubicin was not associated with hair loss or decrease in cardiac ejection fraction. However, hand-foot syndrome or stomatitis was frequent. These studies suggest that liposomal doxorubicin be further evaluated in combination with other active agents in treatment of patients with advanced ovarian cancer.

R.F. Ozols, M.D., Ph.D.

Secondary Cytoreductive Surgery at Second-Look Laparotomy in Advanced Ovarian Cancer: A Gynecologic Oncology Group Study

Williams L, Brunetto VL, Yordan E, et al (Vanderbilt Univ, Nashville, Tenn; Roswell Park Cancer Inst, Buffalo, NY; Rush–Presbyterian St. Luke's Med Ctr, Chicago, et al)

Gynecol Oncol 66:171–178, 1997 4–10

Objective.—One of the potential advantages of second-look laparotomy (SLL) for patients with advanced ovarian cancer is to provide an opportunity for debulking a macroscopic tumor if found. The effect on survival of this procedure has not been studied. Results of a study of the technical feasibility of secondary cytoreduction and the effect of this surgery on survival were presented.

Methods.—Second-look laparotomy was performed on 153 women, aged 20–79 years, with Stage III or IV epithelial ovarian cancer. Cytoreduction was performed on 36 patients. Tumor size before and remaining after cytoreduction was estimated. Survival estimates were determined using the Kaplan-Meier method, and risk factors for survival were evaluated using Cox's proportional hazards model.

Results.—There were 66 patients 60 years of age and older and 36 of these had stage IV disease. There were 127 women with no clinically measurable disease at the time of SLL. At SLL, 69 patients were found to have a tumor larger than 1 cm; this was cytoreduced to leave a microscopic residual in 15 patients and macroscopic small tumor in 18 patients. At SLL, 55 patients had a tumor of 1 cm which was cytoreduced to macroscopic small tumor in 21 patients. At SLL, 29 patients were found to have microscopic disease. Cytoreduction to microscopic disease was accomplished in 36 of 124 patients (29%) found to have macroscopic tumor. Survival depended on tumor size found at SLL and on residual tumor size after debulking. Patients whose debulked tumor was larger than 1 cm had significantly shorter survival times than patients in other categories. Survival was unaffected in patients with microscopic disease and those cytoreduced to microscopic disease. Risk of death was decreased in patients whose tumors were cytoreduced to a lower category. There were few intraoperative complications. Postoperative complications were not evaluated.

Conclusion.—Whether cytoreductive surgery is beneficial and improves outcomes cannot be determined. A randomized, prospective trial is necessary to answer these questions.

▶ A debate surrounding the potential benefit of SLL for ovarian cancer continues, without any new data from randomized trials. Retrospective studies, such as this one, tend to support the role of secondary cytoreduction at SLL. Unfortunately, prospective, randomized trials of secondary cytoreduction and second-look procedures are not likely to be performed. As chemotherapeutic agents improve in efficacy, the importance of surgical cytoreduction may diminish—in the same manner as occurred in testicular cancer. Until that time, it appears that patients with ovarian cancer followed by gynecologic oncologists will likely continue to have more second looks than patients treated by medical oncologists. The Gynecologic Oncology Group no longer mandates that a second-look be done after initial chemotherapy.

R.F. Ozols, M.D., Ph.D.

Predictors of Response to Subsequent Chemotherapy in Platinum Pretreated Ovarian Cancer: A Multivariate Analysis of 704 Patients

Eisenhauer EA, Vermorken JB, van Glabbecke M (Queen's Univ, Kingston, Canada; Univ Hosp Antwerp, Edegem. Belgium; EORTC Data Ctr, Brussels, Belgium)

Ann Oncol 8:963–968, 1997 4–11

Objective.—Whereas the probability of response by patients with ovarian cancer to subsequent chemotherapy with platinum compounds is directly related to the interval between first-line treatment and relapse, serous histology, tumor bulk, and baseline hemoglobin were the only significant predictors of response to second- and third-line paclitaxel treatment. To determine whether these latter observations were unique, a multivariate analysis of factors predictive of response was performed on results of trials of 1,185 platinum-treated patients with ovarian cancer receiving paclitaxel, epirubicin, docetaxel, carboplatin, irinotecan, or gemcitabine.

Methods.—Thirteen studies involving 6 agents were investigated. The agent administered, response to last chemotherapy, number of prior chemotherapy regimens, baseline hemoglobin, tumor histologic findings, liver metastases, performance status, time since last therapy, tumor size, and number of disease sites were subjected to univariate and logistical regression analysis.

Results.—The response rates were 17.3% for paclitaxel, 25.9% for epirubicin, 27.4% for docetaxel, 19% for carboplatin, 14% for gemcitabine, and 24% for irinotecan. Patients with serous histology, normal baseline hemoglobin, tumor size 5 cm or less, and/or more than 6 months

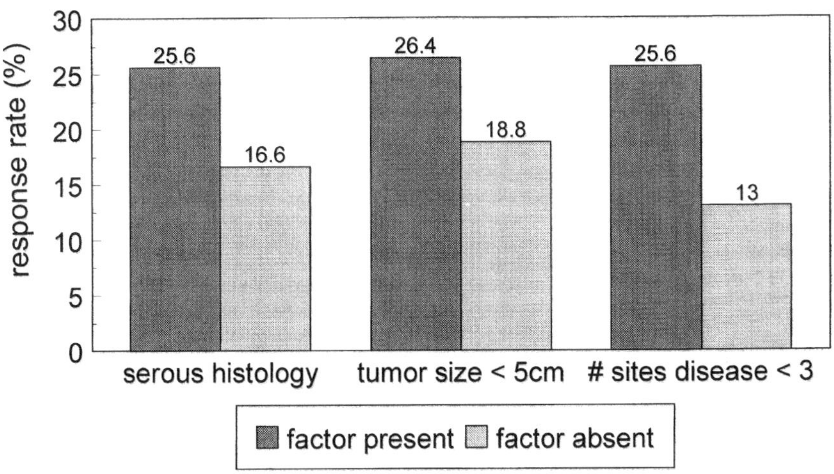

FIGURE 1.—Response rates in pooled data set of 704 patients by factors significant in the final model. (Reprinted by permission of Kluwer Academic Publishers, from Eisenhauer EA, Vermorken JB, van Glabbecke M: Predictors of response to subsequent chemotherapy in platinum pretreated ovarian cancer: A multivariate analysis of 704 patients. *Ann Oncol* 8:963–968, 1997.)

from their last chemotherapy had higher response rates. In the final regression analysis, only serous histology, number of disease sites, and tumor size were significant predictors of response (Fig 1). Time from last chemotherapy was significantly and inversely correlated with tumor size.

Conclusion.—Tumor size, number of disease sites, and serous histology are significant predictors of response to subsequent chemotherapy in platinum-treated patients with ovarian cancer.

▶ Ovarian cancer has been a fertile ground for evaluating the activity of new antineoplastic agents. In fact, the practicing oncologist can select from a menu of at least 8–10 drugs that all have shown "activity" as second-line agents in previously treated patients with ovarian cancer. This large study examines the predictors of response to subsequent chemotherapy in platinum-treated patients. It is of interest that only serous histology, tumor size less than 5 cm, and number of disease sites (less than 2 or more than 2) were independent variables in determining response. The other important factor to consider in this group of patients is the nature of the prior response to platinum-based therapy. It has been established in the past that the platinum-free interval is highly predictive for a response to retreatment with a platinum agent. Consequently, if one considers the activity of second-line agents in ovarian cancer, the response rates must be compared to response rates that could be achieved if the patient was retreated with platinum. Drugs that produce significant activity in patients who are platinum-resistant (i.e., no response to cisplatin or carboplatin, or duration of response less than 6 months) would be the most exciting candidates for inclusion in novel induction regimens for previously untreated patients with advanced disease.

R.F. Ozols, M.D., Ph.D.

Randomised Study of Radical Surgery Versus Radiotherapy for Stage Ib–IIa Cervical Cancer

Landoni F, Maneo A, Colombo A, et al (Univ of Milan, Italy; Istituto di Scienze Biomediche S Gerardo, Monza, Milan, Italy)

Lancet 350:535–540, 1997 4–12

Background.—Though radical surgery and radiotherapy are equally effective treatments for stage 1b and IIa cervical carcinoma, the 2 procedures differ in associated morbidity and type of complications. Five-year survival rates, complications, and recurrences associated with each treatment were determined in the current study.

Methods.—Three hundred forty-three women with newly diagnosed stage Ib or IIa cervical carcinoma were assigned randomly to surgery or radical radiotherapy between 1986 and 1991. Adjuvant radiotherapy was administered postoperatively to women with surgical stage disease of pT2b or greater, less than 3 mm of safe cervical stroma, cut-through, or positive nodes.

Findings.—At a median follow-up of 87 months, the 5-year overall and disease-free survival rates were 83% and 74%, respectively, in both groups. Twenty-five percent of the women undergoing surgery and 26% undergoing radiotherapy had recurrent disease. Univariate and multivariate analyses identified cervical diameter, positive lymphangiography, and adenocarcinomatous histotype as significant factors for survival. Twenty-eight percent of the patients undergoing surgery and 12% undergoing radiotherapy had severe morbidity.

Conclusions.—In these patients with early-stage cervical carcinoma, neither radical surgery nor radiotherapy was superior in overall or disease-free survival rates. The combination of surgery and radiotherapy resulted in the most severe morbidity, especially urologic complications. When determining optimal treatment for individuals with early-stage cervical carcinoma, clinicians should consider factors such as menopausal status, age, medical illness, histologic type, and cervical diameter.

► This large, well-conducted randomized trial of radical surgery vs. radiotherapy as initial treatment for stage Ib–IIa cervical cancer should, but probably will not, resolve the controversy regarding the relative merits of these two modalities in the treatment of cervical cancer. While there was absolutely no difference in survival, mortality was markedly worse in patients randomized to surgery, particularly in those who received postoperative radiation therapy. There does not appear to be agreement regarding clinical criteria, which could potentially be used to select patients who would not require postoperative adjuvant therapy. Clinical trials are in progress to determine whether postoperative chemotherapy may decrease the morbidity associated with the combination of surgery followed by radiation therapy. Such studies have had trouble accruing their required large number of patients. This current study did demonstrate the adverse prognostic effect of adenocarcinoma cell type, which was associated in almost a three-fold increase in risk of relapse. Not only should these patients be stratified in prospective trials but new treatment approaches should be considered for patients with this adverse histologic type of cervical cancer.

R.F. Ozols, M.D., Ph.D.

5 Prostate Cancer

Patient-reported Symptoms After Primary Therapy for Early Prostate Cancer: Results of a Prospective Cohort Study

Talcott JA, Rieker P, Clark JA, et al (Dana-Farber Cancer Inst, Boston; Brigham and Women's Hosp, Boston; Joint Ctr for Radiation Therapy, Boston; et al)

J Clin Oncol 16:275–283, 1998 5–1

Introduction.—In the United States, prostate cancer is the most common and rapidly increasing cancer diagnosis. The choice of treatment will depend upon information about treatment-related complications. After treatment, most men with early prostate cancer will survive for 5 years or more. Radical prostatectomy and radical radiotherapy are the most common treatment and cause serious long-term urinary, bowel, and sexual dysfunction. The complications of therapy for early (nonmetastatic) prostate cancer were assessed.

Methods.—There were 279 men who sought treatment advice and completed required pretreatment forms. Before therapy, and at 3 and 12 months after therapy, the men self-reported symptoms and other measures of quality of life.

Results.—Uncommon before treatment were bowel and bladder symptoms. At 34 months after radiotherapy, patients frequently reported irritative bowel and bladder symptoms, although at 12 months, these subsided somewhat. At 12 months after surgery, substantial urinary incontinence was reported by 11% and wearing of absorptive pads was reported by 35%; this varied little by age. After radiotherapy, incontinence occurred infrequently, and only in men older than 65 years. At 3 months after surgery, inadequate erection was nearly universal and was present in one third of men before treatment. At 12 months, some improvement was seen, primarily in men younger than 65 years. Through 12 months, sexual dysfunction after radiotherapy increased less but continually, suggesting that observed treatment-related differences would decline with further follow-up.

Conclusion.—Bowel and bladder irritability, increasingly severe sexual dysfunction, and, in men older than 65 years, occasional urinary incontinence can occur after external-beam radiotherapy of early prostate cancer. In the year after radical prostatectomy, greater sexual dysfunction and urinary incontinence occur. These complication rates after surgery are greater than were previously reported.

▶ The optional therapy for early-stage prostate cancer is unclear. Patients seeking "treatment of choice" are actually getting advice on the "treatment of chance." By this, I mean that more men with early-stage prostate cancer will die with and not of this malignancy. Our inability to adequately predict the natural history of prostate cancer and evaluate the true impact of our therapeutic interventions leaves the patient to ponder his chances of early vs. late intervention. When men receive diagnoses of early-stage prostate cancer through screening procedures, they are referred to urologists and/or radiation oncologists for therapeutic options. Human nature dictates that these physicians will usually recommend therapy within their own field with biased opinions regarding the morbidity of treatment. This article by Talcott is coauthored by medical, surgical, and radiation oncologists and serves as a useful assessment of self-reported symptoms in patients treated with surgery or radiation therapy. Substantial higher rates of urinary and sexual dysfunction than previously reported occur in both groups of patients. This is an important piece of literature in a controversial area.

P.J. Loehrer, Sr., M.D.

Patient-reported Impotence and Incontinence After Nerve-sparing Radical Prostatectomy

Talcott JA, Rieker P, Propert KJ, et al (Harvard Med School, Boston; Harvard School of Public Health, Boston)

J Natl Cancer Inst 89:1117–1123, 1997 5–2

Objective.—Direct surveys of radical prostatectomy patients show a higher rate of urinary and sexual dysfunction after radical prostatectomy than physician surveys indicate, primarily because the studies are performed retrospectively. Results of a cohort study assessing treatment-related impotence and urinary incontinence reported by patients were assessed.

Methods.—Before and 3 and 12 months after radical prostatectomy, 49 men filled out a questionnaire assessing sexual and urinary function. Results were compared statistically with the surgical technique used: non-nerve-sparing (n = 12), unilateral nerve-sparing (n = 18), or bilateral nerve-sparing (n = 19).

Results.—Of the men who underwent the non–nerve-sparing technique, one quarter were completely impotent before surgery and three quarters had inadequate erections before surgery. Of men who received nerve-sparing surgery, only 8% were completely impotent before surgery and 19% had inadequate erections before surgery. Regardless of the type of surgery, 33 of 47 men were completely impotent 12 months after surgery. Whereas 4 of 37 men who had nerve-sparing surgery were fully potent at 1 year, 62% were completely impotent, and 89% had inadequate erections

1 year after surgery. Inadequate erections after surgery were reported by 26 of 27 patients who underwent non–nerve-sparing surgery, by 36 of 37 who had unilateral nerve-sparing surgery, and by 23 of 28 who had bilateral nerve-sparing surgery. Of 11 patients with adequate erections before surgery, only 4 had adequate erections after bilateral nerve-sparing surgery. Both incontinence and wearing of pads were more frequent 3 months after nerve-sparing than after non–nerve-sparing surgery, although patients having nerve-sparing surgery reported fewer postoperative problems and less incontinence at 12 months.

Conclusion.—Postoperative sexual dysfunction after nerve-sparing radical prostatectomy is more frequent than previously reported. Symptoms of urinary incontinence persist, even at 12 months after surgery.

▶ If there is a lull in conversation among radiation oncologists and urologists, just mention the topic of early-stage prostate cancer. There is no more greatly debated subject in urologic oncology. Not only has the diagnosis of prostate cancer risen exponentially in the last several years, there has been a sixfold increase in the number of radical prostatectomies performed between 1984 and 1990. For a patient with early stage prostate cancer, the decision regarding the optimal treatment is confusing and frightening. In large part, decisions are often made based upon which physician sees the patients.

Whereas many urologists quote a low incidence of impotence and incontinence after radical prostatectomy compared with radiation therapy, this prospective evaluation of urologic symptoms presents an alternative view. As the authors state, many of the physician surveys conducted on prostate cancer are conducted retrospectively. This oftentimes results in selection bias. For example, patients who are sexually active are more likely to seek out nerve-sparing radical prostatectomy than are those patients who are impotent prior to their cancer diagnosis. As a consequence, retrospective reviews of patients treated with radiation therapy or non–nerve-sparing procedures are likely to have larger cohorts of patients with sexual dysfunction than those with nerve-sparing procedures.

These authors prospectively studied men with early-stage prostate cancer to evaluate sexual and urinary functions before and after surgery. The study points out that the incidence of incontinence and impotence is much greater than has been reported by other investigators. On behalf of those patients with prostate cancer who are struggling over the optimal therapy for early-stage disease, this paper provides some valuable insight.

P.J. Loehrer, Sr., M.D.

Immediate Versus Deferred Treatment for Advanced Prostatic Cancer: Initial Results of the Medical Research Council Trial

Kirk D, for the Medical Research Council Prostate Cancer Working Party Investigators Group (Gartnavel Gen Hosp, Glasgow, Scotland)

Br J Urol 79:235–246, 1997 5–3

Background.—Hormonal therapy is a basic component of the management of patients with advanced prostate cancer. Such treatment induces a temporary response, and patients with metastatic disease normally relapse within 2 years. If the relapse occurs after hormonal therapy, death usually occurs within months. It is unclear whether hormonal therapy should be started at diagnosis or when symptoms occur. In 1985, the Medical Research Council trial compared the effects of immediate and deferred hormonal treatment in patients with prostate cancer. The first results of this trial are reported.

Methods.—Immediate or deferred hormonal treatment was administered to 938 patients with locally advanced or asymptomatic metastatic prostate cancer. Treatment consisted of an orchidectomy or a luteinizing hormone–releasing hormone analogue. Data were collected annually on local and distant disease progression, major complications, and survival rates.

Results.—Follow-up data were obtained for 934 patients. Before treatment was started, 29 patients died of prostate cancer and 51 patients died of other causes. Treatment was started in cases of local progression almost as often as for metastatic disease. Progression from M0 to M1 disease and metastatic pain occurred more often in patients given deferred treatment. Transurethral resections were performed for local progression in 141 patients given deferred treatment and in 65 patients given immediate treatment. Patients given deferred treatment had pathologic fractures, spinal cord compression, ureteric obstructions, and development of extraskeletal metastases twice as often as patients given immediate treatment. Of the patients who died after treatment began, 67% died of prostate cancer: of the 361 patients given deferred treatment who died, 257 died of prostate cancer; and of the 328 patients given immediate treatment who died, 203 died of prostate cancer. Of patients with M0 disease, 119 patients died, and 81 of these died of prostate cancer.

Conclusions.—Although it is too early for an absolute recommendation, these findings suggest that immediate hormonal treatment in patients with prostate cancer is more beneficial than deferred treatment. More rapid local and distant disease progression was noted with deferred treatment. Deferred treatment may still be an option for elderly patients with nonmetastatic disease.

► Should hormonal therapy be instituted as soon as possible after the diagnosis of prostate cancer? If one looks at the older data from the Veterans Administration Cooperative Research Group trials, the answer is no. However, the toxicity of therapy with diethylstilbestrol (DES) and the presentation of patients with more advanced disease suggest that a different population of patients is seen today. In addition, leutinizing hormone-releasing hormone agonists are associated with less severe acute toxicities than DES. This paper by the Medical Research Council supports the premise that delaying initiation of hormonal therapy in previously untreated patients with advanced prostate cancer is associated with a worse outcome with respect to progression-free survival rates, sites of metastases, and overall survival rates. This study had some design problems with respect to the type of hormonal therapy and prestudy staging but provides provocative data supporting early hormonal therapy in advanced disease.

P.J. Loehrer, Sr., M.D.

Phase II Trial of Suramin, Leuprolide, and Flutamide in Previously Untreated Metastatic Prostate Cancer

Dawson NA, Figg WD, Cooper MR, et al (Natl Cancer Inst, Bethesda, Md)
J Clin Oncol 15:1470–1477, 1997 5–4

Objective.—Interest in new nonsteroidal antiandrogens for treating prostate cancer is increasing because the death rate from metastatic prostate cancer continues to rise. A pilot trial of a combination of leuprolide, flutamide, and suramin in patients with poorly differentiated (Gleason grade 7 or higher) stage D1 or any stage D2 prostate cancer evaluated tumor response rates, declines in prostate-specific antigen (PSA) levels, time to disease progression, overall survival, and toxicity.

Methods.—Fifty men, aged 42–79 years, with advanced prostate cancer and no prior hormonal therapy or chemotherapy received 250 mg oral flutamide 3 times/day to disease progression, 7.5 mg depot leuprolide IM every 4 weeks indefinitely, and suramin by continuous infusion to a plasma concentration of 175–300 μ/mL on days 1–5 and thereafter as needed to maintain a plasma concentration of 175–300 μ/mL for 8 weeks. Hydrocortisone was orally administered twice daily, 20 mg in the morning and 10 mg in the evening.

Results.—The Karnofsky performance status was 100% in 31 patients. There were 40 patients with stage D2 disease and 2 with stage D1 disease; 45 had bony metastases and 25 had soft tissue metastases. Three patients had complete remission for 19, 37, and 42 months; 30 patients had a partial remission for as long as 61 months. The overall response rate was 67%. There were 18 deaths, and 36 patients have progressed. Median progression-free survival is 12.8 months and was presaged by an increase in PSA levels. The median survival time has not yet been reached, but the median potential followup duration is 44 months. One, 2, and 3 year survival estimates are 92%, 79%, and 63%, respectively. Grade 3 or 4 toxicity, experienced by 19 patients, included reversible severe thrombocytopenia and neutropenia, pain, infection, elevation of transaminases, acute renal failure, disseminated intravascular coagulopathy, weight loss, and vortex keratopathy.

Conclusion.—Survival was excellent in this group of patients with prostate cancer with poor prognoses who received suramin, hydrocortisone, leuprolide, and flutamide. Toxicity was moderate but reversible and resulted in no deaths. A phase III/randomized trial comparing suramin with hormonal therapy alone is recommended.

► Prostate cancer is the most common malignancy in the United States. Not only has the incidence apparently dramatically increased (secondary to screening), the death resulting from this disease has also increased. Since the 1940s when Huggins and Hodges reported the relationship of androgens to prostate growth, hormone therapy has been the cornerstone of advanced disease. Various agents, including combined androgen blockade, have yet to have a significant impact on the progress of such patients. Chemotherapy has been disappointing, with suramin the most active drug noted in numerous phase II trials.

Is primary chemotherapy a reasonable strategy for patients with advanced prostate cancer? The answer is uncertain. However, the results of this trial demonstrate not only the feasibility of such an approach, but also durable remissions which are worthy of further evaluation. Perhaps such approaches will break an impass in the myriad of trials evaluating various agents of total androgen blockade.

P.J. Loehrer, Sr., M.D.

Phase III Trial of Androgen Suppression Using Goserelin in Unfavorable-Prognosis Carcinoma of the Prostate Treated With Definitive Radiotherapy: Report of Radiation Therapy Oncology Group Protocol 85-31

Pilepich MV, Caplan R, Byhardt RW, et al (Catherine McAuley Health Systems, Ann Arbor, Mich; Fox Chase Cancer Ctr, Philadelphia; Mercy Hosp. Scranton, Pa; et al)

J Clin Oncol 15:1013–1021, 1997 5–5

Objective.—Whereas androgen suppression is an effective treatment for prostate cancer, its value as adjuvant therapy to surgery and radiotherapy is unknown. Results of a randomized, phase III clinical trial conducted by the Radiation Therapy Oncology Group and using adjuvant goserelin after radiotherapy in patients with prostate cancer were reported.

Methods.—The effect of adjuvant goserelin on disease progression and survival was evaluated in 945 patients with prostate cancer with clinical stage T1 and T2 disease and a tumor dimensions product of less than 25. Patients received radiotherapy and goserelin (n = 477) (arm I) or radiotherapy alone (n = 468) (arm II). Goserelin was administered during the final week of radiotherapy in arm I or at relapse in arm II.

Results.—In arm I there were 78 local failures, 82 distant metastases, 271 survivors with no evidence of disease (NED), 251 survivors with NED and prostate-specific antigen (PSA) less than 4.0, and 232 survivors with NED and PSA less than 1.5. In arm II there were 135 local failures, 136 distant metastases, 125 survivors with NED, 127 survivors with NED and PSA less than 4.0, and 86 survivors with NED and PSA less than 1.5. All differences were significant. There was no significant difference in total survival at 5 years between arm I and arm II (346 vs. 330). Adjuvant goserelin significantly improved survival in patients with Gleason scores of 8 to 10 compared with patients receiving radiotherapy alone (66 vs. 55%) and marginally improved survival in patients with metastatic disease. The rate of local regression was significantly lower in patients receiving adjuvant goserelin.

Conclusion.—The addition of adjuvant androgen suppression to radiation therapy decreases the rate of local progression but has no impact on overall survival to date. A possible therapeutic advantage exists for patients with Gleason scores of 8 to 10.

▶ There are 4 principle ways to treat prostate cancer: surgery, radiation therapy, hormonal therapy, and observation. Over the past half century, it remains confusing as to which approach or combination of approaches is optimal. In large part, this is the result of differing behaviors of prostate cancer in which many men die "with it rather than from it." This trial, conducted by the Radiation Therapy Oncology Group, evaluates the role of the luteinizing hormone-releasing hormone agonist, goserelin, as adjuvant therapy with definitive radiotherapy in patients with locally advanced (T1, N1, M0 to T3, N1, MO) prostate cancer. Goserelin was administered during the last week of radiation and continued until disease progression. Patients who were treated with radiation therapy alone were given hormonal therapy upon recurrence. No information was given by the authors regarding toxicity, although 31 patients who were assigned to receive goserelin never received the drug.

This trial of immediate vs. delayed hormonal therapy yielded results that might have been anticipated. In other words, freedom from distant metastases, disease-free survival (especially if one uses PSA as a sign of progression), and local control all favored the immediate hormonal therapy arm. However, this trial failed to demonstrate a significant difference between the 2 arms with respect to 5-year survival (75% vs. 71%; $P = 0.52$), although a survival advantage was elucidated for patients with Gleason scores of 8–10 (66% vs. 55%; $P = 0.03$).

Does this trial establish the role of adjuvant hormonal therapy in localized prostate cancer? I don't think so. Does adjuvant therapy benefit patients with high grade lesions? Perhaps. Further studies are needed which not only focus on survival, but also on quality of life and the financial aspects of treatment.

P.J. Loehrer, Sr., M.D.

Interstitial Iodine-125 Radiation Without Adjuvant Therapy in the Treatment of Clinically Localized Prostate Carcinoma

Ragde H, Blasko JC, Grimm PD, et al (Pacific Northwest Cancer Found, Seattle; Univ of Washington, Seattle; Northwest Tumor Inst, Seattle; et al)

Cancer 80:442–453, 1997 5–6

Background.—Prostate brachytherapy for prostate carcinoma was popular for a short time during the 1970s after Whitmore, et al. introduced a method of retropubic implantation of iodine-125 radionuclides. Follow-up showed that the implant had a high rate of local failure, which was attributed to several causes. In the 1980s, various technological advances helped correct the original problems of the open-implantation technique. These advances include transrectal US planimetry for accurate prostate volume determination, transrectal US and template guidance to help implant the prostate transperineally, radiation treatment planning computers, and the availability of palladium-103 for needle insertion.

Methods.—Iodine-125 radionuclides were implanted in 126 consecutive patients with T1 and T2 prostate adenocarcinoma. The minimum radiation dose was 160 Gy. Prebiopsy prostate specific antigen values were obtained for all patients. Clinical biochemical and pathologic studies were performed after implantation. Surgical staging was not performed, and androgen deprivation treatment was not used. Morbidity was graded using the Radiation Therapy Oncology Group grading scale. Prostate specific antigen failure was defined as (1) prostate specific antigen proges-

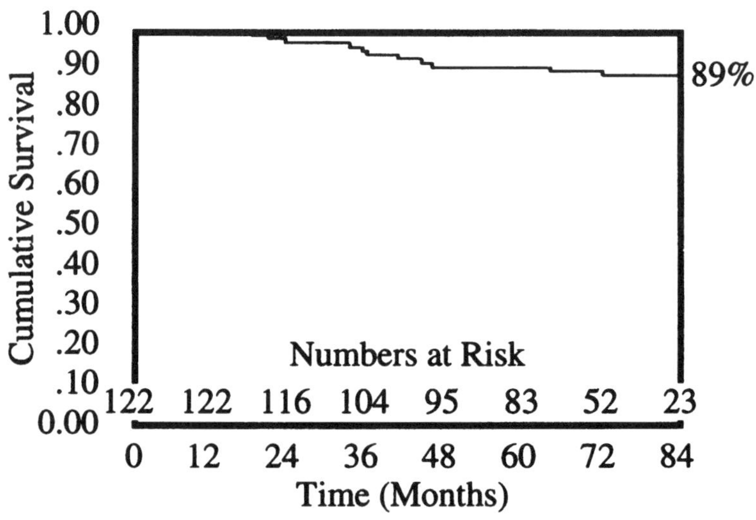

FIGURE 1.—Plot of Kaplan–Meier data to 7 years demonstrates 89% prostate specific antigen progression-free survival. (Courtesy of Ragde H, Blasko JC, Grimm PD, et al: Interstitial iodine-125 radiation without adjuvant therapy in the treatment of clinically localized prostate carcinoma. *Cancer* 80:442–453, 1997. Copyright © 1997 American Cancer Society. Reprinted by permission of Wiley-Liss, Inc., a subsidiary of John Wiley & Sons, Inc.)

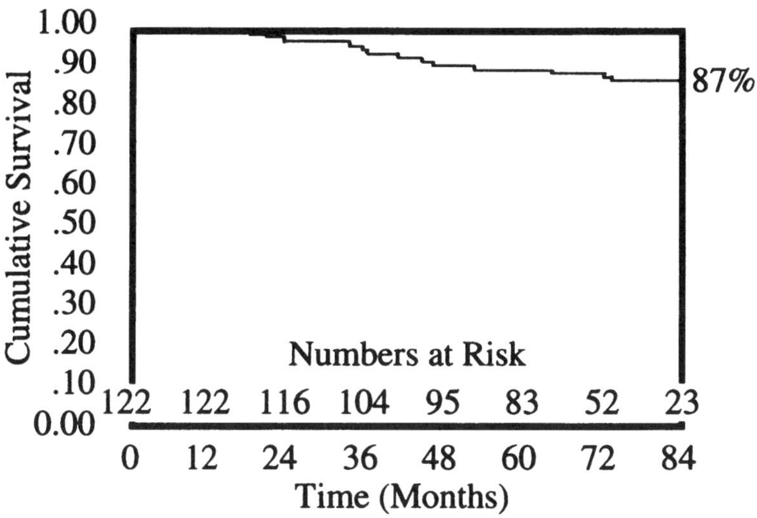

FIGURE 2.—Plot of Kaplan–Meier data to 7 years demonstrates 87% freedom from prostate specific antigen > 1.0 ng/mL failure. (Courtesy of Ragde H, Blasko JC, Grimm PD, et al: Interstitial iodine-125 radiation without adjuvant therapy in the treatment of clinically localized prostate carcinoma. *Cancer* 80:442–453, 1997. Copyright © 1997 American Cancer Society. Reprinted by permission of Wiley-Liss, Inc., a subsidiary of John Wiley & Sons, Inc.)

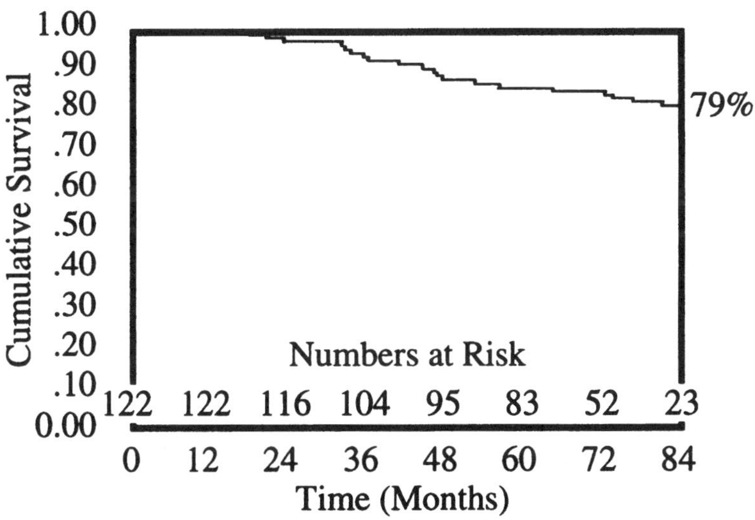

FIGURE 3.—Plot of Kaplan–Meier data to 7 years demonstrates 79% freedom from prostate specific antigen > 0.5 ng/mL failure. (Courtesy of Ragde H, Blasko JC, Grimm PD, et al: Insterstitial iodine-125 radiation without adjuvant therapy in the treatment of clinically localized prostate carcinoma. *Cancer* 80:442–453, 1997. Copyright © 1997 American Cancer Society. Reprinted by permission of Wiley-Liss, Inc., a subsidiary of John Wiley & Sons, Inc.)

sion of 2 consecutive increases from a nadir value and (2) failure to attain a serum prostate specific antigen value of 1.0 ng/mL or 0.5 ng/mL. Follow-up time was 69.3 months.

Results.—Evaluations were completed in 122 of 126 patients; 4 men died less than 1 year after implantation. At 7 years, overall survival was 77%. No patient died from prostate carcinoma. At 7 years, prostate specific antigen progression-free survival was 89% (Fig 1). The outcome for prostate specific antigen of no more than 1.0 ng/mL was 87% (Fig 2). When prostate specific antigen of no more than 5 ng/mL was the outcome measure, and the prostate specific antigen values of these patients were compared with the values proposed for disease-free survival after radical prostatectomy, the 7-year disease-free survival was 79% (Fig 3). There were few complications. Posttreatment incontinence occurred only in patients who had undergone transurethral prostate resection.

Discussion.—Patients with T1 or T2 prostate carcinoma treated with iodine-125 prostate brachytherapy had biochemical outcomes similar to outcomes expected from radical prostatectomy and external beam radiation. This single-session, outpatient procedure causes minimal morbidity and has high patient acceptance. Although the long, natural history of prostate carcinoma has required 10–15 years to assess treatment results, sequential evaluation of serum prostate specific antigen and biopsy may allow treatment results to be assessed sooner than was thought possible.

▶ There are some people who still wish to question whether the brachytherapy approach to prostate cancer is really established or still investigational. I do not think there is any question but that it is an established curative treatment. This series from Seattle shows an excellent survival rate up to 7 years and shows that the biochemical relapses appear to be comparable to patients undergoing radical prostatectomy or external beam, depending on the level of prostate specific antigen elevation that was present initially. Because this is outpatient treatment, it has an economic advantage over the prostatectomy. With more and more emphasis on managed care, that may become pivotal in recommending treatment in the future.

E. Glatstein, M.D.

Posttreatment Biopsy Results Following Interstitial Brachytherapy in Early-Stage Prostate Cancer

Prestidge BR, Hoak DC, Grimm PD, et al (Wilford Hall Med Ctr, San Antonio, Tex; Pathology Associates Inc, Spokane, Wash; Northwest Tumor Inst, Seattle; et al)

Int J Radiat Oncol Biol Phys 37:31–39, 1997 5–7

Background.—Several technological advances have prompted renewed interest in prostate brachytherapy. The pathologic control rate of permanent interstitial brachytherapy using contemporary techniques was reported.

TABLE 2.—Comparison of Presentation Characteristics by Postimplant Biopsy Status (n = 201)

	PostImplant biopsy		
	Positive (%) n = 6	Indeterminate (%) n = 34	Negative (%) n = 161
Stage			
T1a	0	0	4 (2)
T1b	0	3 (9)	3 (2)
T1c	1 (17)	8 (24)	32 (20)
T2a	3 (50)	23 (68)	99 (61)
T2b	2 (33)	0	20 (12)
T2c	0	0	3 (2)
Gleason Score			
2 to 4	3 (50)	10 (29)	56 (35)
5 to 6	3 (50)	19 (56)	90 (56)
≥7	0	4 (12)	11 (7)
ungraded	0	1 (3)	4 (2)
Presentation PSA (ng/ml)			
median	13.1	5.5	6.7
range	0.7–32.4	1.4–29	0.7–32.4
0.1 to 1.0	0	0	5 (3)
1.1 to 4.0	0	11 (32)	43 (27)
4.1 to 10.0	2 (33)	16 (47)	78 (48)
> 10.0	4 (67)	7 (21)	35 (22)

Abbreviation: PSA, prostate-specific antigen.

(Courtesy of Prestidge BR, Hoak DC, Grimm PD, et al: Posttreatment biopsy results following interstitial brachytherapy in early-stage prostate cancer. *Int J Radiat Oncol Biol Phys* 37:31–39. Copyright 1997, Elsevier Science Inc. Reprinted by permission.)

Methods.—Between 1988 and 1994, 402 patients with early stage prostatic carcinoma received permanent ^{125}I or ^{103}Pd interstitial brachytherapy as primary treatment. Two hundred one patients consented to biopsy 12 or more months after implantation, with a median follow-up of 40 months. None had undergone hormonal manipulation. Three hundred sixty-one biopsies were done on these patients.

Findings.—At the last biopsy, 80% of the patients had negative findings on histologic assessment; 17%, indeterminate; and 3%, positive. Only 2 of the 186 patients with a prostate-specific antigen (PSA) level of less than 4 ng/mL at the time of biopsy were positive. Twenty-eight of the 33 patients with indeterminate findings who underwent a subsequent biopsy had negative results, and 2 had positive results. In 3 patients, findings continued to be indeterminate (Table 2; Fig 2).

Conclusions.—The pathologically confirmed local control rate after permanent interstitial brachytherapy for early-stage prostate cancer is at least 80%. With further follow-up, the local control rate is expected to be greater, because most indeterminate biopsies convert to negative over time. These data support the use of modern interstitial brachytherapy methods for selected patients with early-stage prostate adenocarcinoma.

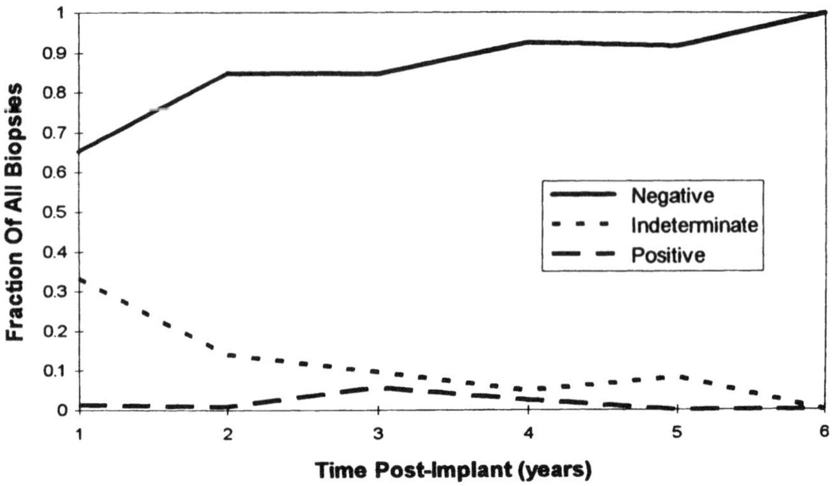

FIGURE 2.—The proportions of negative, indeterminate, and positive prostate biopsies as a function of the postimplant time interval. (Courtesy of Prestidge BR, Hoak DC, Grimm PD, et al: Posttreatment biopsy results following interstitial brachytherapy in early-stage prostate cancer. *Int J Radiat Oncol Biol Phys* 37:31–39. Copyright 1997, Elsevier Science Inc. Reprinted by permission.)

▶ The efficacy of radiation therapy for prostatic carcinoma has been complicated by the interpretation of biopsies. Because these cancers tend to be fairly indolent, it is not always easy to understand what the biopsy findings mean, especially if the biopsies are performed within just a few months of treatment. This series looks at 402 patients who received permanent brachytherapy for early-stage prostatic carcinoma. There is a follow-up of 6 or more years. Half of these patients consented to a biopsy 12 or more months after implant; this group had a median follow-up of 40 months. None received hormonal manipulation. Eighty percent had negative pathologic findings, 17% remained "intermediate," and only 6 (3%) had positive findings. Of 186 patients with a PSA level of less than 4 ng/mL at the time of biopsy, only 2 had positive biopsies.

E. Glatstein, M.D.

6 Genitourinary Cancer

International Germ Cell Consensus Classification: A Prognostic Factor-based Staging System for Metastatic Germ Cell Cancers

Mead GM, for the International Germ Cell Cancer Collaborative Group (Royal South Hants Hosp, Southampton, England)

J Clin Oncol 15:594–603, 1997 6–1

Background.—The incidence of seminomatous and nonseminomatous germ cell tumors (GCT), the most frequent cancers of young men, is increasing rapidly. Mortality from metastatic GCTs was high until the introduction of cisplatin-containing chemotherapy. Now, overall GCT cure rates are better than 80%. A simple prognostic factor-based staging classification system for metastatic GCTs was developed for use in clinical practice and collaborative trials.

Methods.—The study included clinical data on 5,202 patients with nonseminomatous GCT (NSGCT) and 660 patients with seminoma, all treated with cisplatin-containing chemotherapy. The patients were treated by collaborative groups from 10 countries; the median follow-up was 5 years. Multivariate analyses were performed to identify prognostic factors for progression and survival. The multivariate models were then validated in an independent data set of more recently treated patients.

Results.—Independent adverse factors for patients with NSGCT were mediastinal primary site, alfa-fetoprotein level, human chorionic gonadotropin level, lactic dehydrogenase level, and the presence of nonpulmonary visceral metastases. The latter was the main adverse prognostic factor for patients with seminoma. A model constructed from these factors identified 3 risk groups. Sixty percent of patients were in the good prognosis group, which had a 5-year survival of 91%. Twenty-six percent were in the intermediate prognosis group, which had a 5-year survival of 79%. The remaining 14% of patients, all of whom had NSGCT, were in the poor prognosis group, which had a 5-year survival of 48% (Table 4).

Conclusions.—A clinically based prognostic classification system for GCT is reported. This system has been agreed to by all major clinical trial groups currently active worldwide. Use of the classification in clinical practice and research will facilitate international communication regarding the assessment and treatment of GCTs.

► Germ cell tumors are the most common solid tumor in men between the ages of 15 and 35. During the past 2 decades, major strides have been taken

TABLE 4.—IGCC Classification: Progression-Free and Survival Rates in NSGCT Patients

Prognostic Group	Test Set						Validation						MRC/EORTC			
	n	%	5-Year PFS (%)	95% CI	5-Year Survival	95% CI	*n*	%	5-Year PFS (%)	95% CI	5-Year Survival	95% CI	*n*	%	2-Year PFS (%)	95% CI
Good	1,169	56	89	87–91	92	90–94	522	56	87	84–90	92	89–95	184	61	88	83–89
Intermediate	600	28	75	71–79	80	76–84	265	28	74	70–80	81	76–86	74	25	72	60–84
Poor	341	16	41	35–47	48	42–54	150	14	53	44–62	57	48–66	42	14	54	37–71

(Courtesy of Mead GM, and the International Germ Cell Cancer Collaborative Group. International germ cell consensus classification: A prognostic factor-based staging system for metastatic germ cell cancers. *J Clin Oncol* 15:594–603, 1997.)

through the mechanisms of clinical trials in the treatment of patients with disseminated disease. Such trials conducted in North America and elsewhere have often relied on institutional staging systems (e.g., Indiana, Memorial, M.D. Anderson, MRIC). Although there is general agreement about many poor risk features, discrepancies in the staging systems have led to problems with interpretation of published data and collaboration among international groups.

This paper, published by the International Germ Cell Cancer Collaborative Group, represents an unprecedented cooperative effort by investigators to create a new classification for patients with disseminated germ cell malignancies. This paper will serve as a reference for future studies of this disease.

P.J. Loehrer, Sr., M.D.

The Prevalence of Familial Testicular Cancer: An Analysis of Two Patient Populations and a Review of the Literature

Dieckmann K-P, Pichlmeier U (Albertines-Krankenhaus, Hamburg, Germany; Universitätskrankenhaus Eppendorf, Hamburg, Germany)

Cancer 80:1954–1960, 1997 6–2

Introduction.—Testicular cancer has been shown to exhibit a high degree of familial clustering, but there have been few systematic evaluations of the prevalence of familial testicular cancer (FTC). Proportions of FTC were analyzed in a large-scale patient population. Relative risk created by family history was estimated.

Methods.—The median ages of 1,692 patients with testicular cancer with and without a family history of that disease were compared. In a second population of 518 patients with testicular cancer and 531 age-matched controls, the frequency of family history was assessed and the relative risk was calculated. A literature survey was conducted to search for previous systematic reports on FTC.

Results.—In the literature, there were 10 previous reports of FTC. In the prospective investigation, 18 patients had a first-degree relative with testicular cancer (prevalence, 1.1%). The mean age at initial visit did not differ between patients with or without a family history. In the retrospective investigation, 13 patients had FTC; of these, 9 were first-degree relatives. The proportion of patients with testicular cancer was 1.7%, a 3:1-fold increased risk for first-degree relatives of patients with testicular cancer. When these and earlier findings were combined, the weighted mean prevalence of FTC was 1.35%.

Conclusion.—Genetic predisposition is a factor in susceptibility to testicular germ cell cancer. Nearly 1.35% of patients with testicular cancer have a family history of that disease. Patients with a first-degree family history of testicular germ cell cancer had a threefold to tenfold increase in relative risk.

▶ Testicular cancer is the most common cancer in young men between the ages of 14 and 35 years. Identification of risk factors for this disease have been elusive. The most important of these are undescended testicles and a contralateral primary testicular cancer. Over the years, several case reports of familial clustering have suggested an increased risk for this disease among family members. This paper presents convincing data linking family history with the subsequent development of germ cell tumors.

P.J. Loehrer, Sr., M.D.

Risk of Testicular Cancer in Cohort of Boys With Cryptorchidism

Swerdlow AJ, Higgins CD, Pike MC (London School of Hygiene and Tropical Medicine, London; Univ of Southern California, Los Angeles)

BMJ 314:1507–1511, 1997 6–3

Objective.—Orchidopexy late in childhood as treatment for cryptorchidism carries an increased risk of malignancy. Studies of risk have not been conducted on large populations. The risk of testicular cancer and related mortality in patients with undescended testis who had orchidopexy at the Hospital for Sick Children, London, were determined.

Methods.—Between 1951 and 1964, 1,075 boys were treated with orchidopexy and/or hormone therapy. The incidence of testicular cancer in this group was compared with that in the general male population.

Results.—There were 12 cases of testicular cancer in 11 men. The relative risk of testicular cancer in males with cryptorchidism is 7.5. Compared with a testis in a man in the general population, the risk of cancer in an undescended testis is 11.3. Ten cancers occurred after orchidopexy and 1 after hormone therapy. The relative risk of cancer was not significantly age related, but the relative risk decreased significantly with length of time after orchidopexy. The relative risk of cancer after testicular biopsy was significant at 66.7. The relative risk of cancer in an unbiopsied testis was 6.7. Risk of cancer is increased in males with bilateral maldescended testes as opposed to males with unilateral maldescended testes. The relative risk of cancer was highest in males with undescended testes submitted to biopsy.

Conclusion.—There is an increased risk of testicular cancer with cryptorchidism. The relative risk of testicular cancer was highest in males who had had biopsy of the testes.

▶ It has long been recognized that a history of cryptorchidism is associated with an increased risk for testicular cancer. Most of the reported literature involves case-control methods. This large cohort study involved 1,182 boys seen at a single hospital who underwent orchiopexy or hormone treatment for cryptorchidism from 1951 through 1964. Long-term follow-up to evaluate the subsequent development of malignancies was able to be performed in 1,075 of these boys.

This paper provides some interesting results. As expected, patients with cryptorchidism are associated with a higher risk of testis cancer (relative risk of about 7.5 over the general population). Orchiopexy at a younger age did not diminish the risk of cancer. Perhaps most surprising was the much greater risk (relative risk, 66.7) of cancer developing in those testes which had undergone a previous biopsy. This interesting phenomenon and the mechanisms which may lead to cancer after biopsy deserve further evaluation.

P.J. Loehrer, Sr., M.D.

A Study of Reproductive Function in Patients With Seminoma Treated With Radiotherapy and Orchidectomy: (SWOG-8711)

Gordon W JR, Siegmund K, Stanisic TH, et al (Clear Lake Regional Med Ctr, Webster, Tex; Washington Univ, Seattle; Affiliated Urology Specialists, Peoria, Ill; et al)

Int J Radiat Oncol Biol Phys 38:83–94, 1997 6–4

Introduction.—Radiation has adverse effects on the nondiseased testicle in healthy hosts or hosts having testicular cancer. A protocol was developed by one oncology group for patients treated with orchidectomy and radiotherapy in which sperm concentration and selected hormonal parameters in patients with testicular cancer were traced as well as the longitudinal effect of the treatment modality used. The pretherapy subfertile state was better defined, as well as the dose-dependent changes in sperm concentration and follicle-stimulating hormone, and the properties of testicular shields now in common use.

Methods.—There were 53 men with seminoma who were treated with orchiectomy and radiotherapy only. The main parameters followed included sperm concentration, follicle-stimulating hormone levels, and sexual satisfaction scores.

Results.—Before receiving radiotherapy, a fraction of the patients were infertile. Time to recovery of fertility is affected by incidental radiation dose to the remaining testicle. Changes in follicle-stimulating hormone mirror changes in sperm concentration over time at an aggregate level. This occurs with patients free from testicular cancer, as well. After orchidectomy, these men characterized their sexual activity as good.

Conclusion.—As a means of providing maximum protection to the remaining testicle, the use of clamshell-type testicular shields is supported. Within the studied dose range, permanent infertility is uncommon. Follicle-stimulating hormone increases as sperm concentration decreases in the aggregate. The testicular shields should be clamshell with a minimal aperture to reduce internal and collimator scatter, and should have a heavily shielded top and a separate scrotal block on the tray holder to reduce head leakage. Sperm concentration was recovered in about 1 year in patients for whom radiation therapy dose was held below 0.8 Gy.

► Modern data are sparse regarding the risk of infertility in patients with seminoma who are treated with primary radiation therapy. This study provides the benchmark for clinicians treating such patients. For patients with low volume disease who wish to maximize the chance of fathering children, sperm banking and shielding of the remaining testis should be considered. It should be noted that a significant portion of patients with newly diagnosed germ cell tumors will be oligospermic or azoospermic before treatment is initiated.

P.J. Loehrer, Sr., M.D.

Feasibility of Transurethral Resection for Muscle Infiltrating Carcinoma of the Bladder: Long-term Followup of a Prospective Study

Solsona E, Iborra I, Ricós JV, et al (Instituto Valenciano de Oncología, Valencia, Spain)

J Urol 159:95–99, 1998 6–5

Introduction.—Radical cystectomy is the customary treatment of patients with invasive bladder cancer. Transurethral resection has been able to control disease in several reported series, especially in patients with lower clinical disease stages. Long-term follow-up of patients treated with radical transurethral resection for muscle infiltrating bladder cancer was prospectively analyzed to determine progression predictive factors.

Methods.—Two groups of patients were followed. One hundred thirty-three patients with invasive bladder cancer treated by radical transurethral resection who had negative biopsy specimens of the muscle layer of the tumor bed constituted group 1. A control group of 76 patients with invasive pathologic stage pT2–3a, NO -3 bladder cancer treated with cystectomy and evaluated in a comparative, randomized trial made up group 2. Group 1 patients were followed for more than 5 years, and 59 patients (44%) were followed for more than 10 years. Group 2 patients were followed for more than 5 years.

Results.—The 5- and 10-year cause-specific survival rates for group 1 patients were 80.5% and 74.5%, respectively; bladder preservation rates were 82.7% and 79.6%, respectively. These rates were similar for group 2 controls. The only independent progression predictive factor observed was the initial presence of associated bladder carcinoma in situ.

Conclusion.—Radical transurethral resection may be considered in patients with invasive bladder cancer when all biopsy specimens of the periphery and depth of the tumor bed show muscular tissue negative for tumor cells. Patients with initial associated bladder carcinoma in situ may be included in this treatment approach but should undergo Calmette-Guerin immunotherapy and be followed very closely.

▶ Bladder cancer affects approximately 50,000 persons in the United States, with about 20% of these patients destined to die from this disease. Most patients are seen with superficial disease, which is generally well controlled with appropriate intravesicular chemotherapy. One of the most controversial areas involves those patients with muscle invasive disease. A variety of approaches have been used to enhance the improvement and survival of such patients, including preoperative chemotherapy and preoperative radiation therapy. Indeed, the outcome measures of success have included a pathologic complete remission (P_0) at the time of cystectomy.

This paper confirms the fact that a cohort of patients with invasive bladder cancer, particularly those with focal muscular invasion, may be treated successfully with radical transurethral resection of the bladder. It should be emphasized that transurethral resection of bladder tumor is not considered optimal therapy for invasive bladder cancer but, in selected cases, long-term disease-free and overall survival may be achieved. *Perhaps* some patients who have undergone multiple transurethral resections to evaluate preoperative (cystectomy) therapy may be rendered disease free by the transurethral resection procedure itself rather than the preoperative therapy (chemotherapy or radiation therapy).

P.J. Loehrer, Sr., M.D.

Risk of Second Malignant Neoplasms Among Long-term Survivors of Testicular Cancer

Travis LB, Curtis RE, Storm H, et al (Natl Cancer Inst, Bethesda, Md; Danish Cancer Society, Copenhagen; Karolinska Univ Hosp, Stockholm; et al)

J Natl Cancer Inst 89:1429–1439, 1997 6–6

Introduction.—One of the major breakthroughs in cancer treatment was the introduction of the heavy metal compound cisplatin into therapy protocols for testicular tumors. Having a 5-year relative survival rate of more than 90%, testicular cancer is now largely curable, and in recent decades radiotherapy fields to treat testicular cancer have decreased in size, with employment of lower doses. Possible late effects may be seen in men who were treated with earlier, more aggressive approaches. Long-term risks of second cancers among survivors have not been quantified. The site-specific risk of second malignant neoplasms among 1-year survivors of testicular cancer, as well as among 20-year survivors, was quantified.

Methods.—There were 28,843 men identified in tumor registries and of these, 3,300 men had survived more than 20 years. A search of registry files was conducted to find new invasive cancers.

Results.—In 1,406 men, second cancers were reported, with statistically significant excesses noted for acute nonlymphocytic leukemia, acute lymphoblastic leukemia, cancers of the stomach, non-Hodgkin's lymphoma, and cancers of the rectum, colon, prostate, pancreas, bladder, kidney, connective tissue, and thyroid. After seminomas or nonseminomatous tumors, the overall risk was similar. After the diagnosis of testicular cancer, the risk of solid tumors increased with time, yielding an observed-expected ratio of 1.54 among 20-year survivors. Radiotherapy and chemotherapy were associated with secondary leukemia. Radiotherapy was associated with excess cancers of the stomach, bladder, and possibly the pancreas.

Conclusion.—For more than 2 decades following initial diagnosis, men with testicular cancer continue to be at significantly elevated risk of second malignant neoplasms, including secondary leukemia, sarcoma, and cancers of the lung, gastrointestinal tract, and other urogenital sites. Although the precise roles of treatment, natural history, diagnostic surveillance, and other influences are yet to be clarified, patterns of excess second cancers suggest that many factors may be involved.

► The risk of secondary cancers is real for those patients previously treated with chemotherapy and radiation. This has been the experience with many childhood malignancies. This article examines a patient population seen from 1935 to 1993 who were treated for testicular cancer, and the results confirm increasing risk of secondary malignancy in this population. The method of treatment today for germ cell tumors is more succinct and less toxic than that performed in the past. Modern-day experience evaluates a mere 9–12 weeks of chemotherapy for patients with disseminated germ cell tumor, and radiation therapy is now limited to the infradiaphragmatic region for patients with stage II testicular cancer. The authors failed to include a population of patients treated by surgery alone, and in addition failed to clarify with specific details the number of patients receiving primary and salvage therapies. Nonetheless, these data are provocative and serve as a valuable benchmark to which we can compare modern-day treatment. They also serve as a cautionary note for those advocating primary chemotherapy in early-stage disease.

P.J. Loehrer, Sr., M.D.

Management of Stage II Seminoma

Warde P, Gospodarowicz M, Panzarella T, et al (Univ of Toronto)

J Clin Oncol 16:290–294, 1998 6–7

Introduction.—In the management of patients with testicular seminoma, there have been a number of significant advances, including tumor markers, histoimmunocytochemical techniques, computed tomography to image retroperitoneal nodes, and curative chemotherapy regimens. The current controversy in the management of stage II seminoma is whether chemotherapy or radiation therapy should be used as primary treatment, especially with the development of curative chemotherapeutic regimens for patients with testicular germ cell tumors. In a group of patients with stage II seminoma, treatment results of chemotherapy and radiation therapy were assessed to determine prognostic factors for relapse.

Methods.—There were 99 patients with stage II seminoma, with a median age of 35 years, who were managed during a 12-year period.

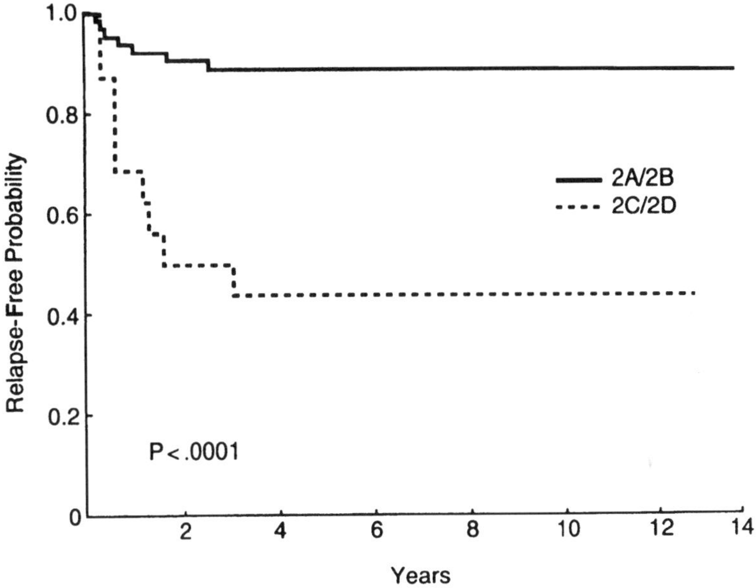

FIGURE 2.—Relapse rate and size of retroperitoneal lymph node disease. (Courtesy of Warde P, Gospodarowicz M, Panzarella T, et al: Management of stage II seminoma. *J Clin Oncol* 16:290–294, 1998.)

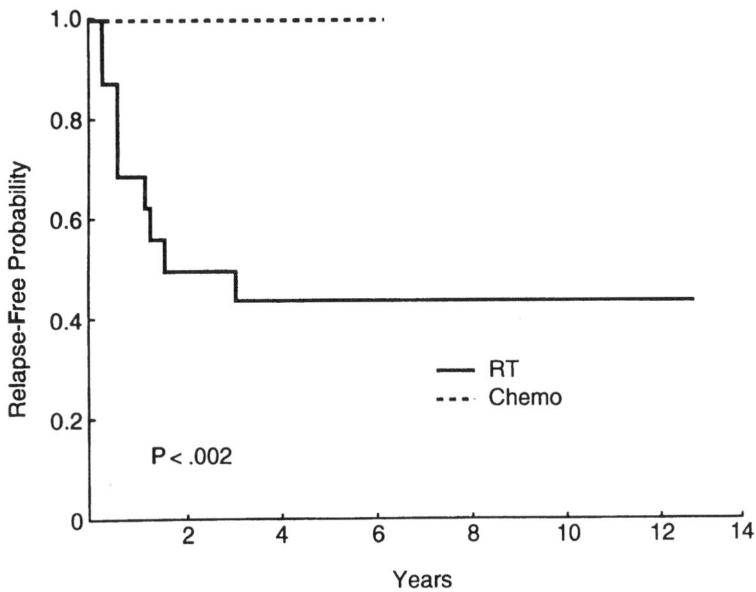

FIGURE 3.—Relapse rate in patients with IIC/D disease based on postorchiectomy treatment. (Courtesy of Warde P, Gospodarowicz M, Panzarella T, et al: Management of stage II seminoma. *J Clin Oncol* 16:290–294, 1998.)

Radiation therapy was performed on 80 patients and chemotherapy was used for 19 patients.

Results.—The 5-year overall actuarial survival rate was 94%, with a median follow-up of 6.7 years. There was a 5-year relapse-free rate of 83% and a 5-year cause-specific survival rate of 94%. Of the 80 patients treated with radiation therapy, 16 (20%) had a relapse, with 9 months the median time to relapse. In all but 2 patients, relapse occurred outside the irradiated area. In patients with a maximum diameter of retroperitoneal lymph node disease of 5 cm (stage IIA and IIB), the relapse-free rate was 89%, and for those with a diameter of nodal disease greater than 5 cm (stage IIC and IID), the relapse-free rate was only 44% (Fig 2). The supraclavicular fossa, bone, and lung-mediastinum were the sites of distant relapse. Disease control was achieved with all 19 patients treated primarily with chemotherapy and none has relapsed. For patients with stage IIA to IIB, the relapse rate at 5-year follow-up was 11% and for those with stage IIC to IID, the relapse rate was 56%. No patient with IIC or IID disease treated with chemotherapy relapsed (Fig 3).

Conclusion.—In patients with stage IIA or IIB seminoma, radiation therapy is highly effective, with a relapse-free rate of 89%. Local control is excellent with radiation therapy in stage IIC or IID, but a 50% risk of distant relapse is unacceptable, and not all patients who relapse can be salvaged. In patients with stage IIC or IID seminoma, chemotherapy should clearly be the primary treatment.

▶ The principal therapeutic difference between seminoma and nonseminomatous germ cell tumors is that the former is much more sensitive to radiation. For the greater part of this century, radiation has been the sole modality of treatment for seminoma. During the past quarter century, it has been recognized that seminoma is also extremely sensitive to cisplatin-based chemotherapy. Which patients should get chemotherapy and which should receive radiation therapy has been confusing for many clinicians.

The Princess Margaret Hospital has had a major impact on the role of radiation therapy in seminoma. Publications by Thomas, et al.[1, 2] led the movement against prophylactic mediastinal radiotherapy for patients with stage II seminoma. This article confirms the excellent prognosis of patients with stage II seminoma. In addition, it helps to define the role of chemotherapy for patients with stage II disease. Treated appropriately, the vast majority of patients with stage II seminoma should be curable.

P.J. Loehrer, Sr., M.D.

References

1. Thomas GM, Rider WD, Dembo AJ, et al: Seminoma of the testis: Results of teatment and patterns of failure after radiation therapy. *Int J Radiat Oncol Biol Phys* 8:165–174, 1982.
2. Thomas GM: Stage I, II seminoma—then and now. *Int J Radiat Oncol Biol Phys* 26:545–546, 1993.

Randomized Trial of Bleomycin, Etoposide, and Cisplatin Compared With Bleomycin, Etoposide, and Carboplatin in Good-Prognosis Metastatic Nonseminomatous Germ Cell Cancer: A Multiinstitutional Medical Research Council/European Organization for Research and Treatment of Cancer Trial

Horwich A, Sleijfer DT, Fosså SD, et al (Med Research Council Testicular Tumour Working Party, London; European Organization for Research and Treatment of Cancer Genitourinary Group, Brussels, Belgium)

J Clin Oncol 15:1844–1852, 1997 6–8

Introduction.—Cisplatin-based chemotherapy is a highly effective treatment for metastatic nonseminomatous germ cell tumors, with good long-term disease-free survival and a presumed cure rate of approximately 85%. Carboplatin has lower toxicity than cisplatin, and was therefore recently introduced for use in patients with metastatic nonseminomatous germ cell tumors. Carboplatin combinations must be evaluated rigorously before they are accepted as standard care. Carboplatin- and cisplatin-based combination chemotherapy were compared for use as first-line chemotherapy in patients with good risk nonseminomatous germ cell tumors.

Methods.—The prospective, randomized, multicenter trial included 598 patients with good-risk nonseminomatous germ cell tumors. The patients were randomized to receive 4 cycles of carboplatin plus etoposide and

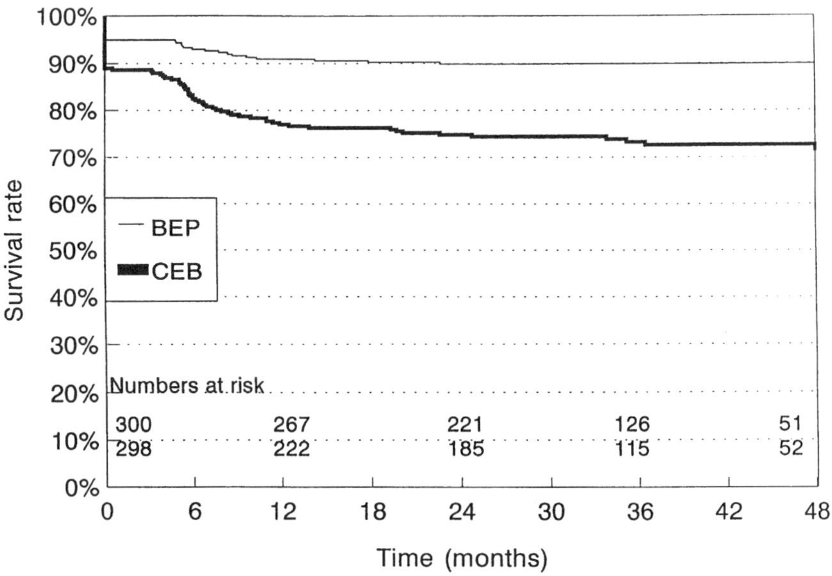

FIGURE 1.—TE09/30896. Failure-free survival by treatment allocated. (Courtesy of Horwich A, Sleijfer DT, Fosså SD, et al: Randomized trial of bleomycin, etoposide, and cisplatin compared with bleomycin, etoposide, and carboplatin in good-prognosis metastatic nonseminomatous germ cell cancer: a multiinstitutional Medical Research Council/European Organization for Research and Treatment of Cancer Trial. *J Clin Oncol* 15:1844–1852, 1997.)

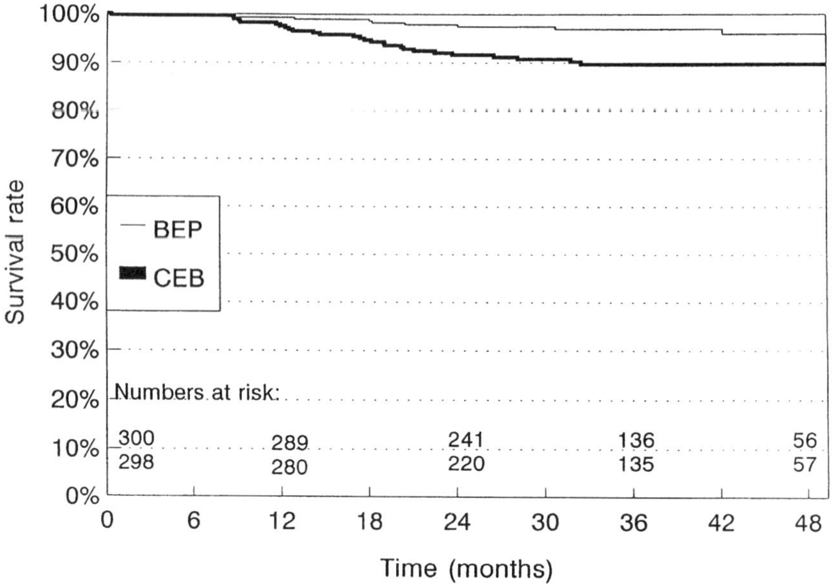

FIGURE 2.—TEO0/30896. Overall survival by treatment allocated. (Courtesy of Horwich A, Sleijfer DT, Fosså SD, et al: Randomized trial of bleomycin, etoposide, and cisplatin compared with bleomycin, etoposide, and carboplatin in good-prognosis metastatic nonseminomatous germ cell cancer: a multiinstitutional Medical Research Council/European Organization for Research and Treatment of Cancer Trial. *J Clin Oncol* 15:1844–1852, 1997.)

bleomycin (CEB) or cisplatin plus etoposide and bleomycin (BEP). Both groups received 120 mg/m^2 of etoposide on days 1, 2, and 3 and 30 U of bleomycin on day 2. Those in the BEP group also received 20 mg/m^2/d of cisplatin on days 1–5 or 50 mg/m^2 on days 1 and 2. Those in the CEB received carboplatin instead; the dose was calculated according to the glomerular filtration rate to achieve a serum concentration × time of 5 mg/mL × minutes. Chemotherapy was given in four 21-day cycles.

Results.—The complete response rate was 94% in the BEP group and 87% in the CEB group. The treatment failure rate was 10% and 26.5%, respectively. The 1-year freedom from failure rate was 91% with BEP and 77% with CEB (Fig 1). Three-year survival was 97% in patients assigned to BEP and 90% in those assigned to CEB (Fig 2).

Conclusions.—The results of carboplatin-based chemotherapy for nonseminomatous germ cell tumors are not as good as those of cisplatin-based chemotherapy, at least in the doses and schedules used in this study. Cisplatin-based chemotherapy, even with moderate doses of etoposide and bleomycin, is confirmed as an effective treatment for these patients. The research groups participating in this study are conducting a further trial to see if the number of cycles of BEP can be reduced from 4 to 3.

► Cisplatin, etoposide, and bleomycin have been the standard therapy for disseminated germ cell tumors. In good-risk patients, attempts to modify therapy to minimize toxicity has been the focus of recent investigators (see Abstract 6–12). One such approach has been to evaluate the substitution of carboplatin for cisplatin. A previous trial conducted by Memorial Sloan Kettering Cancer Center and the Southwest Oncology Group compared 4 cycles of cisplatin plus etoposide to 4 cycles of carboplatin/etoposide. Twenty-four percent of carboplatin/etoposide patients compared to 13% of platinum/etoposide patients had incomplete response or relapse ($P = 0.02$), also with an increased incidence of toxicity noted for the carboplatin arm. At the time of publication, however, no difference in overall survival was reported.

This much larger prospective trial, authored by Horwich et al. and conducted by the EORTC evaluated BEP (note difference dosages for etoposide and bleomycin compared to United States version) vs. CEB (using an A.U.C. of 5 for carboplatin). The difference in complete response rate, failure-free survival, and overall survival all favored the cisplatin arm.

Carboplatin is felt to be a "kinder, gentler" cisplatin and is routinely supplemented by physicians for cisplatin for the treatment of various malignancies. The data from this trial demonstrated that carboplatin is inferior to cisplatin in the treatment of patients with disseminated germ cell tumors. Further modifications of regimens in good-risk patients should be made with extreme caution.

P.J. Loehrer, Sr., M.D.

Paclitaxel Plus Carboplatin in Advanced Carcinoma of the Urothelium: An Active and Tolerable Outpatient Regimen

Vaughn DJ, Malkowicz SB, Zoltick B, et al (Univ of Pennsylvania, Philadelphia)

J Clin Oncol 16:255–260, 1998 6–9

Introduction.—For patients with metastatic carcinoma of the urothelium, cisplatin-based combination chemotherapy regimens are the standard treatment. A search continues for new active chemotherapy agents and combinations for urothelial carcinoma. A novel antimicrotubule agent is paclitaxel, which has demonstrated significant activity against human bladder cancer cell lines in previous studies. In patients with advanced carcinoma of the urothelium, a phase I/II trial of 3-hour paclitaxel plus carboplatin was performed to develop a well-tolerated and active outpatient chemotherapy treatment that would be an alternative to the cisplatin-based regimens.

Methods.—Every 3 weeks, paclitaxel 150–225 mg/m^2 over 3 hours followed by carboplatin (targeted area under the concentration-time curve, 6 mg/mL/min) was administered to patients. Sixteen patients were treated during phase I accrual, and at the phase II dose, an additional 17 patients were enrolled. Patients had a median age of 70 years and a median serum creatinine concentration of 1.1 mg/dL, with a median estimated creatinine clearance at 52 mL/min.

Results.—The maximum tolerated dose of the regimen was not defined during phase I accrual. At the paclitaxel 225 mg/m^2 dose level, phase II accrual occurred. There were 156 cycles administered in all, and the median number of cycles received was 5 with a range of 1–8. The principal nonhematologic toxicity was sensorimotor neuropathy. Significant thrombocytopenia was not common, but significant granulocytopenia was common. At all dose levels, objective responses were demonstrated. The objective response rate was 50% at the phase II dose (paclitaxel 225 mg/m^2 followed by carboplatin at the targeted area under the concentration-time curve 6 mg/mL).

Conclusion.—For patients with advanced carcinoma of the urothelium, paclitaxel plus carboplatin is an active and tolerable outpatient treatment. Patients with advanced age and abnormal renal function can withstand this combination over multiple cycles, making it well suited for this patient population.

Phase II Study of Single-Agent Gemcitabine in Previously Untreated Patients With Metastatic Urothelial Cancer

Stadler WM, Kuzel T, Roth B, et al (Univ of Chicago; Northwestern Univ, Chicago; Indiana Univ; et al)

J Clin Oncol 15:3394–3398, 1997 6–10

Introduction.—The standard of care for metastatic bladder cancer is cisplatin-based therapy. The most commonly administered regimen is the combination of methotrexate, vinblastine, doxorubicin, and cisplatin, but this combination has been questioned recently, as only 3.2% of patients treated with it have more than 5 years of disease-free survival. This combination is also associated with significant toxicities, including severe nausea and vomiting, grade-3 or greater neutropenia, grade-3 or greater mucositis, and significant renal insufficiency. Exploration of additional novel single agents with activity in metastatic bladder cancer is needed. One agent is gemcitabine (difluorodeoxycytidine). The activity of single-agent gemcitabine in previously untreated patients with metastatic transitional cell cancer was determined.

Methods.—In a 19-month period, 40 patients with measurable disease and a Karnofsky performance status of 60% or greater were treated with gemcitabine at 1,200 mg/m^2 3 times weekly on a 4-week cycle. All investigators and an independent radiologist confirmed all responses, which were maintained for at least 54 weeks.

Results.—There was an overall response rate of 28%, with 4 complete and 7 partial responses. Responses were seen at all sites, including the liver. The overall survival time was 54 weeks and the medial progression-free survival time was 20 weeks. There was mild toxicity with 2 grade-4 toxicities. Grade-3 neutropenia or thrombocytopenia was experienced by 25% of patients, and this was rapidly reversed.

Conclusion.—In metastatic transitional cell cancer, gemcitabine exhibits significant activity with minimal toxicity, but survival time remains short. Trials should be conducted of gemcitabine with other active agents. A combination of gemcitabine and cisplatin has already been initiated in another trial, and other agents that could be combined are paclitaxel, ifosfamide, and various antifolate agents. A more effective and less toxic regimen can be developed for patients with metastatic urothelial carcinoma.

▶ Over a decade ago, investigators at Memorial Sloan Kettering Cancer Center, led by Dr. Alan Yagoda, developed the methotrexate, vinblastine, doxorubicin, and cisplatin (MVAC) regimen for patients with advanced bladder cancer. Subsequent prospective trials confirmed its activity by proving superiority over single-agent cisplatin and over the combination regimen of cisplatin, cyclophosphamide, and doxorubicin. Despite this, drug delivery of full dosages of MVAC has been limited in an often elderly patient population who have mild to moderate renal insufficiency.

In the past few years, several drugs have been discovered to have single-agent activity that is comparable if not superior to that of single-agent cisplatin (once considered the cornerstone of treatment of this disease). These 2 articles by Stadler et al. and Vaughn et al. (Abstracts 6–9 and 6–10) are noted examples of novel trials of this disease. In previously untreated patients, gemcitabine and taxol have response rates which exceed 25%. Logically, carboplatin plus taxol has been evaluated and also confirmed to have a reasonably high objective response rate in this disease. It remains to be seen whether or not this regimen is superior to MVAC. Prospective randomized trials are currently underway which are evaluating cisplatin plus gemcitabine vs. MVAC, and carboplatin plus taxol vs. MVAC. The endpoint of these trials is to look not only at response rate and survival, but also importantly at quality of life.

P.J. Loehrer, Sr., M.D.

Salvage Chemotherapy With Vinblastine, Ifosfamide, and Cisplatin in Recurrent Seminoma

Miller KD, Loehrer PJ, Gonin R, et al (Indiana Univ, Indianapolis)

J Clin Oncol 15:1427–1431, 1997 6–11

Background.—About one fourth of patients with disseminated germ cell tumors of any histologic subtype are cured by vinblastine, ifosfamide, and cisplatin (VeIP). The activity of VeIP in patients with recurrent seminoma was investigated.

Methods.—Twenty-four patients with recurrent seminoma treated with VeIP as second-line chemotherapy were included in the retrospective review. All patients had been given cisplatin-containing regimens as primary therapy and 7 had received pelvic radiotherapy. Four courses of VeIP were delivered to all patients. The median follow-up was 7 years, with a minimum of 2 years.

Findings.—Eighty-three percent of the patients achieved a complete remission after VeIP alone. Another patient became disease free after the resection of residual carcinoma. Relapses occurred in 8 patients. Four of 6 patients with extragonadal primary tumors and 2 of 4 who did not have a complete remission after initial chemotherapy are now disease free with VeIP. Overall, 54% of the patients are long-term survivors with VeIP salvage chemotherapy.

Conclusion.—This chemotherapeutic regimen has significant curative potential in patients with recurrent seminoma. It appears to result in a greater complete remission rate, with more long-term survivors, than is achieved in patients with nonseminomatous disease.

► Seminoma is a highly chemosensitive tumor. Although most patients with seminoma are seen with early-stage disease and are cured with radiation alone, a significant portion of patients will have recurrent disease or widely disseminated disease which will require systemic chemotherapy. The investigators at Indiana University, headed by Dr. Lawrence Einhorn, have been responsible for developing curative regimens for nonseminomatous germ cell tumors. When these same combinations and principles of treatment have been applied to seminoma, even better results have been observed.

This study reports a dramatic effect of second-line chemotherapy with VeIP in patients with recurrent seminoma who already had progressed after receiving a cisplatin-based regimen as primary chemotherapy. More than 80% of the patients achieved a complete remission, and there is a plateau on the survival curve. It appears that more then 50% of these patients will be cured. These investigators now rightfully recommend this combination as initial salvage therapy for seminoma.

R.F. Ozols, M.D., Ph.D.

Importance of Bleomycin in Combination Chemotherapy for Good-Prognosis Testicular Nonseminoma: A Randomized Study of the European Organization for Research and Treatment of Cancer Genitourinary Tract Cancer Cooperative Group

de Wit R, Stoter G, Kaye SB, et al (Univ Hosp, Rotterdam, The Netherlands; Academic Hosp Groningen, The Netherlands; Netherlands Cancer Inst, Amsterdam; et al)

J Clin Oncol 15:1837–1843, 1997 6–12

Introduction.—Of patients with good-prognosis testicular nonseminoma, about 90% have a complete response to cisplatin combination chemotherapy, with relatively few relapses. It has been suggested that deleting bleomycin from the treatment regimen might reduce treatment toxicity in this group. This approach was tried in a prospective, randomized trial.

Methods.—The study included 419 patients with good-prognosis nonseminomatous testicular cancer. All received 4 cycles of cisplatin (20 mg/m^2 on days 1–5) and etoposide (120 mg/m^2 on days 1, 3, and 5). They were randomly assigned as to whether they received bleomycin (30 mg weekly) or not. Treatment outcomes and toxicity were compared.

Results.—A total of 395 patients proved eligible for the study. The complete response rate with chemotherapy alone or chemotherapy followed by surgery was 87% in the etoposide plus cisplatin (EP) group vs. 95% in the bleomycin, etoposide, and cisplatin (BEP) group, a significant difference (P = 0.0075). Each group was followed up for a median of 7 years, and each had a relapse rate of 4%. Only 11% of patients had unfavorable outcomes; there were no significant differences in time to progression or survival. Patients receiving BEP had significantly more acute and late pulmonary toxicity, and were the only ones to have Raynaud's phenomenon. There were 2 deaths from pulmonary toxicity in the BEP group.

Conclusions.—In patients with disseminated nonseminomatous testicular cancer, BEP remains the most effective chemotherapy regimen. Even in patients with good prognosis, bleomycin cannot be deleted without a reduction in treatment efficacy. Bleomycin is associated with increased toxicity, especially pulmonary toxicity. Further study is needed to address this problem.

► Since the early 1970s, bleomycin has been an important component of therapy for patients with advanced germ cell tumors. Samuels at M.D. Anderson Hospital demonstrated synergy of vinblastine and bleomycin in germ cell tumors. Later, Einhorn at Indiana and others incorporated cisplatin, which resulted in a dramatic improvement in the complete remission rate and cure in patients with disseminated disease. With the advent of etoposide therapy, numerous investigators questioned the continuing role of bleomycin as part of combination therapy. To date, several trials have been conducted evaluating the role of bleomycin. One such trial compared the Memorial trial of VAB-6 vs. four cycles of cisplatin and etoposide in good risk disease. No differences between these two regimens were found.

Several other groups, however, have looked at the role of bleomycin. The Australasian Germ Cell Tumor Trial Group compared 4 cycles of cisplatin and vinblastine with or without bleomycin and found a slightly higher remission rate for the Cisplatin, Vinblastine, Bleomycin arm (94% vs. 89%) with the tumor-related mortality significantly greater for patients who did not receive bleomycin. The Eastern Cooperative Oncology Group looked at 3 cycles of cisplatin and VP-16 with or without bleomycin and found a significantly worse outcome in failure-free survival (86% vs. 69%) and overall survival (95% vs. 86%) in patients not receiving bleomycin.

This article by de Wit. et al. reports the third such trial that suggests an inferior outcome when bleomycin is omitted from cisplatin combination therapy. Patients eligible for this trial had good risk (as defined by the diagnostic factors of the European Organization for The Research & Treatment of Cancer and the British Medical Research Council) and were randomized to 4 cycles of EP vs. 4 cycles of BEP therapy. The BEP arm was associated with a higher complete remission rate (95% vs. 87%; $P = 0.0075$). No significant differences were detected in terms of time to progression and overall survival. Acute and late pulmonary toxicity was significantly greater for patients receiving bleomycin. These authors treated the BEP patients to a total bleomycin dosage of 360 mg/m^2, which may account for the increased pulmonary toxicity. A previous Southeastern Cancer Study Group (SECSG) trial proved that 3 and 4 cycles of BEP (270 IV vs. 360 IV, respectively) were therapeutically equivalent with only a 1% incidence of pulmonary toxicity for the 3-cycle arm. As a consequence, the added toxicity of bleomycin (to a total dose of 360 mg/m^2) is probably not necessary. Although not compared directly, it is likely that 4 cycles of EP and 3 cycles of BEP would yield a comparable survival, but perhaps a lower response rate as suggested by this prospective trial. But if 3 cycles of therapy are to be administered, bleomycin should be included.

P.J. Loehrer, Sr., M.D.

Radiotherapy After Chemotherapy for Metastatic Seminoma: A Diminishing Role

Duchesne GM, for the MRC Testicular Tumour Working Party (UCL Med School, London)

Eur J Cancer 33:829–835, 1997 6–13

Background.—Some authorities advocate a policy of observation after chemotherapy for metastatic testicular seminoma, whereas others recommend radiotherapy to prevent progression, even though no effect on overall survival has been documented. The uncertainty about the role of radiotherapy in this setting was reflected in the inconsistent use of postchemotherapy irradiation among the centers participating in the MRC Trial TE12. To determine optimal management, the risk of relapse associated with different management strategies for patients with seminoma at the MRC United Kingdom and Norwegian centers was calculated.

Methods and Findings.—Data on 302 patients with metastatic testicular seminoma treated at 10 centers between 1978 and 1990 were analyzed. The primary end point—the progression-free survival rate after chemotherapy with or without additional radiotherapy—was correlated with type of primary chemotherapy, the sites and sizes of masses before and after chemotherapy, extent of surgical resection after chemotherapy, and the use of radiotherapy. At the completion of chemotherapy, 174 patients had residual disease. The presence of any visceral metastases or increased lactate dehydrogenase before chemotherapy and the presence of residual disease at visceral sites after chemotherapy were the most important prognostic factors for progression. About half the patients with residual disease had radiotherapy after chemotherapy. Selection was based mainly on institutional practice. Among patients given platinum-based chemotherapy, the delivery of radiotherapy did not significantly affect progression-free survival. The progression-free survival rate among patients given bleomycin, etoposide, and cisplatin was 88% and was also unaffected by the use of radiotherapy after chemotherapy. Among patients with residual masses limited to the abdomen after platinum-based chemotherapy, radiotherapy had an estimated absolute benefit of 2.3%.

Conclusion.—Postchemotherapy radiotherapy appears to have only minimal potential benefit in patients with metastatic seminoma. Thus, the use of adjuvant radiotherapy to residual masses after platinum-based chemotherapy for metastatic seminoma is not necessary.

Residual Mass Following Chemotherapy of Seminoma

Horwich A, Paluchowska B, Norman A, et al (Royal Marsden NHS Trust and Inst of Cancer Research, Sutton, England)

Ann Oncol 8:37–40, 1997 6–14

Objective.—After chemotherapy for large-volume seminoma, CT will reveal a residual mass in one third to two thirds of patients. The management of residual disease is controversial. The purpose of this analysis was to evaluate the need for additional therapy in such patients.

Methods.—Between October 1978 and May 1994, 45 patients were treated with cisplatin-based chemotherapy for advanced seminoma. Eleven patients had been previously treated with radiotherapy and had relapsed. Following chemotherapy 33 patients had residual radiographic disease. Management of these patients included surgical resection (of fibrosis) in 4 patients, radiation therapy to residual disease in 15 patients and observation only in the remaining 14 patients. Patients were followed from 10 to 202 months and evaluated every 3 months for 2 years, every 6 months for 2 years, and annually thereafter.

Results.—At follow-up, 41 patients were still alive and 4 had died of cancer. Five- and 10-year survival rates were 93%. Of the survivors, 39 were disease-free and 2 had relapsed but were in remission after second-line treatment. When tumor size was less than 5 cm, 7 of 9 patients attained complete remission with chemotherapy. When tumor size exceeded 5 cm, only 5 of 34 patients achieved complete remission after chemotherapy. Three of these 12 responders also received adjuvant radiotherapy, and none have relapsed. Four of 33 patients with residual masses had exploratory surgery that revealed fibrotic masses but no malignancy; 15 of them received adjuvant radiotherapy, and 14 were observed. Of the 15 receiving radiotherapy for whom data are available, there were no recurrences among 4 patients with residual masses of less than 3 cm, and there was 1 recurrence among 6 patients with residual masses of 3 cm or larger. Of the 14 observed patients, there was 1 recurrence among the 3 patients with residual masses of less than 3 cm and 1 recurrence among the 10 patients with residual masses of 3 cm or larger.

Conclusion.—In 73% of patients with seminoma, a residual mass remained after cisplatin-based combination chemotherapy. The risk of recurrence of seminoma after chemotherapy was not related to size of residual mass or to use of adjuvant radiotherapy.

► One of the few controversies in the field of germ cell tumors is the optimal management of patients with seminoma who have a persistent residual mass after cisplatin-based combination chemotherapy. Investigators at Memorial Sloan-Kettering Cancer Center suggested that residual masses 3 cm or larger have an approximate 27% incidence of persistent seminoma. Yet at Indiana University and elsewhere, the incidence of persistent seminoma in residual masses has been 10% or less.

These papers together with several others dispute the significance of residual masses in patients with serologically negative pure seminoma after chemotherapy. In patients with nonseminomatous germ cell tumors, resection of residual disease after chemotherapy will reveal necrosis (45%), teratoma (45%), or persistent carcinoma (10%). In contrast, residual disease after chemotherapy for seminoma does not consist of teratoma, but numerous series now show an approximately 10% relapse rate (or less) when such patients are treated with appropriate cisplatin-based combination chemotherapy. Indeed, Duchesne and his co-authors believe that the absolute benefit of radiotherapy to the residual mass is about 2.3%.

It is clear that an occasional patient with persistent disease will have residual seminoma. Further mechanisms to identify these patients are warranted. A previous trial investigating gallium scans did not prove useful, and an ongoing trial at Indiana University is evaluating positron emission tomography scans to help further delineate the residual disease process.

P.J. Loehrer, Sr., M.D.

Residual Masses After Chemotherapy for Metastatic Testicular Cancer: The Clinical Implications of the Association Between Retroperitoneal and Pulmonary Histology

Steyerberg EW, for the Re-analysis of Histology in Testicular Cancer (ReHiT) Study Group (Erasmus Univ, Rotterdam, The Netherlands)

J Urol 158:474–478, 1997 6–15

Introduction.—Histologic findings at retroperitoneal lymph node dissection are reported to be predictive of the residual pulmonary histologic status after chemotherapy for metastatic testicular cancer. One-hundred fifty-nine patients with metastatic nonseminomatous testicular cancer who underwent retroperitoneal lymph node dissection and thoracotomy were evaluated to determine the relationship between retroperitoneal and pulmonary histology.

Methods.—All patients received cisplatin-based induction chemotherapy. The relationship between retroperitoneal and lung histologic status was examined. Well-known predictors for residual histologic status (necrosis, mature teratoma, and cancer) were analyzed.

Results.—Necrosis was detected more often at retroperitoneal lymph node dissection when the primary tumor was negative for teratoma, the residual mass was small, or the reduction in size was great. Residual mass size and decrease in size were not predictive of the histologic status of the residual lung lesion. There was a strong association between histologic findings in the retroperitoneum and the lungs. Necrosis at retroperitoneal lymph node dissection was correlated with an 89% probability of necrosis in the lung.

Conclusion.—These findings show that retroperitoneal lymph node dissection should be performed before thoracotomy. If necrosis only is detected on dissection, the necessity for thoracotomy is doubtful. Histologic status at retroperitoneal dissection is a strong predictor of histologic status at thoracotomy.

▶ Treatment of disseminated germ cell tumor is associated with several nuances which often plague the clinician. One of these is the optimal management of patients with residual radiographic disease after systemic chemotherapy. This paper helps define the proper sequence of surgical procedures in patients with residual infradiaphragmatic and supradiaphragmatic disease. In patients without teratoma in the primary specimen, the results of the retroperitoneal lymph node dissection is highly predictive of the findings at thoracotomy. Thus, one may spare selected patients from 2 major operations by avoiding a thoracotomy. If teratoma is present in the primary specimen, both procedures are still indicated.

P.J. Loehrer, Sr., M.D.

Intensive Induction-sequential Chemotherapy With BOP/VIP-B Compared With Treatment With BEP/EP for Poor-prognosis Metastatic Nonseminomatous Germ Cell Tumor: A Randomized Medical Research Council/European Organization for Research and Treatment of Cancer Study

Kaye SB, Mead GM, Fossa S, et al (Univ of Glasgow, Scotland; Royal South Hants Hosp, Southampton, England; Univ Hosp Birmingham, England; et al)

J Clin Oncol 16:692–701, 1998 6–16

Introduction.—One of the outstanding success stories of modern cancer treatment is the management of metastatic testicular teratoma with the bleomycin/etoposide/cisplatin schedule; however, up to 20% of patients are not cured by this regimen. More intensive schedules have been reported, but comparisons have not been conducted. A minor modification is the schedule of bleomycin, vincristine, and cisplatin/etoposide, ifosfamide, cisplatin, and bleomycin. Whether treatment with the more intensive regimen was more effective than treatment with bleomycin, etoposide, and cisplatin was investigated.

Methods.—There were 380 patients who had one or more of the following: mediastinal or supraclavicular mass 5 cm or greater in diameter; a retroperitoneal mass 10 cm or greater in diameter; liver, bone, or brain metastases; at least 20 lung metastases (any size); and serum beta human chorionic gonadotropin 10,000 IU/L or more or alfa fetoprotein 1,000 IU/L or more.

Results.—In the proportion of patients who achieved a complete response with chemotherapy alone, there was no significant difference between the 2 arms with 54% achieving a response in the intensive bleomycin, vincristine, cisplatin/etoposide, ifosfamide, cisplatin, and bleomycin therapy arm, and with 54% achieving a response in the bleomycin, etoposide, and cisplatin/etoposide and cisplatin arm. A total of 107 patients (28%) had progressive disease, with a median follow-up of 3.1 years. Between the 2 arms, there was no significant difference in time to first disease progress, or failure-free or overall survival. For bleomycin, etoposide, and cisplatin/etoposide and cisplatin, the 1-year failure-free survival rate was 60% and for intensive bleomycin, vincristine, cisplatin/etoposide, ifosfamide, cisplatin, and bleomycin therapy, it was 53%. With intensive bleomycin, vincristine, cisplatin/etoposide, ifosfamide, cisplatin, and bleomycin therapy, grade 3 or 4 myelosuppression, febrile neutropenia, and weight loss were more pronounced and there were more toxic deaths than with bleomycin, etoposide, and cisplatin/etoposide and cisplatin.

Conclusion.—Compared to treatment with bleomycin, etoposide, and cisplatin/etoposide and cisplatin, the intensive bleomycin, vincristine, cisplatin/etoposide, ifosfamide, cisplatin, and bleomycin therapy was associated with more toxicity, but there was no evidence of an improvement in response rate or survival.

► Over the past several years, various approaches have been undertaken to improve the therapeutic outcome of patient trials for poor risk germ cell tumors. Cisplatin, etoposide, and bleomycin (BEP) has been compared to more dose intense regimens with cisplatin (200 mg/m^2 vs. 100 mg/m^2 per course), substitution of ifosfamide for bleomycin, and alternating "non-cross"-resistant regimens. This prospective randomized trial evaluated the bleomycin, vincristine, cisplatin/etoposide, ifosfamide, cisplatin, and bleomycin regimen that was promulgated by our British colleagues as a novel regimen and has a flavor of all 3 of the aforementioned strategies. This regimen, however, like others tested, failed to demonstrate a therapeutic advantage over BEP alone. Until future trials prove otherwise, BEP is the treatment of choice in patients with advanced disease.

P.J. Loehrer, Sr., M.D.

Prevalence of Carcinoma In Situ of the Testis in 207 Oligozoospermic Men From Infertile Couples: Prospective Study of Testicular Biopsies

Giwercman A, Thomsen JK, Hertz J, et al (Rigshospitalet, Copenhagen; Herlev Hosp, Copenhagen; Gentofte Hosp, Copenhagen; et al)

BMJ 315:989–991, 1997 6–17

Introduction.—Carcinoma in situ of the testis is considered a preinvasive lesion observed in all types of testicular germ cell tumors. Male infertility is a suspected risk factor for carcinoma in situ. There is speculation that testicular biopsy for carcinoma in situ should be offered as a screening to men who are infertile. The magnitude of risk needs to be determined before screening is recommended. The need for screening for carcinoma in situ in infertile males was evaluated prospectively.

Methods.—The age range of 207 oligozoospermic males from infertile couples was 18–50 years. All except 6 men underwent bilateral biopsies; unilateral biopsies were performed when only 1 gonad was present in the scrotum. The estimated relative risk of carcinoma in situ of this cohort was compared with that of a corresponding normal population of Danish males. The calculated risk was based on data from the Danish Cancer Registry.

Results.—None of the biopsy specimens revealed carcinoma in situ among the infertile males. The calculated risk for the population of Danish males matched for age and year of birth was 0.8.

Conclusion.—Moderately oligozoospermic males of couples referred for infertility are at no increased risk for carcinoma in situ of the testis. Further prospective investigation is needed to determine whether males with severe oligozoospermia and pronounced testicular atrophy with very irregular echo patterns are at increased risk for carcinoma in situ of the testis.

► Carcinoma in situ (CIS) is believed to be the preinvasive lesion that antedates development of testicular cancer. Several authors have reported retrospective reviews suggesting that male infertility is a risk factor for the development of carcinoma in situ. As 20% to 80% of patients presenting with testicular carcinoma have oligospermia or azospermia, this relationship seems plausible. This prospective study, however—written by a well-respected group who previously defined the importance of CIS in testicular carcinoma—fails to support the hypothesis that infertility, by itself, is a risk factor for CIS.

P.J. Loehrer, Sr., M.D.

7 Gastrointestinal Cancer

Pelvic Exenteration for Locally Advanced Rectal Carcinoma: Factors Predicting Improved Survival

Meterissian SH, Skibber JM, Giacco GG, et al (Univ of Texas, Houston)

Surgery 121:479–487, 1997 7–1

Introduction.—Extensive surgery for complete tumor extirpation is required in up to 10% of rectal cancers. The most important treatment factor in determining patient outcome is the ability of the surgeon to accomplish tumor-free resection margins, which could involve en bloc removal of the rectum, bladder, distal ureters, and reproductive organs. The 5-year survival rate was found to be up to 50% for patients with rectal cancer. The use of preoperative radiotherapy has improved the resectability status of patients. To aid in the selection of patients most likely to benefit from this extensive surgical procedure, biological markers that may predict outcome and guide the use of preoperative adjuvant therapy are needed. Whether any clinicopathologic factors—such as age, gender, type of exenteration, tumor extent, adjuvant therapy, tumor DNA ploidy, and S-phase fraction—could predict survival in patients having pelvic exenteration for rectal cancer was determined.

Methods.—Pelvic exenteration for rectal adenocarcinoma in which tumor-free pathologic margins were obtained was performed in 40 patients in a 9-year period. Primary tumors were seen in 29 patients and 11 had recurrent disease. Twenty patients had a total exenteration, 18 had a posterior exenteration, and 2 had an anterior exenteration.

Results.—Significant predictors of survival were age, preoperative chemoradiation therapy, and an S phase of 10% or more. A relative risk for cancer-related death was 0.13 with age older than 55 years. A relative risk for cancer-related death of 0.05 was associated with chemoradiation. These 2 factors have a beneficial effect. Poor survival was indicated by an S-phase fraction of 10% or greater, which had a relative risk of cancer-related death of 16.97. A 5-year survival rate of 65% (low risk) was found with a prognostic index of less than 1.37. A 5-year survival rate of 20% (high risk) was found in patients with a prognostic index of less than 1.37.

Conclusion.—In patients who require pelvic exenteration for resection of locally advanced rectal carcinoma, adjuvant chemoradiation may significantly improve survival. A predictor of poor outcome is an S-phase fraction of 10% or greater.

▶ Locally advanced or recurrent rectal cancer poses a significant problem for the surgeon involved in treatment decisions. Unrelenting pelvic extension of rectal cancer—even in the absence of systemic disease—causes pain, infection, bleeding, and fistula, and will lead to a rapid progressive decline in quality of life for the patient. Radical pelvic surgery for patients with locally advanced rectal cancer is a considerable surgical procedure and can be associated with significant morbidity. This paper addresses a prognostication scheme in an attempt to predetermine those patients who will subsequently benefit from an aggressive surgical approach. The difference in cancer-related survival of patients with an S-phase fraction of 10% or greater is dramatic. The usefulness of predictive outcome information, as presented in this paper, is that it provides a valuable quantitative method for evaluating patient risk profiles before consideration of radical salvage pelvic surgery.

B.L. Eisenberg, M.D.

Hospital Volume Influences Outcome in Patients Undergoing Pancreatic Resection for Cancer

Glasgow RE, Mulvhill SJ (Univ of California, San Francisco)

West J Med 165:294–300, 1996 7–2

Objective.—Although resection of pancreatic cancer has traditionally resulted in high rates of morbidity and mortality, some centers report mortality rates of less than 5% and major morbidity rates about 30%. The relation between hospital volume and postoperative outcome in patients undergoing major pancreatic resection for malignancy in California was retrospectively evaluated using data from the Office of Statewide Health Planning and Development.

Methods.—After assessment of the predictive role of patient characteristics, the relationship between hospital volume and operative morbidity and mortality was studied using logical regression analysis.

Results.—Between 1990 and 1995, 1,910 patients had a pancreaticoduodenectomy (n = 1,424), proximal subtotal pancreatectomy (n = 158), total pancreatectomy (n = 123), or distal (Whipple) pancreatectomy (n = 205) with respective mortalities of 9.4%, 8.9%, 16.3%, and 1.0%. Mortality for total pancreatectomy was significantly higher than for the Whipple procedure. Of the 1,705 assessable patients, 70% were 60 years of age or older. Operative mortality was significantly associated with the number of comorbid factors, older age, male sex, and the need for total pancreatectomy. The incidence of postoperative intra-abdominal infection and decreasing hospital volume also increased mortality significantly. Hospitals treating fewer than 2 patients per year accounted for 88% of reporting institutions. Larger volume hospitals had significantly lower hospital charges, less resource usage, less mortality, fewer complications, and were more likely to discharge patients home.

Conclusion.—There is a significant relationship between patient outcome and hospital volume for patients undergoing pancreatic resection for cancer. These data support regionalization for high-risk procedures.

▶ This article addresses an aspect for the quality concerns and costs analysis of difficult and complex surgical care. In this instance, they report on patients undergoing pancreatic resection for pancreatic cancer in a statewide survey of volume vs. outcome from participating hospitals. Those hospitals that perform the majority of pancreatic surgery document a decreased procedure-related morbidity and mortality, and a subsequent decrease in overall costs per patient compared to those hospitals performing only a few pancreatic resections per year. This is the latest study to observe that cost and quality can be paired in considering complex and time-consuming surgical procedures. It also has been noted that those hospitals where resident housestaff perform complex procedures such as major pancreatic resections with a teaching surgeon attending do not report any substantial increase in adverse operative or postoperative events. At least on these outcome evaluations, one can make a logical case for cost-effective quality care involving the limitation of certain technologically demanding surgical procedures to centers of excellence. These issues will become increasingly controversial as health care dollars are divided up on the basis of patient care outcomes variables.

B.L. Eisenberg, M.D.

Prospective Randomized Study of Laparoscopic *Versus* Open Colonic Resection for Adenocarcinoma

Stage JG, Schulze S, Moller P, et al (Frederiksberg Hosp, Copenhagen; Sundby Hosp, Copenhagen; Hvidovre Hosp, Copenhagen)

Br J Surg 84:391–396, 1997 7–3

Objective.—Whereas laparoscopic surgery is as good as or better than conventional surgery for many operations, retrospective and prospective studies have not proved it to be unequivocally superior to conventional surgery for all patients with colorectal cancer. Laparoscopic and open colonic resection were compared in a randomized fashion with respect to outcome, complications, and immunomodulation.

Methods.—Either laparoscopy (n = 15) or open surgery (n = 14) was performed on 29 patients (16 women) aged 48–93 years with colorectal cancer. Results of the 2 groups were compared statistically.

Results.—Whereas length of stay after surgery was significantly shorter for the laparoscopy group than for the open surgery group (5 vs. 8 days), duration of surgery was significantly longer for the laparoscopy group than for the open surgery group (150 vs. 95 minutes). The laparoscopy group experienced significantly less pain at rest, during coughing, during mobilization, and at rest throughout the study than did the open surgery group. Pulmonary function and fatigue were similar in both groups. Plasma interleukin-6 levels were significantly higher in the laparoscopy group than in the open surgery group. Pneumonia and esophagitis developed in 1 patient who had laparoscopy, and 1 patient who had laparoscopy was reoperated upon for hypotension and abdominal pain.

Conclusion.—Laparoscopic surgery is a safe and acceptable alternative to open surgery, although the differences are not marked.

► Minimally invasive surgical techniques have advanced rapidly in the last few years. Therapeutic operative procedures and laparoscopic surgery have gone beyond cholecystectomy and are now being incorporated into treatment paradigms for abdominal malignancies. The safety and efficacy of oncologic laparoscopic extirpative surgery is unclear, however, and this will hopefully be addressed in a systematic scientific manner before developing care standards. This article from Denmark reviews a prospective randomized trial of laparoscopic vs. open colon resection for cancer. The important points in this well conducted (but quite small in patient number) clinical trial are that the radicality of surgery was the same in both groups and the complications were similar, but the laparoscopic group had earlier discharge and less postoperative pain. As data accumulate, laparoscopic colectomy trials of this type will be important in evaluating the clinical usefulness of a laparoscopic approach. One must caution that long-term oncologic results of laparoscopic colon resection for cancer are not yet known and there remains the question of port site recurrences. Additionally, unless there proves to be a decided advantage of therapeutic laparoscopic surgery over open procedures for colorectal cancers, because the learning curve for performing a laparoscopic resection is quite steep, this procedure may not be routinely advisable in the surgical management of this disease.

B.L. Eisenberg, M.D.

The National Cancer Data Base Report on Carcinoma of the Anus

Myerson RJ, Karnell LH, Menck HR (Washington Univ, St Louis, Mo; Univ of Iowa, Iowa City; American College of Surgeons, Chicago)

Cancer 80:805–815, 1997 7–4

Objective.—Anal carcinoma is rare and carries a low mortality rate. Management of the disease centers around preserving anorectal function. Disease characteristics, care, and outcome based on data from the National Cancer Data Base were reviewed.

Methods.—Patterns of care, long-term outcome, and trend data for anal carcinoma patients from 1988 (n = 1,050) to 1993 (n = 1,289) were analyzed statistically.

Results.—The average age at diagnosis declined from 62.8 years in 1988 to 61.8 years in 1993. About half the patients were female throughout the study; 87.2% were non-Hispanic whites in 1993. The use of the "cloacogenic zone" category increased from 0.3% in 1988 to 8.9% in 1993, and "overlapping lesion" decreased from 29.2% to 18.8%. The proportion of epidermoid carcinoma increased from 74.3% to 79.1%, whereas the percentage of adenocarcinomas declined from 21.9% to 16.5%. The proportion of early-stage carcinomas increased from 66.6% to 73.4%, and the number of cases not staged decreased from 43.9% to 17.8%. Patients with epidermoid carcinoma were 67.1% female, whereas patients with adenocarcinoma were 42.0% female.

The use of resection decreased during this period, whereas the use of radiation therapy increased from 67.4% to 72.6% and the use of chemotherapy increased from 57.4% to 64.8%. The overall use of surgery declined from 53.8% in 1988 to 49.1% in 1993 but increased for adenocarcinoma. Overall 5-year survival was 53.9% for 1988 cases. This was broken down to 57.6% for epidermoid carcinoma and 41.3% for adenocarcinoma, 56.2% for females and 49.6% for males, 71.3% for stage I disease and 23.1% for stage IV disease, and 64.0% for nonsurgical treatment of stage I-II epidermoid carcinoma and 65.4% for surgical treatment.

Conclusion.—Radiochemotherapeutic treatment of epidermoid carcinoma of the anus is increasing. Surgery plus radiotherapy and/or chemotherapy is becoming more common. Studies confirm the efficacy of conservative radiation plus chemotherapy for treatment of epidermoid carcinoma. Early-stage epidermoid carcinoma and female sex favor increased 5-year survival.

► This paper reports the results of data collected in the National Cancer Data Base for the management of carcinoma of the anus. Treatment trends nationally within the last 15 years have been heavily weighted toward radiochemotherapy and a nonsurgical approach for squamous cancer of the anus. It is now generally accepted that radical surgery for patients with epidermoid carcinoma of the anus should be considered only as salvage therapy in those patients in whom first-line radiochemotherapy or second-line chemotherapy cannot adequately provide local disease control. This is in contradistinction to adenocarcinoma in which surgery continues to play an important role in a multimodality approach that frequently includes radiochemotherapy treatment paradigms as well.

B.L. Eisenberg, M.D.

Locally Advanced Rectal Carcinoma: Pelvic Control and Morbidity Following Preoperative Radiation Therapy, Resection, and Intraoperative Radiation Therapy

Kim HK, Jessup JM, Beard CJ, et al (Harvard Med School, Boston)

Int J Radiat Oncol Biol Phys 38:777–783, 1997 7–5

Objective.—Six percent to 14% of patients with rectal cancer have locally advanced and initially unresectable tumors. The effect of combined preoperative external beam radiotherapy (EBRT) and 5-fluorouracil with surgical resection and intraoperative radiotherapy (IORT) at 1 institution was reviewed.

Methods.—Between October 1982 and October 1993, 40 patients (19 women), aged 36 to 78 years, received preoperative EBRT at a median dose of 50.4 Gy delivered in 1.8 to 2 Gy fractions 5 days/week, and 30 received IV 5-FU. Thirteen patients had recurrent disease and 27 had primary tumors. Of the 33 patients having curative resection, 26 with questionable margins had IORT at a median dose of 12.5 GY delivered to the tumor bed to a depth of 1 to 2 cm. Patients were typically followed for 33 months.

Results.—At follow-up, 20 patients were alive and 12 were disease free. Fourteen of 19 patients having a complete resection were alive and 9 were disease free at a median of 34 months. Fourteen of 22 patients with locally advanced disease were alive and 9 were disease free (Fig 2). The 5-year actuarial local control and overall survival rates for patients having com-

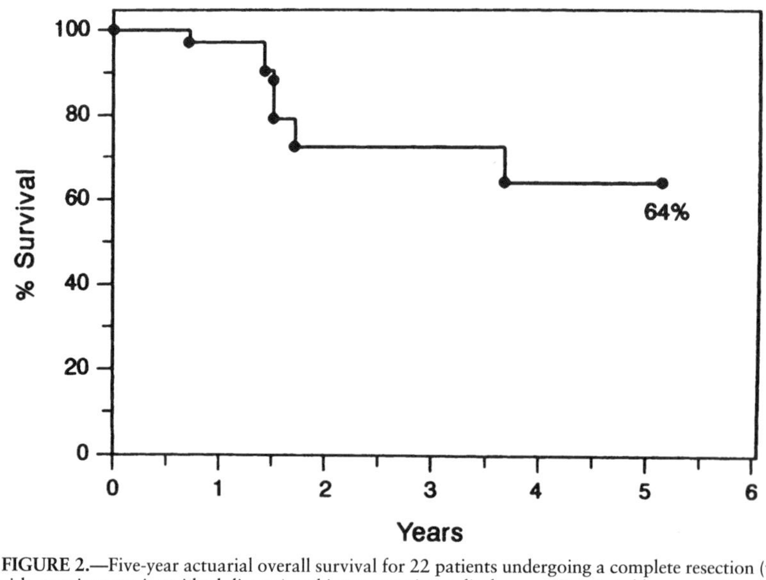

FIGURE 2.—Five-year actuarial overall survival for 22 patients undergoing a complete resection (with or without microscopic residual disease) and intraoperative radiotherapy. (Reprinted by permission of the publisher from Kim HK, Jessup JM, Beard CJ, et al: Locally advanced rectal carcinoma: Pelvic control and morbidity following preoperative radiation therapy, resection, and intraoperative radiation therapy. *Int J Radiat Oncol Biol Phys* 38:777–783, copyright 1997 by Elsevier Science Inc.)

TABLE 4.—Local Control for Patients Receiving Preoperative External Beam Radiotherapy and Curative Resection With/Without Intraoperative Radiotherapy

Extent of resection	+IORT *n*	+IORT Local control	−IORT *n*	−IORT Local control
Complete resection	13	92%	6	33% ($p = 0.017$)
Microscopic residual	9	67%		
Gross residual	4	0%	1*	1/1
Total	26		7	

*Received presacral interstitial implant with ^{125}I sutures.

(Reprinted by permission of the publisher from Kim HK, Jessup JM, Beard CJ, et al: Locally advanced rectal carcinoma: Pelvic control and morbidity following preoperative radiation therapy, resection, and intraoperative radiation therapy. *Int J Radiat Oncol Biol Phys* 38:777–783, copyright 1997 by Elsevier Science Inc.)

plete resection with and without IORT were 75% and 64%, respectively. The local control rate for patients having IORT was significantly higher than for patients not having IORT (Table 4). There were no treatment-related deaths. Pelvic soft-tissue complications developed in 17 of 26 patients having a curative resection and IORT and in 2 patients who did not have IORT. None of the 7 patients who received a myocutaneous thigh flap after multiple episodes of perineal/pelvic complications or delayed wound healing had additional complications. Seven of 11 patients with recurrent tumors and 16 of 22 with primary cancer had complications. No patient had osteoradionecrosis.

Conclusion.—Combined modality therapy with preoperative radiotherapy and IORT improves local control of locally advanced or initially unresectable rectal cancer. Use of a myocutaneous flap improved the complication profile for the 65% of patients with perineal/pelvic complications or delayed wound healing in this series.

▶ These investigators from Boston have been using intraoperative radiation therapy after preoperative radiation therapy for locally advanced colorectal cancer thought to be initially unresectable. They had a series of 40 cases of which 27 were primary presentations. What is interesting is that the authors used a 300 kVp orthovoltage unit for the treatment, prescribing to a depth of 1–2 cm. Thirty-three of the patients were able to undergo what was thought to be a curative resection after the preoperative radiation; 5 had gross residual disease. The local control rate for the intraoperative radiation therapy was an outstanding 92% when the margins were negative. Unfortunately, intraoperative orthovoltage radiation therapy was not effective for gross residual disease. For those with primary disease, the actuarial local control rate was 73%.

These investigators have achieved excellent results. They have pointed out, from a curative point of view of this kind of treatment, that the real value will be in patients seen with locally advanced disease. Perhaps a megavoltage beam would be more effective against gross disease, but that is a relatively minor issue. The authors believe that the intraoperative approach has a great deal of merit, and it probably does. However, to establish this requires a prospective study, which, up until now, has not been done. It would be nice if the advocates of this treatment could get their act together and work as a group to establish the benefit of this therapy one way or another.

E. Glatstein, M.D.

Survival After Repeat Hepatic Resection for Recurrent Colorectal Hepatic Metastases

Bines SD, Doolas A, Jenkins L, et al (Rush-Presbyterian-St Luke's Med Ctr, Chicago)

Surgery 120:591–596, 1996 7–6

Introduction.—Hepatic metastases from colorectal cancer is associated with poor prognosis. Initial surgical resection offers the only curative therapy currently available. Recurrent disease after hepatic resection is confined to the liver in up to 30% of patients. These patients are potential candidates for repeat hepatic resection. Survival of patients undergoing repeat hepatic resection for recurrent colorectal hepatic metastases was retrospectively evaluated.

Methods.—Of 131 patients who underwent hepatic resection for metastatic colorectal cancer, 107 underwent curative resection. Of these, 31 had recurrences confined to the liver. Thirteen of 107 patients (12%) underwent repeat hepatic resection and were followed to evaluate survival data.

Results.—The site of the first hepatic metastasis could be compared with the site of hepatic recurrence in 10 patients; recurrent cancers were in the same area of original resection in 3 patients (30%) and at sites remote from the site of first resection in 7 patients (70%). At resection, all patients were free of extrahepatic disease and had negative resection margins. Procedures were as follows: 6 wedge resections, 2 left lateral segmentectomies, 3 right lobectomies, and 2 trisegmentectomies. The average hospital stay was 17.2 days. The morbidity rate was 23% (3/13) and the mortality rate was 8% (1/13). Four patients died of recurrent disease. The mean disease-free survival was 9.7 months and the mean total survival was 39 months. One patient underwent second resection for recurrent disease at 21 months and lived an additional 78 months. At a mean follow-up of 34.9 months, 7 patients were alive and disease free. The actual 5-year survival rate was 23% (3/13) and the actual disease-free survival rate was 15% (2/13).

Conclusion.—The survival rate for patients with recurrent colorectal hepatic metastases is improving. In this series of 13 patients with recurrent disease confined to the liver after initial hepatic resection, the median survival was 24 months following re-do hepatic resection. A delay of several months is suggested before repeat resection to allow the full spectrum of a patient's recurrence to become apparent.

▶ Hepatic resection is the only treatment that provides long-term survival for patients with metastatic colorectal cancer. In the natural history of metastatic colorectal disease, disease will be confined to the liver in approximately 30% of patients. There is a great deal of information in the literature regarding positive selection factors for patients who undergo hepatic metastasectomy. However, it must be realized that approximately one third of the patients who undergo this operative procedure will eventually experience recurrence within the liver.

This article addresses the potential for repeat surgical resection in patients with a second recurrence confined to the liver. Obviously, selection factors are most important, and, in this retrospective study, clearly those patients who have disease confined to the liver in small anatomical areas are the best candidates for repeat hepatic resection. It is also noteworthy that those patients who eventually undergo resection have a reported median survival in the range of 2–4 years.

It is prudent that patients with a recurrent hepatic metastasis have a delay of several months before undergoing repeat resection to allow for any potential additional disease to become radiographically apparent. The value of this article lies in the fact that patients who have hepatic-only recurrence after initial hepatic metastasectomy should at least be considered for repeat hepatic resection, and in a carefully selected subset of these patients, long-term survival can be achieved.

B.L. Eisenberg, M.D.

Significance of Lymph Node Involvement at the Hepatic Hilum in the Resection of Colorectal Liver Metastases

Beckurts KTE, Hölscher AH, Thorban ST, et al (Technische Universität München, Germany; Univ of Cologne, Köln, Germany)

Br J Surg 84:1081–1084, 1997 7–7

Objective.—Technical feasibility and expected prognostic benefit are important considerations in deciding whether to perform hepatectomy for colorectal liver metastases. The frequency and prognostic significance of regional lymph node involvement of the hepatoduodenal ligament were prospectively evaluated using univariate and multivariate analysis.

Methods.—Hepatectomy for liver metastases, after hepatic hilar nodal sampling removal, was performed in 126 consecutive patients (49 women), aged 38 to 80 years, with hepatic metastases documented by CT and ultrasonography. Patients were followed every 3 months during the first year and every 6 months thereafter. Kaplan-Meier survival curves and 5-year survival rates were determined.

Results.—Postoperative complications occurred in 26 patients. There were 2 early deaths. Complete resection was achieved in 119 patients. Infiltrated lymph nodes in the hepatoduodenal ligament were detected in 35 patients. The 3- and 5-year survival rates of all patients were 31% and 14%, respectively. Multivariate analysis identified significant prognostic

TABLE 2.—Multivariate Analysis of Significant (Univariate) Prognostic Factors in 119 Patients With Complete Resection of Colorectal Liver Metastases

Variable	Relative risk	χ^2	Degrees of freedom	*P*
Colorectal carcinoma				
pN_0 *versus* pN_{1-3}		2·50	1	n.s.
Grade (G1,G2/ G3, G4)		0·80	1	n.s.
Liver metastases				
No. of metastases (single/multiple)		3·60	1	n.s.
Metachronous/ synchronous	1·40 (1·10–1·77)	7·60	1	0·0052
Lymph nodes of hepatoduodenal ligament (infiltrated/ not infiltrated)	1·84 (1·41–2·42)	19·20	1	0·0001

Note: Values in parentheses are 95% confidence intervals.
Abbreviations: pN, pathologic node; *n.s.*, not significant.
(Courtesy of Beckurts KTE, Hölscher AH, Thorban ST, et al: Significance of lymph node involvement at the hepatic hilum in the resection of colorectal liver metastases. *Br J Surg* 84:1081–1084, 1997. Publisher, Blackwell Science Ltd.)

factors (Table 2). Survival rates for patients with infiltrated lymph nodes were significantly lower than for patients without lymph node metastases (Fig 1).

Conclusion.—Patients with infiltrated hepatic lymph nodes had a significantly reduced survival, compared with patients without lymph node metastases.

▶ Evaluation for hepatic resection in those patients with metastatic colorectal cancer isolated to the liver has become an important consideration for therapy. Although many reviews have been written on this subject, it is not yet entirely clear as to the ideal patient variables that will provide a select benefit from hepatic metastasectomy, as evidenced by long-term survival.

This paper indicates, in a rather dramatic fashion, that lymph node involvement in the hepatic hilum precludes curative hepatic resection for patients with metastatic colorectal cancer. Unlike patients in other retrospective reviews, all patients in this series were subject to hepatic hilar lymph node sampling, and histologic diagnosis was confirmed in all patients with positive nodes. This negative prognostic factor holds true for patients who have microscopic, as well as macroscopic, metastatic disease within the hepatic hilar nodes.

The implication is that patients who undergo laparotomy and consideration for a liver resection for metastasectomy should also have hepatic hilar lymph node sampling as part of their procedure. However, nodal disease may not be predictable by gross appearance. I have personally seen patients with 5-mm lymph nodes in the hepatic hilum that were positive for metastatic adenocarcinoma. Obviously, any method (such as radioimmuno-guided

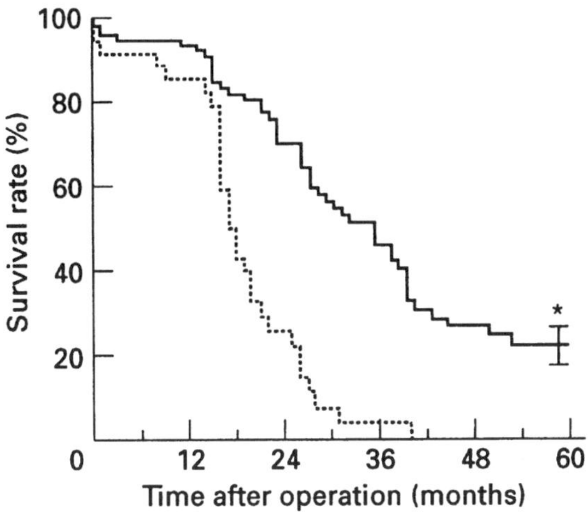

No. at risk

Nodes not infiltrated	84	67	47	26	13	9
Nodes infiltrated	35	27	7	1	0	0

FIGURE 1.—Five-year survival curves of 119 patients after complete removal of colorectal liver metastases, depending on the nodal involvement of the hepatoduodenal ligament. *Dashed line* indicates nodes involved; *solid line* indicates nodes not involved; *asterisk* indicates 95% confidence interval. *P* less than 0.0001 (Kaplan-Meier test). (Courtesy of Beckurts KTE, Hölscher AH, Thorban ST, et al: Significance of lymph node involvement at the hepatic hilum in the resection of colorectal liver metastases. *Br J Surg* 84:1081–1084, 1997. Publisher, Blackwell Science Ltd.)

biopsy) that could be used to examine these lymph nodes in a directed fashion might eventually increase cure rates for those individuals who actually undergo hepatic resection.

B.L. Eisenberg, M.D.

Cost of Open Versus Laparoscopically Assisted Right Hemicolectomy for Cancer

Philipson BM, Bokey EL, Moore JWE, et al (Univ of Sydney, Concord, Australia)

World J Surg 21:214–217, 1997 7–8

Introduction.—The technical feasibility of laparoscopic colonic resection has been reported, but there has been little information on the cost of this procedure. The cost of open right hemicolectomy (ORHC) and that of laparoscopically assisted right hemicolectomy (LARHC) were evaluated in a retrospective review of 61 patients with colon cancer.

Methods.—A cost analysis (based on Australian dollars) was performed on 33 patients who underwent ORHC and 28 patients who underwent LARHC. Cost was assessed from the date of surgery to the date of discharge.

Results.—The LARHC was significantly more expensive than the ORHC ($9,064 vs. $7,881) and was associated with significantly longer operating room use (261 vs. 203 minutes). The cost of disposables was significantly greater for LARHC than for ORHC ($854 vs. $189).

Conclusion.—There was no cost benefit for LARHC compared to ORHC in patients undergoing surgery for colon cancer.

▶ This article from Australia represents a large series of patients from a single hospital experience undergoing either ORHC for colon cancer or a laparoscopically assisted technique involving the same operation for the same indications. With the introduction of LARHC, there was anticipation that this procedure would result in less postoperative pain; a shortened hospital stay; more rapid return of the patient to normal daily activities; and, most importantly, an overall cost benefit for patients undergoing the laparoscopic procedure.

In this instance, we have a single institutional experience with 1 operation, namely right hemicolectomy with indication that there is no cost benefit for the laparoscopically assisted procedure, and, in point of fact, the laparoscopic procedure was significantly more expensive to perform. In addition, there was no other apparent benefit, most notably there was no significant shortening of postoperative recovery or time of hospitalization. Obviously, these economic considerations do not address the scientific questions, namely, whether an LARHC for cancer is clinically sound, as judged by recurrence and survival statistics.

The answer to the latter question is not yet known; however, if the driving impetus here is cost containment, there appears to be no difference—or even a negative factor—in major LARHC for cancer. The scientific questions await further evaluation through cooperative group studies and long-term follow-up.

B.L. Eisenberg, M.D.

Follow-up of Patients After Resection for Colorectal Cancer: A Position Paper of the Canadian Society of Surgical Oncology and the Canadian Society of Colon and Rectal Surgeons

Richard CS, McLeod RS (Univ of Toronto)

Can J Surg 40:90–100, 1997 7–9

Objective.—Whereas there is widespread agreement that there should be colorectal surveillance programs to detect local or distant recurrences when they are still operable, there is uncertainty regarding the best follow-up strategy. Because many believe that guidelines should be evidence based rather than developed from expert opinion and consensus, follow-up strategies for patients with colorectal cancer treated by curative resection were reviewed and evaluated.

Methods.—A MEDLINE search identified survival analysis studies on colorectal cancer published between 1966 and February 1996. The relationships between types of surveillance strategy and survival were compared statistically.

Results.—There is little evidence to indicate a significant survival benefit from postoperative surveillance programs, primarily because of the small size of the studies reviewed. The overall potential benefit is estimated at 10% or less.

Conclusion.—There is little evidence for justifying postoperative surveillance of patients with colorectal cancer. Large studies evaluating the effectiveness of follow-up are necessary.

► Outcomes research and the economic impact of treatment profiles are becoming an increasingly important aspect of health care delivery. Although the follow-up of patients successfully treated for colorectal cancer is widely practiced and usually extensive, there is no standardization or specific recommendations for follow-up care based on a statistically proven survival benefit. This paper summarizes the recent literature evaluating intensive follow-up evaluation (frequent history and physical examination, liver function tests, fecal occult blood test, chest x-ray studies, imaging scans, carcinoembryonic antigen determination, and colonoscopy) compared with minimal follow-up or no follow-up.

The conclusion from this manuscript—which utilizes and analyzes a number of prospective and retrospective patient series—is that there is no conclusive survival evidence either to support or to refute the value of follow-up surveillance programs for detecting recurrence of colorectal cancer. However, in evaluating any surveillance program, the infrequency of isolated recurrences that can be cured by surgical intervention can, at best, only be expected to provide an overall potential survival benefit of 10% or less. Therefore, large patient numbers in a prospective database would be necessary to establish both the frequency and intensity of cost-effective follow-up for patients with high-risk colorectal cancer.

The problem of equating cost-benefit for large population-based studies vs. cost-benefit for any particular individual remains an ethical dilemma. Most clinicians feel an obligation to follow fairly closely patients with a prior diagnosis of colorectal cancer, and practice patterns would most surely benefit from standardization of the interval and duration of such follow-up.

B.L. Eisenberg, M.D.

Extended Resection for Locally Advanced Colorectal Carcinoma

Rowe VL, Frost DB, Huang S (Kaiser Permanente Med Group, Los Angeles)

Ann Surg Oncol 4:131–136, 1997 7–10

Objective.—Because 10% of colorectal cancers have penetrated adjacent structures, surgeons must weigh the benefit of multivisceral resection. Results were presented of a review of MVRs to determine which locally advanced tumors are potentially curable and which are not.

Methods.—The review covered the records of 118 patients with colorectal cancer (52 men), aged 25 to 85 years, with stage B3 or C3 tumors and invasive (B3+, C3+) or inflammatory (B3−, C3−) adhesions. Survival estimates and comparisons were analyzed statistically.

Results.—Of the 58 stage B3 tumors, 54 stage C3 tumors, and 6 equivocal tumors, 69% had carcinomatous adhesions; stage C tumors were significantly more likely than stage B tumors to have carcinomatous adhesions. A total of 174 organs or structures were removed in 59% of patients including 1 adjacent secondary organ structure (ASOS) in 64 patients, 2 in 33 patients, 3 in 11 patients, and 4 in 1 patient. Carcinomatous adhesions—most commonly bladder, small bowel, uterus, vagina, and abdominal wall—were present in 63% to 77% of patients having an ASOS. Five-year actuarial survival rates were 62% for stage B3 tumors, 38% for stage C3 tumors, 78% for stage B3− tumors, 58% for stage B3+ tumors, 34% for stage C3+ tumors, and 64% for stage C3− tumors. Patients with B3−/C3− tumors had a better 5-year survival rate than did patients with B3+/C3+ tumors (71% and 47%, respectively). Stage was the most significant predictor of survival according to multivariate analysis.

Conclusion.—Resection of ASOS can extend the 5-year survival of patients with locally advanced colorectal cancer. Lymph node spread predicted decreased 5-year survival.

► Surgeons are often faced with intraoperative decision making regarding treatment of locally advanced colorectal cancer. Many times this concerns potential disease extension beyond the confines of the colon or rectal wall. This article confirms the fact that those patients who have stage B3 or C3 colorectal cancer can have a favorable long-term outcome, with extended resection involving contiguous organs. It is notable that there was no distinguishing significant survival difference between those patients who had inflammatory adhesions as compared with those with carcinomatous adhesions. The main principle of surgical oncology here is en bloc resection and—within the guidelines of this principle—any dissection that violates dense adhesions between contiguous organs involved in a primary or recurrent colorectal cancer can potentially leave disease behind and result in a significant survival disadvantage.

B.L. Eisenberg, M.D.

Hepatic Resection for Noncolorectal, Nonneuroendocrine Metastases: A Fifteen-Year Experience With Ninety-Six Patients

Harrison LE, Brennan MF, Newman E, et al (Mem Sloan-Kettering Cancer Ctr, New York)

Surgery 121:625–632, 1997 7–11

Introduction.—The role of hepatic resection in noncolorectal, nonneuroendocrine (NCNN) metastases is not well defined. Predictive factors

TABLE 2.—Distribution of Primary Tumors

Genitourinary	*(n = 34)*	*Soft tissue*	*(n = 41)*	*Gastrointestinal*	*(n = 7)*	*Miscellaneous*	*(n = 14)*
Testicular	9	Sarcoma	27	Gastric	5	Unknown	8
Adrenal	7	Melanoma	7	Pancreas	2	Head & neck	2
Ovary	7	Breast	7			Parotid	1
Renal	5					Thyroid	1
Uterine	4					Brain	1
Cervix	2					Sweat gland	1

(Courtesy of Harrison LE, Brennan MF, Newman E, et al: Hepatic resection for noncolorectal, nonneuroendocrine metastases: A fifteen-year experience with ninety-six patients. *Surgery* 121:625–632, 1997.)

TABLE 3.—Results of Analysis for Factors Predictive of Outcome

Factor	Univariate *p* value	Multivariate *p* value
Type of liver resection	NS	—
Other organ resected	NS	—
Extrahepatic disease	NS	—
Symptoms	NS	—
Age	NS	—
Disease-free interval	<0.05	<0.05
Primary tumor type	<0.05	<0.05
Curative resection	<0.05	<0.05

Abbreviation: NS, not significant.
(Courtesy of Harrison LE, Brennan MF, Newman E, et al: Hepatic resection for noncolorectal, nonneuroendocrine metastases: A fifteen-year experience with ninety-six patients. *Surgery* 121:625–632, 1997.)

for survival were evaluated in a large series of patients with hepatic resection for NCNN metastases to determine whether outcome justified the surgery.

Methods.—Records of 96 patients who underwent liver resection for metastatic NCNN cancer from 1980 to 1995 at a single institution were retrospectively examined. Predictive factors for survival were assessed.

Results.—Primary tumors for NCNN cancer were as follows: 34 genitourinary, 41 soft tissue, and 21 metastases from other primary cancers (Table 2). Thirty-two patients underwent wedge resection, 44 received formal lobectomy, and 20 required an extended hepatic lobectomy for tumor clearance. There were no surgical deaths. At 1, 3, and 5 years after hepatic surgery, the overall survival rates were 80%, 45%, and 37%, respectively. Survival did not differ according to type of liver resection, bilateral vs. unilateral disease, or resection of extrahepatic disease. Predictors of significantly better survival were a disease-free interval greater than 36 months before discovery of liver metastases, curative resection, and primary tumor group (genitourinary tumor outcome was better than soft tissue; soft tissue was better than gastrointestinal) (Table 3).

Conclusion.—Primary tumor type, disease-free interval, and curative resection were predictive of patients with NCNN metastases who could benefit from hepatic resection. Quality of life and cost effectiveness should be evaluated in a prospective series of patients with NCNN metastases for whom hepatic resection and chemotherapy are assessed.

► As more experience is gained regarding hepatic resection for metastatic disease, the technical aspects of the procedure have been better defined, and the potential morbidity/mortality has declined. There is a substantial body of literature supporting the use of hepatic resection in metastatic colorectal cancer as well as in certain neuroendocrine tumors. However, the use of selective hepatic resection for metastatic tumors other than those from these primary sites is not generally considered.

This paper from the Memorial Sloan-Kettering Cancer Center investigates a large group of patients who underwent resection for hepatic metastases associated with a number of different types of primary cancers. Results support selective use of hepatic resection in these patients. This is notable, as many of these patients had metastatic tumors from such diverse histologies as soft tissue sarcomas, melanoma, and breast cancer. Obviously, the point here is that very careful selection factors for surgical intervention can result in survival that exceeds the expected norm for the primary cancer in question.

One must also realize that natural selection factors and disease biology come into play in the long-term survival of these patients. Perhaps, in the future, specific molecular indicators will allow us to select out patients with disease confined solely to the liver from among those patients with a variety of primary cancers who are generally considered to have diffuse systemic disease.

B.L. Eisenberg, M.D.

Hepatic Resection for Metastatic Colorectal Cancer Results in Cure for Some Patients

Jamison RL, Donohue JH, Nagorney DM, et al (Mayo Clinic and Mayo Found, Rochester, Minn)

Arch Surg 132:505–511, 1997 7–12

Introduction.—In patients given a diagnosis of colorectal carcinoma, 25% will have synchronous hepatic metastases, and in another 25%, metastases will develop during follow-up. Surgical resection is the only hope for cure. Some experts believe that careful patient selection, not alteration of the natural history of the disease, is responsible for long-term survival. Long-term disease-free and overall survivals for patients undergoing hepatic resection for colorectal cancer metastases were calculated. Significant predictors of improved survival were assessed.

Methods.—Hepatic resection for colorectal cancer metastases was performed on 280 patients from the Mayo Clinic between 1960 and 1987. There were 85 survivors at the time this retrospective trial was published in 1992. The disease-free interval after initial hepatic resection was calculated and is now reported for survivors followed for a mean of 11.3 years.

Results.—There were no new prognostic indicators of long-term survival among the features of metastatic disease analyzed at the time of the initial report. Significant risk factors for long-term survival continued to be clinical presentation of metastatic disease by physical examination or abnormal liver enzymes, satellite configuration of hepatic lesions, extrahepatic lymph node involvement, presence of resectable extrahepatic disease, and need for any perioperative blood product transfusion. The overall 5-year survival rate of this patient series was 27%; 10-year actuarial survival was 20%. At 10 years after surgery, 28 patients were alive. Two patients alive and free of disease at 5-year follow-up had recurrent disease. There were no cancer-related deaths in any other patients free of disease at 5 years.

Conclusion.—Patients who were alive and disease-free 5-years after resection of hepatic resection rarely experienced disease recurrence. These findings support those of earlier reports.

▶ This article from the Mayo Clinic presents a large, single-institution experience over 27 years. It is significant in that it indicates that surgical resection in these patients provides the only opportunity for potential cure and, in this series, afforded 10-year survival rates. The indication here is that those patients surviving 5 years after hepatic metastasectomy for colorectal cancer will be long-term survivors. This is an important concept considering the fact that we are often asked by patients of the chance of long-term survival should they undergo this extensive surgery.

Additionally, there clearly are risk factors associated with recurrence that have been reported in a number of other studies. This study supports the fact that the following variables represent significant risk factors in long-term survival: disease presentation as a clinical manifestation rather than a rising carcinoembryonic antigen or an asymptomatic radiological finding; hepatic tumors presenting multiple scattered or satellite lesions; the presence of extrahepatic disease, particularly within the portal lymph nodes; and the use of blood transfusions. All are factors linked to a decreased 5-year survival rate. The message here is that, in the absence of these unfavorable characteristics, the majority of patients who undergo hepatic resection for metastatic colorectal cancer should have an even better survival than the usual reported 25% to 30% at 5 years and 20% at 10 years.

B.L.Eisenberg, M.D.

Laparoscopy in the Management of Gastric Adenocarcinoma

Burke EC, Karpeh MS Jr, Conlon KC, et al (Mem-Sloan Kettering Cancer Ctr, New York)

Ann Surg 225:262–267, 1997 7–13

Objective.—Because most patients with gastric cancer have advanced disease, they are at high risk for abdominal metastases. Laparoscopy is significantly better than imaging techniques for diagnosing metastatic disease. The prevalence, sensitivity, specificity, and accuracy of laparoscopy, and the number of patients spared open exploration without resection and the outcome of patients with exploration but not resection were studied.

Methods.—Laparoscopy was attempted at Memorial-Sloan Kettering Cancer Center in 111 consecutive patients with gastric adenocarcinoma from December 1990 to December 1995 to assess metastatic disease. Results were compared with those from 60 control patients. Kaplan-Meier survival curves were calculated.

Results.—Laparoscopy was successful in 110 patients, and accurately staged presence or absence of metastatic disease in 94% of patients. There were 32 true positive, 65 true negative, 0 false positive, and 6 false positive results for a sensitivity of 84% and a specificity of 100%. Laparoscopy only was performed in 24 patients who had a significantly shorter hospital stay than patients who also had exploratory surgery (1.4 vs. 6.5 days). Patients with laparoscopy only had fewer complications and less operating room time, and none required subsequent laparotomy.

Conclusion.—Laparoscopy can help diagnose metastatic disease in patients with gastric cancer with a sensitivity of 84% and a specificity of 100% and avoids unnecessary laparotomy.

▶ The place of diagnostic laparoscopy in the staging of gastrointestinal (GI) malignancies remains the subject of controversy. Questions have arisen regarding efficacy and accuracy with the routine use of this technique. In this report from Memorial Sloan Kettering Cancer Center, the use of staging laparoscopy in patients with operable gastric cancer detected occult metastatic disease in more than one third of the patients. This has significant implications in this disease, because preoperative staging can often underestimate the extent of the GI malignancy. The important point is the laparoscopy performed by an experienced surgeon can prove quite sensitive in detecting occult peritoneal disease as well as liver metastasis in upper GI malignancy, most notably in gastric and pancreatic cancer. This can be very useful in the accurate staging of patients entered into preoperative neoadjuvant treatment trials and in preventing unnecessary laparotomy in asymptomatic patients with metastatic GI cancer. Ultimately, laparoscopy may prove more useful as a diagnostic rather than a therapeutic tool in the management of GI malignancy.

B.L. Eisenberg, M.D.

Vessel Counts and Expression of Vascular Endothelial Growth Factor as Prognostic Factors in Node-Negative Colon Cancer

Takahashi Y, Tucker SL, Kitadai Y, et al (Univ of Texas MD Anderson Cancer Ctr, Houston)

Arch Surg 132:541–546, 1997 7–14

Introduction.—Only 15% of patients with node-positive colon cancer who undergo adjuvant chemotherapy have improved survival. Vessel counts and expression of vascular endothelial growth factor (VEGF) have been shown to be correlated with synchronous metastatic formation in colon carcinoma. Whether vessel counts and VEGF expression can be used as prognostic factors for development of distant recurrence in patients with node-negative colon cancer was determined.

Methods.—Paraffin-embedded tumor specimens from 27 patients with Dukes' stage B colon cancers who underwent surgery between 1988 and 1989 were examined for factor VIII, VEGF, basic fibroblast growth factor, proliferating cell nuclear antigen, mucin production, and the presence of vascular, lymphatic, or perineural invasion. The development and interval to recurrence were observed.

Results.—At a median of 24 months, 8 patients had liver, lung, or lymph node metastases. The median follow-up for patients with no recurrence was 60 months. Patients with no recurrence had a significantly lower mean tumor vessel count, compared with patients with recurrent disease (20 vs. 33). Perineural invasion, vessel count, and VEGF expression were correlated with time to recurrence by univariate analysis. Multivariate analysis revealed only vessel count was significantly related to differences in time to recurrence. Expression of VEGF was associated with vessel count.

Conclusions.—Vessel counts and expression of VEGF in patients with primary colon cancer were significantly related to shortened times to recurrence at distant sites.

► Establishing predictors of metastatic potential for solid tumors is important in designing treatment schemes for adjuvant therapy. High-risk patients can usually be identified by positive nodal status. However, patients with either breast or colorectal cancer can have distant recurrence in the absence of nodal metastases.

In this paper, the authors explore the validity of examining new vessel density and VEGF expression in patients with node-negative colon cancer as a corollary to risk of distant disease recurrence. There was a strong correlation between increased average vessel density and disease recurrence as has been reported by other groups evaluating both colorectal cancer and breast cancer. In addition, there was a positive correlation in this paper between VEGF intensity and elevated vessel counts. This information may have clinical relevance as more multi-institutional patient data become available to evaluate and standardize these diagnostic parameters to patient outcomes.

B.L. Eisenberg, M.D.

Identifying Stage B Colorectal Cancer Patients at High Risk of Tumor Recurrence and Death

Mulcahy HE, Toner M, Patchett SE, et al (St Vincent's Hosp, Dublin; Univ College Dublin)

Dis Colon Rectum 40:326–331, 1997 7–15

Introduction.—Clinical features have not been helpful in distinguishing poor prognosis in patients with stage B colorectal cancer. A wide range of clinical and pathologic variables were assessed in 117 patients with stage B colorectal cancer to determine whether poor outcome could be identified.

Methods.—Medical records of 117 patients with stage B cancer who underwent curative surgery were assessed for age, gender, symptom duration, bowel obstruction, tumor size, tumor differentiation, mucin production, necrosis, lymphocytic infiltrate, perineural invasion, vascular invasion, tumor margin, and invasion through bowel wall. Histologic slides were analyzed by a pathologist "blinded" to clinical details and outcome.

Results.—Significant correlations were observed between bowel obstruction and poor prognosis. Perineural invasion was associated with decreased survival. In the subgroup of patients with rectal but not colonic cancer, vascular invasion was correlated with poor long-term outcome. Tumor necrosis and perineural invasion were independently correlated with outcome in multivariate regression analysis.

Conclusions.—Long-term outcome in patients with stage B colorectal cancer can be related to discrete clinicopathologic variables. This is important because adjuvant therapy has been shown to enhance survival in patients at high risk for tumor recurrence.

► Adjuvant therapy has become the accepted standard for high-risk patients with colorectal cancer. There is good clinical trial data to support its use in patients with node-positive colon cancer and, by virtue of this fact, it has become routine to offer adjuvant therapy to patients with node-positive rectal cancer as well. However, between 20% and 40% of patients with T3 node-negative colorectal cancer will have recurrent disease. Risk factors in this group of patients other than obstruction and perforation have not been standardized for the purpose of inclusion into clinical trials.

This paper evaluates risk factors in a large group of patients with stage B colorectal cancer. Multivariate analysis indicates that perineural invasion and tumor necrosis are both independent risk factors associated with decreased survival. Until we can establish a reproducible molecular basis for prognostication or better identification of micrometastatic nodal involvement, clinical trials should include stratification schemes based on standard risk factors for node-negative colorectal cancer such as the ones presented in this paper. This will enable us to develop future treatment paradigms for patients at higher risk for recurrent disease.

B.L. Eisenberg, M.D.

Cryosurgical Ablation of Hepatic Metastases From Colorectal Carcinomas

Yeh KA, Fortunato L, Hoffman JP, et al (Fox Chase Cancer Ctr, Philadelphia)
Am Surg 63:63–68, 1997 7–16

Objective.—Almost half of the individuals with colon or rectal cancer will die of their disease. Because curative resection is contraindicated in patients with hepatic metastases or close surgical margins, cryoablation has been used. Outcomes in these patients were reviewed.

Methods.—Between February 1992 and May 1995, 24 patients (10 women), aged 34–84 years, with metastatic colon and rectal carcinoma underwent cryoablation of metastatic tumors (n = 12) or cryoablation for close resection margins (n = 12). Surgery was palliative in 3 patients and curative in 21. Disease-free and overall survival rates were calculated.

Results.—The average hospital stay was 8.4 days. Pleural effusions developed in 7 patients in each group, 1 cardiac dysrhythmia in each group, stroke in 1 patient, and line sepsis in 1 patient who underwent cryoablation of central lesions, atelectasis in 1 patient, and myocardial infarction in 1 patient who underwent cryoablation for close or positive surgical margins. Overall survival was 31 months and disease-free survival was 19.5 months for patients receiving cryoablation for close surgical margins. The overall survival for patients with central lesions was 31 months and the mean disease-free survival period was 23 months. At last follow-up (37 months), there were 20 survivors, with 2 patients dying of complications and 2 of their disease. Nine survivors were disease-free and 11 were alive with their disease, including the 3 palliatively treated patients. Recurrent disease that developed in 10 patients included extrahepatic in 6, hepatic in 2, and combined in 2. The median time to recurrence in these patients was 9.5 months and median survival was 14 months. Overall survival and disease-free survival for all patients were 32.7 and 23.5 months, respectively.

Conclusion.—In patients with metastatic colon and rectal cancer, cryoablation of hepatic metastases or close resection margins is a safe alternative that increases survival and has an acceptable complication rate.

► Surgical resection in selected patients with metastatic colorectal hepatic metastases has now become an accepted procedure and has been documented to provide long-term survival in up to 30% to 40% of patients. Cryosurgical ablation of hepatic metastases utilizes a developing technology to provide for in situ tumor destruction in selected patients who are not otherwise candidates for hepatic resection. This procedure is applicable to those patients who have colorectal metastases confined to the liver and who are otherwise not candidates for resection by virtue of the number and location of the hepatic metastases, or co-morbid conditions of the patient that would preclude major hepatic resection. This procedure is also applicable to those patients who have primary hepatocellular carcinoma that is small, focal, and surrounded by cirrhotic liver, thereby precluding resection. Review of recent literature now substantiates the fact that patients can be treated with cryoablation and, in some instances, manifest long-term survival. This article also demonstrates that cryoablation may be used as an adjuvant to patients who undergo major hepatic resections and yet still have less than ideal margins. Larger patient numbers and more clinical experience will be necessary before the actual role of hepatic cryoablation therapy can be fully realized in treatment paradigms. However, this can be a safe method of treatment and it has already proved to be successful in selected groups of patients.

B.L. Eisenberg, M.D.

Rectal Cancer Risk in Hereditary Nonpolyposis Colorectal Cancer After Abdominal Colectomy

Rodriguez-Bigas MA, and the International Collaborative Group on HNPCC (Roswell Park Cancer Inst, Buffalo, NY)

Ann Surg 225:202–207, 1997 7–17

Background.—The recommended treatment for hereditary nonpolyposis colorectal cancer (HNPCC) is total abdominal colectomy (TAC) or subtotal abdominal colectomy (STC). This procedure is fairly new, and the risk for rectal cancer after TAC or STC has not yet been determined. This study investigated this risk.

Method.—Data were gathered by means of a questionnaire mailed to the members of the International Collaborative Group on HNPCC. The goal was to locate patients with rectal cancer who had had TAC or STC performed. Data were analyzed by the Kaplan-Meier method, the Cox's proportional hazards method, and the log-rank test.

Results.—Seventy-one patients who had undergone HNPCC were located. The median follow-up was 158 months (range, 38 to 282 months) after initial treatment. In 8 of these patients, cancer of the rectum developed, 6 of them were being carefully observed. Significant variables for rectal cancer risk, as determined by multivariate analysis, include age at treatment and postprocedural observation. Following TAC or STC, the risk of rectal cancer is 3% each 3 years for years 0–12.

Conclusion.—Because patients with HNPCC have a rectal cancer risk factor of 12% twelve years after abdominal colectomy, and because there is also a direct correlation between age at colectomy and rectal cancer risk, it is important to maintain aggressive surveillance by using endoscopy of the rectum after colectomy.

▶ Genetic linkage studies and the development of a molecular progression model for colorectal cancer have provided insights into the inheritance of increased risk for the development of colorectal cancers in individual patients. This article reports on the overall incidence of rectal cancer after TAC in patients who fulfill the Amsterdam criteria for HNPCC. Because most patients with HNPCC have right-sided colon cancer, there has been little emphasis on overall risks for the subsequent development of rectal cancer. This HNPCC registry group reported a 12% incidence of metachronous rectal cancer within 12 years of an abdominal colectomy. Notably, this is similar to reports of subsequent rectal cancer in patients with adenomatous familial polyposis colon cancer. Further emphasis is placed on the necessity for yearly endoscopic surveillance of patients with HNPCC, particularly those patients with previously excised adenomatous polyps of the rectum. This is important because these patients appear to have a more rapid progression from polyp to cancer than the patients with sporadic colon cancer.

B.L. Eisenberg, M.D.

Diagnostic Workup of Patients With Suspected Pancreatic Carcinoma: The University of California-Los Angeles Approach

Gloor B, Todd KE, Reber HA (Univ of California, Los Angeles)
Cancer 79:1780–1786, 1997 7–18

Background.—The authors of this study were concerned with the overuse and misuse of diagnostic procedures used to determine the presence of pancreatic malignancy. These procedures include laparoscopy, endoscopic retrograde cholangiopancreatography (ERCP), fine-needle aspiration (FNA), and CT.

Method.—Researchers reviewed literature and relied upon personal experience to depict the assumptions inherent in a diagnostic workup for a patient with suspected pancreatic carcinoma in a university medical center.

Results.—The best overall patient assessment method in this situation is helical CT. This is frequently the only test necessary. First, the physician should check to see whether pancreatic carcinoma is indicated by the patient's blood test and history. Next should be a check for a mass at the head of the pancreas in the helical CT scan that appears excisable. If both of these conditions are met, the patient should be prepared for surgery. Without the mass present, an ERCP should be used for further testing. To gain diagnostic proof that could prevent surgery, an FNA for cytology is needed. If other methods fail to confirm resectability, laparoscopy should be performed.

Conclusion.—These indications for test order are based on cost effectiveness and overall effectiveness.

► This paper presents a single institutional experience outlining preference relative to the workup and diagnosis of patients with obstructive jaundice for resolving clinical suspicion of pancreatic cancer. Among experts in the management of pancreatic cancer, there continues to be controversy involving the extent and cost of diagnostic studies (both invasive and noninvasive) in the initial evaluation of patients with suspected pancreatic cancer. Clearly, there will be variations in the approach depending on the clinical circumstances, the need for tissue diagnosis, the initial assessment of operability, and the experience of the surgeon involved.

The University of California at Los Angeles group makes a convincing argument for the helical CT scan being, in many cases, the only diagnostic test necessary for the diagnosis and assessment of patients with extrahepatic biliary obstruction, thus surplanting the necessity for ERCP, US, FNA cytology, MRI, or visceral angiography. Obviously, the accuracy and interpretation of this diagnostic test and 3-dimensional vascular-enhanced imaging are operator dependent. Additionally, where clinical studies using neoadjuvant treatment for pancreatic cancer are concerned, there is generally a requirement for both tissue diagnosis (FNA cytology) and bile duct temporary stenting because any planned surgery for these patients is delayed during the preoperative therapy phase of treatment.

As technological advances in diagnostic imaging are developed, the clinical paradigm will continue to undergo evolution. However, individual institutional preferences will still depend on the close interaction among the pancreatic surgeon, the diagnostic radiologist, and the gastroenterologist.

B.L. Eisenberg, M.D.

Suppression of Human Colorectal Mucosal Prostaglandins: Determining the Lowest Effective Aspirin Dose

Ruffin MT IV, Krishnan K, Rock CL, et al (Univ of Michigan, Ann Arbor; East Tennessee State Univ, Johnson City; Univ of California, San Diego; et al)

J Natl Cancer Inst 89:1152–1160, 1997 7–19

Introduction.—The incidence of or mortality from colorectal cancer could be reduced with aspirin, but previous human studies that explored the relationship have been observational or interventional. Aspirin was developed as a chemopreventive agent for human colorectal cancer. To select a chemopreventive dose and schedule for aspirin, the relationship of aspirin dose, pharmacokinetics, and prostaglandin concentration in human colorectal mucosa was defined.

Methods.—There were 65 participants of whom 10 received placebo, 10 received 40.5 mg of aspirin, 10 received 81 mg of aspirin, 10 received 162 mg of aspirin and 10 received 324 mg of aspirin, while 15 received 648 mg of aspirin. By using a competitive enzyme immunoassay, the biopsy specimens were assayed for prostaglandins E_2 and $F_{2\alpha}$. High-performance liquid chromatography was used to determine plasma concentrations of acetylsalicylic acid and salicylic acid.

Results.—The lowest dose to significantly suppress colorectal mucosal prostaglandin E_2 concentrations from baseline at 24 hours after the first dose was 162 mg. There was a significant suppression for those receiving 81 mg at 72–78 hours after the last dose. The lowest dose to significantly suppress colorectal mucosal prostaglandin $F_{2\alpha}$ concentrations from baseline at 24 hours after the first dose was 324 mg. At 24–30 hours and at 72–78 hours after the last dose, the lowest dose causing a marked reduction in the level of prostaglandin $F_{2\alpha}$ was 40.5 mg. At any of the biopsy time points, no detectable amounts of acetylsalicylic acid or salicylic acid were present in the plasma.

Summary.—To significantly suppress concentrations of colorectal mucosal prostaglandin E_2, the lowest dose of aspirin taken daily was 81 mg, and to suppress colorectal mucosal prostaglandins $F_{2\alpha}$, the lowest dose was 40.5 mg. The plasma at the time points studied did not have detectable amounts of aspirin or salicylic acid when the suppression occurred. A single daily dose of 81 mg of aspirin in future studies of this drug as a chemopreventive agent for colorectal cancer is recommended on the basis of these observations.

► During the last 2 decades, we medical oncologists have lived in an era of "dose intensity." Thus, it is refreshing to see work that focuses on the minimal amount of therapy needed. Support of the finding that aspirin and nonsteroidal anti-inflammatory agents (NSAIDs) have the ability to inhibit development of colon cancer and colon polyps has prompted several trials. Numerous retrospective trials have shown a reduction in colorectal cancer risk, but data from prospective trials have been conflicting. The mechanism action of NSAIDs and aspirin in preventing colorectal cancer is unknown, but leading candidates include the inhibition of cyclo-oxygenase and the diminution of prostaglandin synthesis. Thus, these are reasonable targets of intermediate end points. This study is a rationale design effort to determine the optimal dosages of aspirin when used as a chemopreventive agent. Future prospective trials are clearly warranted.

P.J. Loehrer, Sr, M.D.

Adjuvant Postoperative Fluorouracil-Modulated Chemotherapy Combined With Pelvic Radiation Therapy for Rectal Cancer: Initial Results of Intergroup 0114

Tepper JE, O'Connell MJ, Petroni GR, et al (Univ of North Carolina, Chapel Hill; Mayo Clinic, Rochester, Minn; Duke Univ, Durham, NC; et al)

J Clin Oncol 15:2030–2039, 1997 7–20

Background.—The currently accepted treatment for rectal adenocarcinomas that puncture the bowel wall (this is also true for those with tumor-positive lymph nodes) is flourouracil (5-FU)-based chemotherapy in combination with radiation therapy. This study investigated the efficacy of adding leucovorin and/or levamisole to this combination.

Method.—Four cycles of bolus 5-FU–based systemic chemotherapy and pelvic radiation were given to the 1,696 patients (Fig 1). Four treatment schemes were used: (1) chemotherapy+5-FU, (2) chemotherapy+5-FU+leucovorin, (3) chemotherapy+5-FU+levamisole, and (4) chemotherapy+5-FU+leucovorin+levamisole.

Results.—The median follow-up was 48 months. Levamisole and leucovorin did not show a significant advantage over 5-FU alone. In fact, gastrointestinal toxicity may have occurred with the 3-drug combination. It is highly unlikely that further research will show a value for these drugs in the treatment of adenocarcinomas of the rectum.

Conclusion.—This study did not show benefit from adding levamisole to the rectal cancer treatment. Further follow-up is necessary to evaluate leucovorin when added to pelvic radiation and 5-FU.

► Over the last 10 years, the adjuvant treatment paradigm for high-risk rectal cancer has changed from empirical use of postoperative radiation

RANDOMIZE

1.	**5-FU** (500 mg/m^2/d, d 1-5, 29-33)	**RT** (5040-5400 cGy) + **5-FU** (500 mg/m^2/d, d 57-59, 85-87)	**5-FU** (450 mg/m^2/d, d 1-5, 29-33)
2.	**5-FU** (425 mg/m^2/d, d 1-5, 29-33) + **leucovorin** (20 mg/m^2/d, d 1-5, 29-33)	**RT** (5040-5400 cGy) + **5-FU** (400 mg/m^2/d, d 57-60, 85-88) + **leucovorin** (20 mg/m^2/d, d 57-60, 85-88)	**5-FU** (380 mg/m^2/d, d 1-5, 29-33) **leucovorin** (20 mg/m^2/d, d 1-5, 29-31) (begin 28 days after end of RT)
3.	**5-FU** (450 mg/m^2/d, d 1-5, 29-33) + **levamisole** (150 mg/d x 3, q 14 d x 4)	**RT** (5040-5400 cGy) + **5-FU** (500 mg/m^2/d, 57-59, 85-87) (begin 28 days after end of RT)	**5-FU** (400 mg/m^2/d, d 1-5, 29-33) **levamisole** (150 mg/d x 3 q 14 d x 4)
4.	**5-FU** (425 mg/m^2/d, d 1-5, 29-33) + **leucovorin** (20 mg/m^2/d, d 1-5, 29-33 + **levamisole** (150 mg/d x 3 q 14 d x 4)	**RT** (5040-5400 cGy) + **5-FU** (400 mg/m^2/d, d 57-60, 85-88) + **leucovorin** (20 mg/m^2/d, 57-60, 85-88)	**5-FU** (380 mg/m^2/d, d 1-5, 29-33) + **leucovorin** (20 mg/m^2/d, d 1-5, 29-33) + **levamisole** (150 mg/d x 3 q 14 d x 4) (begin 28 days after end of RT)

FIGURE 1.—Treatment schema. (Courtesy of Tepper JE, O'Connell MJ, Petroni GR, et al: Adjuvant postoperative fluorouracil-modulated chemotherapy combined with pelvic radiation therapy for rectal cancer: Initial results of Intergroup 0114. *J Clin Oncol* 15:2030–2039, 1997.)

therapy alone to a combination of postoperative chemotherapy and radiation therapy. These results have improved both local control (an important aspect of rectal cancer treatment) and overall survival.

In this report from an intergroup rectal adjuvant trial describes a 4-arm study with the objective of comparing modulated 5-FU with or without levamisole to 5-FU alone combined with radiation therapy (see Fig 1). With only a median follow up of 48 months, the results of the study indicate that 5-FU bolus/radiation therapy alone was just as efficacious as the other treatment arms. I believe this study clearly indicates that there is no role for levamisole in the adjuvant therapy of rectal cancer because its addition enhanced toxicity without improving response. Local recurrence was noted in 11% of the patients. This, again, demonstrates the effectiveness of a combination regimen in providing improved local control in patients with advanced but resectable rectal cancer.

Of note, the combination of 5-FU/leucovorin and radiation therapy produced a 3-year disease-free survival rate of 68% which may yet prove—with longer follow-up data—to be superior to bolus 5-FU and radiation therapy alone. In addition, continuous venous infusion of 5-FU with radiation therapy has been proven to be more efficacious than bolus 5-FU. However, this information did not come to light until this 4-arm study was nearly one half completed. Therefore, future studies with continuous venous infusion of 5-FU vs. other adjuvant regimens may yet prove it to be the superior choice of therapy.

B.L. Eisenberg, M.D.

Aggressive Surgical Management of Recurrent Rectal Cancer: Is It Worthwhile?

Ogunbiyi OA, McKenna K, Birnbaum EH, et al (Washington Univ, St Louis)
Dis Colon Rectum 40:150–155, 1997 7–21

Introduction.—The incidence of recurrent disease in patients who undergo curative surgery for primary rectal cancer ranges from 3.5% to 30% (2.6% to 30% for local recurrence; 7% to 24% for systemic recurrence). Patients with recurrent rectal cancer after potentially curative surgery for primary rectal tumor were assessed retrospectively to determine whether radical surgery in appropriately selected patients can yield significant disease-free survival.

Methods.—All 489 patients underwent preoperative external beam radiation therapy and curative surgery. Patients with recurrent disease were carefully selected to undergo potentially curative or palliative surgery, as determined by staging criteria.

Results.—Of the initial curative surgery group, 44 (9%) had recurrent disease at a median of 18 months. Twenty-eight patients (5.7%) had local pelvic recurrence alone. The overall survival rate at a median of 15 months was 41% (18/44). Fourteen of 18 patients underwent curative resection; the disease-free survival rate at a median of 25 months was 86%. Patients who underwent palliative surgery had a mean survival of 12 months. Of 6 patients in the curative group with second recurrences, 4 underwent further curative surgery and were disease-free at a median of 19.5 months. Eleven patients who underwent palliative surgery had good symptomatic relief and improved quality of life. There was no survival advantage for these patients, compared with 19 patients who underwent nonsurgical palliative treatment.

Conclusion.—An aggressive surgical approach provided significant disease-free survival for this carefully selected group of patients with recurrent rectal cancer. Good symptomatic relief and improved quality of life were found in patients who underwent palliative surgery.

▶ The incidence of overall recurrence of rectal cancer still remains in the 20% to 30% range, with isolated pelvic recurrences accounting for approximately 10% to 20% of these. Obviously, factors specifically associated with rectal cancer, such as nodal involvement and extramural extension, will dictate the probability of local or systemic recurrence in these patients. Most of these patients, however, will have adjuvant therapy consisting of radiation and/or chemotherapy as dictated by the severity of their initial disease. Therefore, treatment considerations for recurrent disease in these patients are limited.

This article reviews a single institutional retrospective experience in the surgical management of recurrent rectal cancer with intent to cure or palliate. The article reaffirms the fact that the selective use of aggressive surgery in these patients can be rewarding in that removal of all gross disease with negative microscopic margins can result in long-term cure rates. This is true whether the rectal cancer recurrence is detected in a symptomatic or an asymptomatic patient and regardless of whether the cancer recurrence is manifested as local disease or systemic disease. Another point of this article concerns the palliative effect of surgical intervention, even if survival advantage cannot be demonstrated. In those patients who have palliative surgery for clear-cut related symptoms without curative attempt, there is an improvement in both symptomatic relief and quality of life compared with the nonoperative patients.

This is a theme that has been expressed in several articles in the recent literature. It is clear that any patient who has a recurrence of a rectal cancer should at least be considered for surgical treatment in the absence of contraindications, either medical or specific disease related.

B.L. Eisenberg, M.D.

Implications of Fine-Needle Aspiration in Patients With Resectable Pancreatic Cancer

Johnson DE, Pendurthi TK, Balshem AM, et al (Fox Chase Cancer Ctr, Philadelphia)

Am Surg 63:675–680, 1997 7–22

Objective.—The debate regarding the value of fine-needle aspiration (FNA) for the diagnosis of pancreatic cancer revolves around its variable sensitivity, high cost, and risk of seeding the peritoneal cavity with malignant cells. Results of a safety and reliability study of FNA biopsy of the pancreas were reported.

Methods.—Records of 32 patients with pancreatic cancer undergoing FNA before having curative pancreaticoduodenectomy were reviewed for results of positive peritoneal cytology, peritoneal recurrences, and survival. The FNA was performed under CT or fluoroscopic guidance, using a 22 gauge Chiba needle. Cytology was performed on peritoneal washings. Fine-needle aspiration and cytologic results were compared statistically. The FNA results were also compared with peritoneal failure and with survival.

Results.—Of the 21 patients who had FNA, results were 14 positive, 3 suspicious, 2 negative, and 2 nondiagnostic. There were 12 single attempts, 8 double attempts, and 1 triple attempt. Sensitivity was 89.5%, and positive predictive value was 100%. Of the 28 peritoneal washes performed, 5 results were positive or suspicious, and 23 were negative. Of the 5 patients with positive results, 3 (16.7%) had both FNA and peritoneal cytology and 2 (20%) had positive peritoneal washings and no FNA. Patients were followed for 5 to 76 months. There were 8 peritoneal failures, 6 (28%) had FNA and 2 (18%) had no FNA. There were no significant differences between positive peritoneal cytology or survival in the FNA and no-FNA groups.

Conclusion.—Fine-needle aspiration appears to be a safe and reliable method for confirming the diagnosis of pancreatic cancer.

► Preoperative diagnosis of pancreatic cancer can be problematic, especially in the clinical setting of a small pancreatic cancer with considerable surrounding inflammation of a secondary pancreatitis. There are a number of developing multimodality treatment schemes for pancreatic adenocarcinoma, some of which involve neoadjuvant treatment. It is, therefore, necessary, in many instances, to obtain a tissue diagnosis before exploratory laparotomy and pancreatic resection. Fine needle aspiration has been recognized as an effective, reasonably sensitive, and safe method of obtaining a tissue diagnosis of pancreatic adenocarcinoma, although concerns arise as to the potential for implantation of tumor cells.

This article reviews a 9-year experience with percutaneous FNA cytology in patients with resectable adenocarcinoma of the pancreas considered for a neoadjuvant treatment protocol. As noted, there was no increase in the incidence of complications either preoperatively or postoperatively, and there was no increase in the number of positive abdominal lavage cytologies or intra-abdominal recurrence of cancer between the FNA and the non-FNA groups. As mentioned in the article, the FNA technique used a percutaneous small-gauge needle under CT guidance, with a cytotechnologist present to immediately evaluate the material for degree of adequate cellularity.

In the future, other methods may be as effective or more so in determining a preoperative diagnosis of pancreatic carcinoma, including the use of endoscopic ultrasound-directed needle biopsy of the pancreas. Nevertheless, this article does establish the fact that patients can receive a diagnosis with a percutaneous FNA of the pancreas without subsequent concerns for mechanical tumor dissemination.

B.L. Eisenberg, M.D.

Preoperative and Postoperative Chemoradiation Strategies in Patients Treated With Pancreaticoduodenectomy for Adenocarcinoma of the Pancreas

Spitz FR, Abbruzzese JL, Lee JE, et al (Univ of Texas MD Anderson Cancer Ctr, Houston)

J Clin Oncol 15:928–937, 1997 7–23

Introduction.—The role of preoperative adjuvant chemoradiation in patients undergoing pancreaticoduodenectomy for adenocarcinoma of the pancreas is unclear. The effects of preoperative vs. postoperative chemoradiation on treatment toxicity, length of treatment, tumor recurrence, and survival in patients who underwent potentially curative therapy for adenocarcinoma of the pancreas were assessed.

Methods.—From July 1990 to July 1995, 142 patients with resectable localized adenocarcinoma of the pancreatic head underwent a multimodality approach that included either preoperative or postoperative chemoradiation. Those patients with biopsy-confirmed adenocarcinoma and low-density mass in the pancreatic head received preoperative chemoradiation. Patients with no mass on CT or negative preoperative biopsy underwent pancreaticoduodenectomy with planned postoperative chemoradiation.

Results.—There was no delay in surgery because of toxicity in patients who received preoperative chemoradiation, compared with 24% of patients (6 of 25) of patients who did not receive postoperative chemoradiation because of delayed recovery after surgery. There were no between-group differences in toxicities from chemoradiation. Patients who received rapid-fractionation preoperative chemoradiation had significantly briefer duration of treatment, compared with patients who received postoperative chemoradiation or standard-fractionation preoperative chemoradiation (62.5, 98.5, and 91.0 days, respectively). There were no significant between-group differences in survival at a median follow-up of 19 months. Local and regional (peritoneal) recurrence, respectively, were observed in 0% and 10% of patients who received preoperative chemoradiation, compared with local or regional recurrence in 21% of patients who received postoperative chemoradiation.

Conclusions.—Toxicity, patterns of tumor recurrence, and survival were similar in patients treated with either preoperative or postoperative chemoradiation and pancreaticoduodenectomy for adenocarcinoma of the pancreatic head. Nearly one fourth of patients with planned postoperative chemoradiation had delayed postoperative adjuvant chemoradiation because of prolonged recovery.

▶ This article from M.D. Anderson Cancer Center reports on a single institutional series of 142 patients with adenocarcinoma of the pancreas. These patients were all potentially resectable and were candidates for either preoperative or postoperative chemoradiation adjuvant therapy. Although survival rates were similar between the 2 groups, the preoperative chemoradiation group did not experience a delay in surgery. In contrast, prolonged recovery after pancreaticoduodenectomy prevented the delivery of adequate adjuvant therapy in 25% of the patients in the postoperative group. One must also note that the preoperative adjuvant group generally had larger tumors and yet none had a positive margin of resection after pancreaticoduodenectomy, and their pathology specimens had a decreased number of positive lymph nodes compared with the postoperative adjuvant therapy group. This suggests therapy-associated tumor downstaging in the neoadjuvant group.

I believe that combined chemoradiation therapy as an adjuvant treatment has become standard for patients with resectable pancreatic cancer. These therapies appear to have a beneficial survival effect as well as a positive effect on local recurrence. It appears from this single institutional experience as well as others that preoperative adjuvant therapy has an advantage over postoperative adjuvant therapy mainly in enhancing patient compliance without evidence of increased toxicity. The obvious goal is to improve drug treatment for microscopic subclinical systemic disease that is already present at the time of surgical resection in the majority of these patients. Trials are underway utilizing such new drugs as gemcitabine in hopes of promoting a therapeutic advantage for systemic effect.

B.L. Eisenberg, M.D.

Outpatient Bowel Preparation for Elective Colon Resection

Le TH, Timmcke AE, Gathright JB Jr, et al (Ochsner Clinic and Alton Ochsner Med Found, New Orleans, La)
South Med J 90:526–530, 1997 7–24

Objective.—Because in-hospital mechanical bowel cleansing before colon resection is a time-consuming and labor-intensive process, outpatient preoperative preparation has been advocated using the safe and effective polyethylene glycol-electrolyte lavage solution. The cost-effectiveness and

TABLE 2.—Surgical Outcome

	Outpatient Bowel Preparation	*Inpatient Bowel Preparation*
Days of hospitalization		
Mean	9 ± 2.7	10.7 ± 4.6
Range	5–25	6–41
Days of nothing by mouth		
Mean	6 ± 2.0	6.8 ± 3.1
Range	3–17	2–21
Days of nasogastric tube		
Mean	5.5 ± 2.0	6.0 ± 2.9
Range	2–15	0–20
Days of gastrostomy tube		
Mean	6.2 ± 1.4	7.2 ± 3.4
Range	4–9	3–20
Discharge-outcome		
Home	144 (99.3%)	170 (97.7%)
Rehabilitation	0	3
Death	1 (0.7%)	1 (0.6%)

(Reprinted by permission from Le TH, Timmcke AE, Gathright JB Jr, et al: Outpatient bowel preparation for elective colon resection. *South Med J* 90:526–530, 1997.)

safety of outpatient and inpatient bowel preparation were assessed retrospectively.

Methods.—Of the 319 patients who had elective segmental or total abdominal colectomy with primary anastomosis (patients needing protective proximal stoma were excluded), 145 had outpatient bowel preparation and 174 had inpatient preparation. Patients were matched for age, sex, preoperative diagnosis, postoperative diagnosis, procedures done, and comorbidity factors. Operative complications and bowel preparation costs were determined.

Results.—Mortality rates for inpatients and outpatients were 0.6% and 0.7%. Morbidity rates were 21% and 19%, respectively. All other outcome measures, including costs, were also lower for outpatients than for inpatients (Table 2 and Table 3).

TABLE 3.—Cost of Preoperative Bowel Preparation

	Outpatient	*Inpatient*
PEG-ELS*	$17.34	$ 16.80
Erythromycin	11.64	9.00
Neomycin	11.64	9.48
Room (semi-private)		360.00
Total	$40.62	$395.28

*Polyethylene glycol-electrolyte lavage solution.

(Reprinted by permission from Le TH, Timmcke AE, Gathright JB Jr, et al: Outpatient bowel preparation for elective colon resection. *South Med J* 90:526–530, 1997.)

Conclusion.—Outpatient bowel preparation is safe and effective and offers a substantial cost savings.

▶ Traditionally, patients with scheduled elective colorectal surgery underwent preoperative bowel cleansing for 1–2 days as a hospitalized inpatient. The advent of better bowel cleansing methods such as polyethylene glycol-electrolyte lavage solution has improved the efficacy of oral cleansing methods and decreased the time necessary for thorough bowel preparation. Nevertheless, most patients continue to have inpatient bowel preparations before surgery. This article from the Ochsner Clinic analyzes a large group of patients retrospectively evaluated for comparison of inpatient vs. outpatient bowel preparation. There was no difference in those areas where most surgeons believe that inpatient preparation provides a decided advantage. These include postoperative infection and other complications, and days hospitalized postoperatively. Obviously, the method of outpatient bowel preparation applies best to patients without evidence of obstruction or renal compromise. In addition, I might add that elderly patients coming from long distances to the hospital for morning surgery likewise may have problems with adequate hydration before open abdominal surgery. Therefore, although in most cases, outpatient bowel preparation is cost-effective and clinically justified, the surgeon's discretion in these decisions is still quite important.

B.L. Eisenberg, M.D.

Randomised Trial of Surgery Alone Versus Surgery Followed by Radiotherapy for Mobile Cancer of the Rectum

Arnott SJ, for the Medical Research Council Rectal Cancer Working Party (St Bartholomew's Hosp, London)

Lancet 348:1610–1614, 1996 7–25

Background.—Local recurrence (LR) often comes after apparently successful surgery for rectal cancer. This study examines the effect of postoperative radiotherapy in reducing LR in mobile Dukes' stage B and C rectal cancer.

Method.—Four hundred sixty-nine randomized patients were studied from 1984 to 1989. Researchers followed these patients from 46 different hospitals for 5 years. Patients were residents of the Republic of Ireland and the United Kingdom. Half of the patients underwent surgery only (235 patients) and the other half underwent both surgery and radiotherapy (234 patients). The radiotherapy followed surgery by 4 to 6 weeks and consisted of 40 Gy in 20 fractions of 2Gy over 4 weeks.

Results.—Researchers found a hazard rate for overall survival of 0.84 (95% confidence interval, 0.65–1.07; $P = 0.17$). This was the result of 284 deaths (145 surgery-only patients and 139 radiotherapy patients). Five years after treatment, 79 surgery-only patients and 48 radiotherapy patients experienced LR (hazard ratio, 0.54 [0.38–0.77], $P = 0.001$). There was distant recurrence in 83 and 75 patients, respectively (hazard ratio, 0.85). Disease-free survival had a 0.85 hazard ratio.

Conclusion.—In patients given radiotherapy, LR was nearly halved in comparison with patients who underwent only surgery. Postoperative radiotherapy seems to curtail LR but further studies on survival outcome are needed. The LR rate found in this study may seem a bit high for today's standards but, as more trials are combined, a more accurate picture will be provided.

Influence of Surgery on Metachronous Distant Metastases and Survival in Rectal Cancer

Köckerling F, Reymond MA, Altendorf-Hofmann A, et al (Univ of Erlangen, Germany)

J Clin Oncol 16:324–329, 1998 7–26

Background.—Survival after optimal surgery using total mesorectal excision (TME) has not been thoroughly investigated as a survival criterion for rectal cancer though it is proven to reduce local recurrence (LR). Part of this uncertainty lies in the incidence of distant postoperative metastases. This study investigated surgery quality gauged by LR and its effects on survival and the incidence of distant metastases.

Method.—For 1,581 patients treated for rectal carcinoma by curative resection between 1974 and 1991, this study monitored recurrence and survival with a medium follow-up of 13 years. Physicians did not treat any test subject with TME, as it was not introduced until 1985. Chemotherapy and radiotherapy were not used.

Results.—During this rather lengthy study period in which many technical advances were made, the LR rate dropped (39.4% to 9.8%; P = 0.0001) and the 5-year survival rate increased (50% to 71%, P less than 0.0001). A five-year survival rate that was significantly lower (P less than 0.0001) was observed in patients in whom LR developed (306 patients). Two hundred seventy-five patients exhibited distant metastases. Better-quality surgery did not curtail initial distant metastases. Throughout the study, distant metastases was consistent (P = 0.44).

Conclusion.—Surgery quality, although a variable for survival of rectal cancer, does not initially influence whether or not distant metastases will occur. Unless the surgeon is considered a risk factor, researchers cannot take LR to be a criterion for adjuvant therapy outcome.

▶ These 2 articles (Abstracts 7–25 and 7–26) address the very important concern of LR in patients with operable rectal cancer. The devastating effect of a local failure, even in the absence of systemic disease, must be an important adjuvant treatment consideration. The large, randomized trial from the United Kingdom using postoperative radiation therapy in patients with T3 or N1/N2 rectal cancers is representative of well-constructed postoperative trials favoring the effect of radiation therapy on decreasing the incidence of

LR. However, in this series, the surgery-alone group had an LR of 33%, which is in contradistinction to the excellent local failure rate of 10% with surgery alone reported from the Erlangen group.

These studies obviously present surgical patient groups that cannot be truly comparable: One presents a prospective, randomized trial of surgery alone vs. surgery-plus–radiation therapy, and the other reports on a retrospective surgical series of patients with rectal cancer, using wide-field TME. It is, however, reasonable to assume that the additional results of radiation therapy in enhancing local disease control should be compared with a control group representing adequate disease-clearing surgery. Postoperative radiation therapy may, in some cases, compensate for inadequate surgical technique. It is also notable from these 2 articles that although disease-clearing surgery alone or surgery plus adjuvant radiation therapy can decrease the expected rate of LR and, thereby, affect quality of life and secondary metastases after LR, neither has an effect on metachronous systemic metastases or, subsequently, on overall survival.

B.L. Eisenberg, M.D.

Value of Carcinoembryonic Antigen Monitoring in Curative Surgery for Recurrent Colorectal Carcinoma

Lucha PA Jr, Rosen L, Olenwine JA, et al (Naval Med Ctr, Portsmouth, Va; Lehigh Valley Hosp, Allentown, Pa)

Dis Colon Rectum 40:145–149, 1997 7–27

Introduction.—The usefulness of carcinoembryonic antigen (CEA) monitoring for decreasing cancer mortality in patients who have undergone surgery for colorectal carcinoma is questionable. The impact on patient survival of a postoperative CEA-monitoring protocol was assessed in a tertiary medical center by 5 board-certified colorectal surgeons.

Methods.—Medical records of 285 patients who underwent operative resection for colon or rectal carcinoma between 1981 and 1985 were reviewed. The CEA levels were evaluated: every 2 months for the first 2 years, every 3 months for the third year, every 6 months for years 4 and 5, and annually thereafter. When CEA levels were above 5 ng/mL, diagnostic imaging and/or endoscopy were performed.

Results.—A total of 280 patients (98.2%) were followed up for an average of 80 months. The sensitivity, specificity, and positive predictive value of CEA monitoring (for a level of 5 ng/mL) for recurrent disease was 67%, 92%, and 71%, respectively. Forty-four of 62 patients (71%) with persistent CEA elevations had documented metastatic recurrence. Of the 44 patients with elevated CEA and recurrence, 11 underwent surgical resection with curative intent. None of the 11 patients with recurrent disease who underwent resection for cure had symptoms associated with elevated CEA. There was no surgical mortality, and 3 of 11 patients (27%) were disease-free at 5 years. Of 223 patients with normal CEA levels, 22

(10%) had recurrent disease. There were no long-term survivors among patients with recurrent disease and normal CEA.

Conclusions.—Careful preoperative evaluation with CEA yielded a 27% (3 of 11 patients) long-term survival rate without surgical mortality. The relatively low yield for cure in following up patients with CEA levels needs further evaluation. It is time—it has been more than 16 years since the National Institutes for Health reviewed this topic.

▶ The value of routine CEA monitoring in follow-up for patients with colorectal cancer remains unproven. Any real benefit should be reflective in long-term survival statistics. Unfortunately, there is no reported substantial data to support this concept.

This article suggests benefit to a small portion of patients in a nonrandomized study. It represents CEA determinations on a frequent regimen within a large patient population with good long-term follow-up. Even within the confines of this tightly controlled study, only 60% of the patients were actually in compliance with CEA determinations. Additionally, only 1% of the total patients in this series were cured as a result of CEA follow-up. This is not inconsistent, however, with other similar series.

It is clear that serial CEA determinations can lead to an earlier investigation in an asymptomatic patient with resectable recurrent disease confined to the liver or lung. This may translate into improved survival in a few selected individuals. Unfortunately, not all patients with recurrence will initially have an elevated CEA value, and most of the patients who do have elevated CEA values will not be resectable with curative intent.

B.L. Eisenberg, M.D.

Radical Surgery and Postoperative Radiotherapy as Combined Treatment in Rectal Cancer: Final Results of a Phase III Study of the European Organization for Research and Treatment of Cancer

Arnaud JP, Nordlinger B, Bosset JF, et al (Centre Hospitalo-Universitaire, Angers, France; CHU, Besancon, France; Hôpital Saint-Antoine, Paris; et al)

Br J Surg 84:352–357, 1997 7–28

Objective.—Whether preoperative or postoperative radiotherapy improves overall survival after radical surgery for rectal cancer is unclear. Results of the European Organization for Research and Treatment of Cancer (EORTC) randomized clinical trial evaluating the role of postoperative irradiation in the patients who had curative surgical resection for locally advanced rectal cancer were summarized.

Methods.—Within 14 weeks after surgery for resection of Dukes B or C rectal cancer, 172 patients were randomly allocated to receive radiotherapy (46 Gy 5 days a week for 30–38 days) (n = 84) or no treatment (n = 88). Patients were followed up for an average of 84.7 months to recurrence or death.

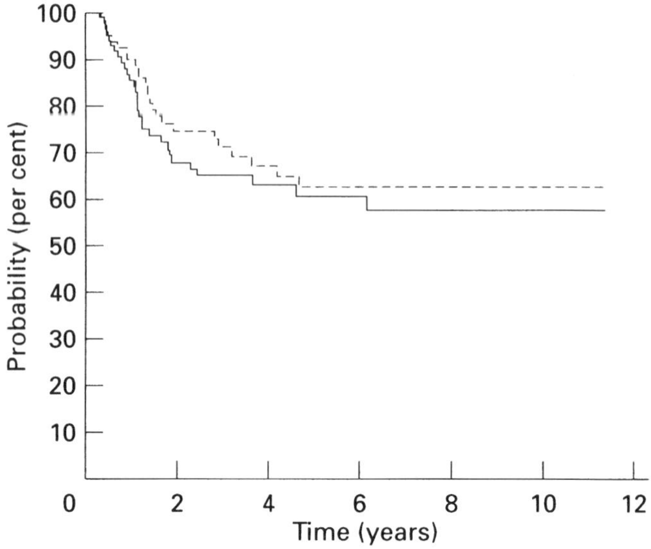

No. at risk						
Control	88	46	32	23	11	3
Radiotherapy	84	47	32	21	11	5

FIGURE 2.—Local disease-free interval in the surgery alone (*solid line*) and postoperative radiotherapy (*dashed line*) groups. $P = 0.46$ (log rank test). (Courtesy of Arnaud JP, Nordlinger B, Bosset JF, et al: Radical surgery and postoperative radiotherapy as combined treatment in rectal cancer: Final results of a phase III study of the European Organization for Research and Treatment of Cancer. *Br J Surg* 84:352–357, 1997. Publisher, Blackwell Science Ltd.)

Results.—Two patients in the radiotherapy group had severe acute complications, 1 patient in the surgery only group died of pulmonary embolism, and 47 patients in the radiotherapy group experienced acute toxicity symptoms. There were no disease-free survival, local disease-free interval, or overall survival differences between groups (Fig 2).

Conclusion.—Postoperative radiotherapy made no difference in disease-free survival, local disease-free interval, or overall survival in patients after radical surgery for rectal cancer.

▶ The importance of this article lies in the fact that it represents a large, well-controlled, prospective evaluation of the efficacy of postoperative radiation therapy in the treatment of locally advanced rectal cancer. There has long been controversy regarding the use of radiation therapy in the treatment of locally advanced rectal cancer as an adjuvant either preoperatively or postoperatively. Obviously, the goal of such treatment would be initially to prevent local recurrence, which in the case of rectal cancer carries considerable morbidity, and hopefully to translate that benefit into an overall survival advantage. Individual anecdotal experience or retrospective institutional reviews generally report a benefit for postoperative radiation therapy in a patient who has low-lying rectal cancer with transmural tumor penetrance or positive nodes. Additionally, there are prospective randomized data relating to the efficacy of preoperative radiation therapy with proven benefit for local control. This European Organization for Research and Treatment of Cancer trial evaluating the use of postoperative adjuvant radiotherapy alone failed to demonstrate any benefit for local control (see Figure 2) or in overall survival. This supports data from previous prospective randomized studies evaluating radiotherapy alone as an adjuvant in the postoperative setting in that no benefit was obtained for local disease control or survival. It is apparent from this report as well as others that there is no important benefit from postoperative radiation as a single treatment modality in patients with high risk rectal cancer. Therefore, it appears that the only compelling prospective data demonstrating enhanced benefit for adjuvant therapy in rectal cancer can be found in patients with either preoperative radiation as a single modality or with a combination of radiation and chemotherapy.

B.L. Eisenberg, M.D.

Randomized Comparison Between Chemotherapy Plus Best Supportive Care With Best Supportive Care in Advanced Gastric Cancer

Glimelius B, Ekström K, Hoffman K, et al (Univ of Uppsala, Sweden; Huddinge Univ, Stockholm; Centralsjukhuset, Karlstad, Sweden; et al)

Ann Oncol 8:163–168, 1997 7–29

Background.—Although chemotherapy is extensively used, the extent to which it relieves tumor-related symptoms, improves quality of life, and prolongs survival in patients with gastric cancer is unknown. The outcomes of chemotherapy plus best supportive care were compared with those of best supportive care alone.

Methods.—Sixty-one patients with advanced gastric cancer were randomly assigned to 1 of these 2 interventions between 1991 and 1995. If supportive measures alone were not palliative, chemotherapy was added. Chemotherapy consisted of 5-fluorouracil, leucovorin, and etoposide or, in elderly patients with poor performance, 5-fluorouracil and leucovorin. The European Organization for Research in Cancer Therapy QLQ-C30 was used to assess quality of life.

Findings.—Forty-five percent of the patients receiving chemotherapy and 20% of those receiving supportive care alone had an improved or prolonged high quality of life for at least 4 months. Similarly, 55% and 20%, respectively, were judged by their treating physicians to be subjectively improved or continuing to do well for at least 4 months. Patients given chemotherapy had a median survival of 8 months, compared with 5 months for those receiving supportive care alone: a nonsignificant difference. However, after adjustments for imbalances in pretreatment characteristics, chemotherapy was associated with a survival benefit. In addition, the quality-adjusted survival time and time to disease progression were longer for those receiving chemotherapy than for those given supportive care alone (medians, 5 and 2 months, respectively).

Conclusion.—Chemotherapy can prolong survival and improve the quality of life of patients with advanced gastric cancer. Unfortunately, the number of patients benefiting from treatment is still somewhat limited.

▶ This paper represents a valid attempt by a Swedish group to address the issue of whether palliative polychemotherapy can prolong duration and quality of life in patients with advanced inoperable gastric cancer. The routine use of chemotherapy is accepted in patients with incurable gastric cancer without substantial data to support any true beneficial effect. It is not likely that ethical considerations will allow a phase III randomized comparison study of chemotherapy vs. best supportive care for any advanced upper gastrointestinal tract cancer. This study, however flawed in its concept (the control group could receive chemotherapy by patient request), still demonstrated a clear difference in quality of life (both subjectively and objectively evaluated) and quality-adjusted survival in favor of the chemotherapy group. Clearly, unbiased and well documented information supporting the routine use of polychemotherapy in patients with advanced gastric cancer to enhance the quality of life and to prolong a quality-improved life is an important contribution to the literature.

B.L. Eisenberg, M.D.

Palliative Reirradiation for Recurrent Rectal Cancer

Lingareddy V, Ahmad NR, Mohiuddin M (Thomas Jefferson Univ, Philadelphia; Univ of Kentucky, Lexington)

Int J Radiat Oncol Biol Phys 38:785–790, 1997 7–30

Objective.—In the 10% to 25% of patients with recurrent rectal cancer after high-dose adjuvant chemoradiation, there are few options for palliation or longterm survival. Results of palliative reirradiation in patients with locally recurrent adenocarcinoma of the rectum were presented.

Methods.—Palliative pelvic reirradiation for recurrent disease was given to 52 patients (21 females), aged 37 to 79 years, with rectal cancer previously treated by surgery. The Karnofsky Performance Score was 70 or less for 17 patients and over 70 for 35. The pathologic disease stage was II or III in 28 patients and I or less in 24. Initially, 5 patients had radiation therapy alone, and the remainder had curative surgery plus radiation therapy. The median initial and reirradiation doses were 50.4 Gy and 30.6 Gy, respectively. Reirradiation doses were given as 1.2 Gy twice daily to 22 patients and 1.8 to 2.0 Gy daily to 30 patients. Twenty patients also received a boost dose of 6.0 to 20.0 Gy. Intravenous 5-fluorouracil, 200 to 300 mg/m^2/day was administered concurrently to 47 patients. Patients were followed every 3 to 4 months for the first year and at least every 6 months thereafter. Eight patients were still alive at 13 to 48 months (Fig 1).

Results.—Sixteen patients (31%) had Radiation Therapy Oncology Group grade 3 toxicity necessitating interruption or termination of treatment. An additional 16 patients experienced grade 1 or 2 toxicity. Twelve

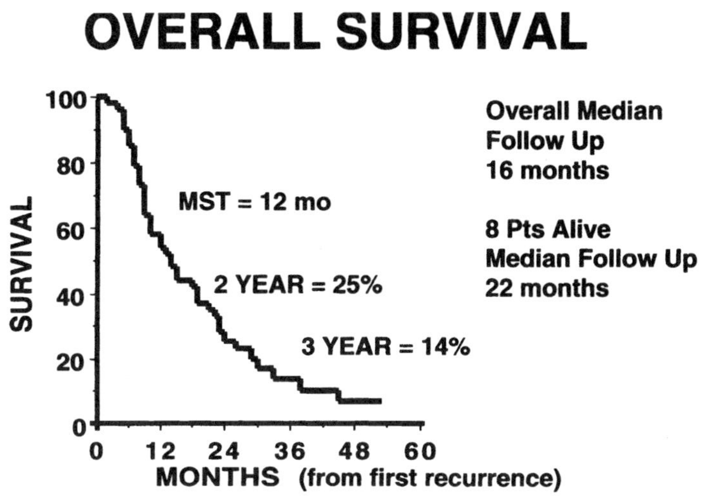

FIGURE 1.—Survival after reirradiation for recurrent rectal cancer. *Abbreviation: MST*, median survival time. (Reprinted by permission of the publisher from Lingareddy V, Ahmad NR, Mohiuddin M: Palliative reirradiation for recurrent rectal cancer. *Int J Radiat Oncol Biol Phys* 38:785–790, copyright 1997 by Elsevier Science Inc.)

patients had late grade 3 toxicity and 4 had late grade 4 toxicity. On univariate and logistic regression analyses, hyperfractionated radiotherapy was associated with less late toxicity. Reirradiation was effective in palliation of symptoms in most patients (Table 5).

Conclusion.—Reirradiation for recurrent rectal cancer increases survival and provides excellent palliation of symptoms, with moderate toxicity.

► It is not that rare for one to face the problem of recurrent rectal cancer that has been previously irradiated. What is unusual is to find data on this subject, and this paper offers some. The results are very acceptable, considering that this involves a retreatment. Grade III and IV late toxicity rates are acceptable for retreatment considering the total doses used. The palliation appears to have been quite good. Obviously, these patients generally have metastatic disease, so their long-term survival is still poor. But it is interesting to find that local problems can be reasonably well palliated with moderate doses.

TABLE 5.—Efficacy of Reirradiation in Palliation of Symptoms

	No. of patients	Complete response	Partial response	Median duration	Palliated until death
Bleeding	15	100%	N/A	10 months	80%
Pain	40	65%	28%	9 months	33%
Mass effect	25	24%	64%	8 months	20%

(Reprinted by permission of the publisher from Lingareddy V, Ahmad NR, Mohiuddin M: Palliative reirradiation for recurrent rectal cancer. *Int J Radiat Oncol Biol Phys* 38:785–790, copyright 1997 by Elsevier Science Inc.)

My experience with this situation is, perhaps, relevant. I have treated at least a couple dozen such patients. If the only thing they had was pelvic recurrence, I have treated them very aggressively with doses of 6,000 rad or more on a twice-daily basis. I have usually used 150 rad twice a day because I think it gives a slight advantage in normal tissue injury—at least, long-term—although these patients have a lot of gastrointestinal symptoms during treatment. It is interesting that virtually all the patients I have treated have been treated for mass or bleeding problems, and the pain that one sees has generally been associated with the mass problem, rather than that peculiar intractable pain syndrome that is traditionally seen as part of pelvic recurrence when the patient has not been previously irradiated. The criteria that I have used for selecting patients for retreatment are that there is at least 1 year between the 2 courses and that the tissues appear to be minimally affected by the first course of treatment. The assessment of tissue appearance includes re-evaluation of the rectal mucosa, as seen through sigmoidoscopy.

E. Glatstein, M.D.

Improved Survival With Preoperative Radiotherapy in Resectable Rectal Cancer

Påhlman L, and the Swedish Rectal Cancer Trial (Univ of Uppsala, Sweden)
N Engl J Med 336:980–987, 1997 7–31

Background.—Although adjuvant radiotherapy for rectal cancer has been studied extensively, no one has shown unequivocably that radiotherapy improves overall survival. However, the local recurrence rate is decreased. It was determined whether preoperative radiotherapy with a 3- or 4-beam technique in patients younger than 80 years could be given without increasing postoperative mortality, to substantiate the previously reported decrease in local recurrence rate with radiotherapy and to document its effects on survival.

Methods.—Between 1987 and 1990, a total of 1,168 patients with resectable rectal cancer were randomly assigned to receive preoperative irradiation followed by surgery within 1 week or to surgery alone. The radiation dose was 25 Gy delivered in 5 fractions in 1 week.

Findings.—Radiotherapy did not increase mortality after surgery. The local recurrence rate after 5 years was 11% in the patients receiving combined treatment and 27% in the group having surgery alone. All subgroups defined by Dukes' stage displayed this difference. Overall 5-year survival was 58% in the combined treatment group and 48% in the surgery-only group. At 9 years, cancer-specific survival rates were 74% and 65%, respectively, among patients treated with curative resection (Fig 3; Table 2).

Conclusions.—In this trial, designed to detect even a small but clinically relevant survival benefit associated with radiotherapy before surgery in patients with resectable cancer, irradiation was found not only to decrease

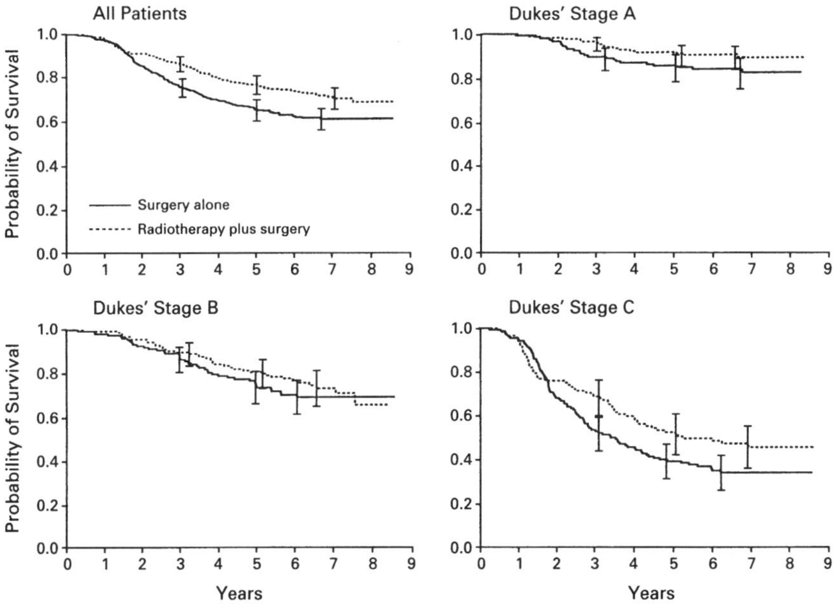

FIGURE 3.—Cancer-specific survival among all patients undergoing curative operations, according to Dukes' stage and treatment assignment. The *bars* indicate 95% confidence limits. (Courtesy of Påhlman L, and the Swedish Rectal Cancer Trial: Improved survival with preoperative radiotherapy in resectable rectal cancer. *N Engl J Med* 336:980–987. Copyright 1997, Massachusetts Medical Society. Reprinted by permission of *The New England Journal of Medicine*. All rights reserved.)

the rate of local recurrence but also to improve survival. The survival benefit was 21%.

▶ I have read this paper carefully, and I find no particular weakness. This study from Sweden looks at patients who had resectable rectal cancer and randomly assigned almost 1,200 patients to 1 week of preoperative radiation (25 Gy) followed by surgery within a week, or surgery alone. There was no increase in postoperative mortality after radiation. At 5 years, the local recurrence rate was only 11% in the group that received 25 Gy, as opposed to 27% in the group treated with surgery alone.

I have never understood why preoperative radiation has been accepted so poorly in this country. I believe part of it has to do with the fact that university services are largely dominated by the chief resident who does not wish to delay the case. Whether that is true remains to be seen.

This study's findings certainly suggest that a quick week of preoperative treatment is indicated. Not only does this appear to be associated with a major improvement in local control, but there is a suggestion that the rate of distant metastatic disease is diminished after preoperative radiation (see Table 2). Is it possible that some of these patients are actually disseminated from the surgery itself if the cells are not treated before surgery?

E. Glatstein, M.D.

TABLE 2.—Rates of Local Recurrence According to Dukes' Stage and Surgical Outcome Among Patients With Resected Tumors Assigned to Radiotherapy Plus Surgery or Surgery Alone

Surgical Outcome	Radiotherapy plus Surgery				Surgery Alone			
	Dukes' Stage A	Dukes' Stage B	Dukes' Stage C	Total	Dukes' Stage A	Dukes' Stage B	Dukes' Stage C	Total
	number with recurrence/total number (percent)							
Distant metastases	0/5	0/11	5/26 (19)	5/42 (12)	1/4 (25)	3/12 (25)	8/25 (32)	12/41 (29)
Locally noncurative surgery	0	3/6 (50)	1/8 (12)	4/14 (29)	0	0/8	10/11 (91)	10/19 (53)
Local cure uncertain	0/2	6/13 (46)	7/28 (25)	13/43 (30)	0/3	5/8 (62)	17/32 (3)	22/43 (51)
Curative surgery	8/174 (5)	11/165 (7)	22/115 (19)	41/454 (9)	17/147 (12)	31/145 (21)	58/162 (36)	105/454 (23)
Total	8/181 (4)*	20/195 (10)†	35/177 (20)‡	63/553 (11)‡	18/154 (12)	39/173 (23)	93/230 (40)	150/557 (27)

*$P = 0.02$ for the comparison with the same subgroup in the surgery-alone group.
†$P = 0.002$ for the comparison with the same subgroup in the surgery-alone group.
‡$P < 0.001$ for the comparison with the same subgroup in the surgery-alone group.
(Courtesy of Påhlman L, and the Swedish Rectal Cancer Trial: Improved survival with preoperative radiotherapy in resectable rectal cancer. *N Engl J Med* 336:980–987.

Importance of Adenomas 5 mm or Less in Diameter That Are Detected by Sigmoidoscopy

Read TE, Read JD, Butterly LF (Lahey-Hitchcock Med Ctr, Burlington, Mass)

N Engl J Med 336:8–12, 1997 7–32

Background.—Authorities disagree on the need for colonoscopy in patients with adenomas of 5 mm or less in diameter detected by sigmoidoscopy. The prevalence of proximal colonic neoplasms was prospectively determined in a large group of asymptomatic patients at average risk for colorectal cancer and with diminutive benign adenomatous polyps on screening flexible sigmoidoscopy.

Methods.—A total of 3,496 consecutive patients underwent sigmoidoscopy, 311 of whom were found to have neoplastic rectosigmoid polyps. One hundred eight were excluded because of a history of colonic neoplasia, symptoms, previous colonic assessment, or incomplete follow-up data. The remaining 203 patients underwent colonoscopy. Rectosigmoid adenomas 5 mm in diameter or less were designated diminutive; 6–10 mm, small; and 11 mm or greater, large.

Findings.—Neoplasms were detected in the proximal colon of 29% of the 137 patients with diminutive index polyps, 29% of the 52 patients with small index polyps, and 57% of the 14 patients with large index polyps. Advanced neoplasms were detected in 6%, 10%, and 29%, respectively. Two patients with diminutive index polyps had proximal carcinoma in situ. Another 2 in this group had proximal stage I carcinomas. Proximal stage III carcinoma was found in a patient with a large index polyp.

Conclusions.—The prevalence of proximal colonic neoplasms, including advanced lesions, in asymptomatic average-risk patients with rectosigmoid adenomas of 5 mm in diameter or less is substantial. Thus colonoscopy is warranted in these patients.

► The sequence of adenomatous polyp progression to adenocarcinoma represents an established risk factor in patients with polypoid adenomas. Therefore, it is advisable to diagnose by biopsy and to remove preferably by endoscopic polypectomy all polyps regardless of size. Recommendations by the American Cancer Society and the American College of Surgeons indicate a need for screening flexible sigmoidoscopy in asymptomatic, fecal occult blood–negative, average-risk patients older than 50 years. This study establishes the necessity of colonoscopy in patients at average risk who are found on screening to have small (less than 5 mm) adenomatous polyps in the rectosigmoid area. Subsequent colonoscopy in these patients revealed a 29% incidence of proximal neoplasm, nearly 10% of which were advanced. This study presents a clear indication for routine colonoscopy in all patients with adenomas found on flexible sigmoidoscopy. This appears to be a cost-effective method for prevention of a subsequent proximal colon cancer, even in patients with diminutive index polyps in the rectosigmoid area.

B.L. Eisenberg, M.D.

A Prospective Randomized Study of Follow-up After Radical Surgery for Colorectal Cancer

Kjeldsen BJ, Kronborg O, Fenger C, et al (Odense Univ, Denmark)

Br J Surg 84:666–669, 1997 7–33

Objective.—Whether there is a survival benefit from follow-up after curative colorectal cancer surgery is unproven. The possible influence of follow-up on survival was examined in a prospective, randomized study.

Methods.—After radical surgery, 597 patients were randomly allocated to frequent follow-up (group 1, N = 290) or follow-up only at 2 and 5 years (group 2, N = 307). Survival differences were analyzed statistically and Kaplan-Meier curves were calculated.

Results.—Recurrences were detected in 76 group 1 patients and 80 group 2 patients. The disease-free survival period was significantly shorter for group 1 patients than for group 2 patients. In patients followed for more than 5 years, there were 49 recurrences in each group. On average, recurrences in group 1 patients were diagnosed 9 months earlier than

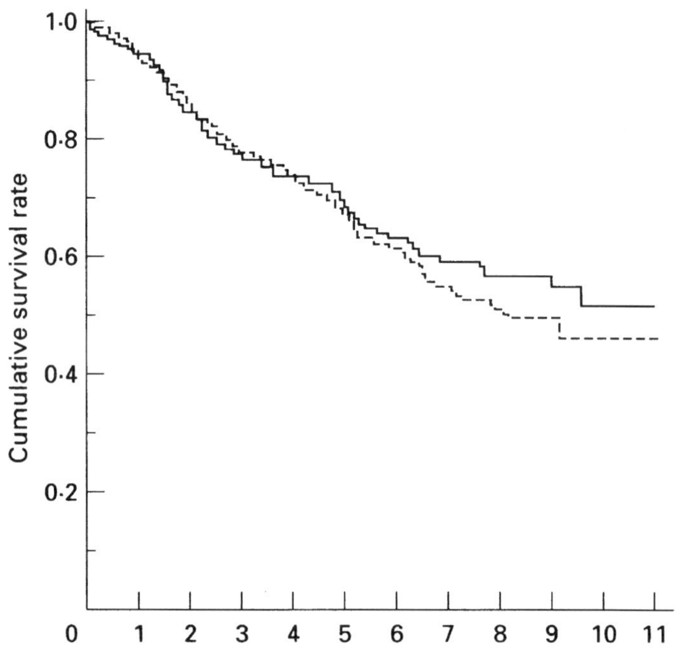

No. at risk						
Group 1	290	203	133	85	43	13
Group 2	307	212	144	78	40	5

FIGURE 3.—Cumulative survival rate in groups 1 (*solid line*) and 2 (*dashed line*). $P = 0.48$ (log rank test). (Courtesy of Kjeldsen BJ, Kronborg O, Fenger C, et al: A prospective randomized study of follow-up after radical surgery for colorectal cancer. *Br J Surg* 84:666–669, 1997. Publisher, Blackwell Science Ltd.)

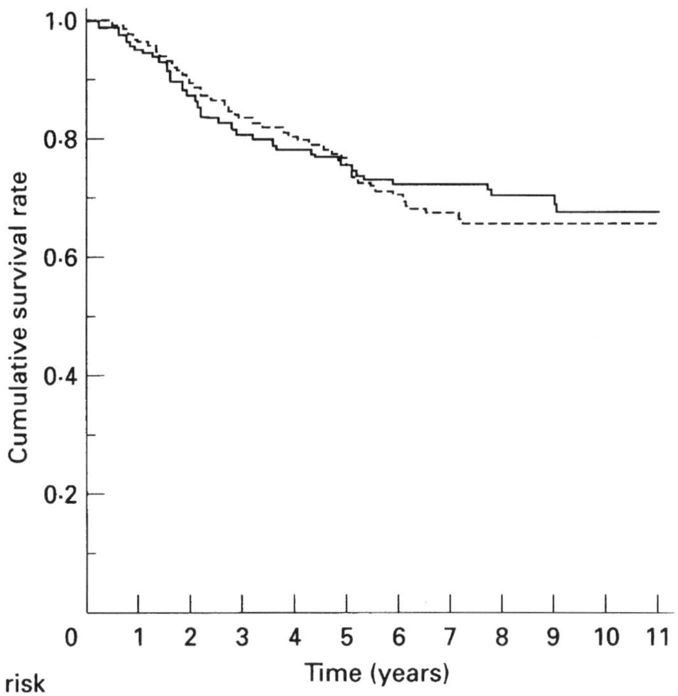

No. at risk						
Group 1	290	203	133	85	43	13
Group 2	307	212	144	78	40	5

FIGURE 4.—Cumulative cancer-related survival rate in groups 1 (*solid line*) and 2 (*dashed line*). P = 0.90 (log rank test). (Patients who died from causes other than colorectal cancer are censored.) Courtesy of Kjeldsen BJ, Kronborg O, Fenger C, et al: A prospective randomized study of follow-up after radical surgery for colorectal cancer. *Br J Surg* 84:666–669, 1997. Publisher, Blackwell Science Ltd.)

recurrences in group 2 patients. More group 1 than group 2 patients had new curative surgery. There was no significant overall survival difference between the groups (Figs 3 and 4).

Conclusion.—Whereas group 1 patients had recurrences diagnosed earlier and underwent new curative surgery more frequently, there was no significant overall survival difference between the groups.

▶ This excellent randomized study attempts to address the question posed in the preceding paper concerning the value of intensive follow-up in patients with a history of colorectal cancer. In a well-controlled, population-based study from Denmark, almost 600 patients underwent randomization over a period of 10 years into intensive vs. nonintensive follow-up evaluation as to whether longer survival would result from an earlier detection for treatment of recurrent, as well as metachronous, colorectal cancer. The findings substantiate the fact that patients in the intensive follow-up group did have earlier detection of recurrent disease and, subsequently, underwent more attempted second-look curative surgery. However, the bottom line in outcomes data evaluating the intensity and duration of follow-up should be survival benefit, and in this study, no survival benefit was demonstrated.

A note of caution should be inserted into the interpretation as the group actually used for statistical analysis was fairly small and the follow-up, although frequent, did not include standard carcinoembryonic antigen determinations or diagnostic imaging studies. The question of standardized paradigms for follow-up in colorectal or any other epithelial cancer still remains subjective and, in many cases, without any valid scientific data. Until such data are conclusively forthcoming, this question of management will be left to individual practices.

B.L. Eisenberg, M.D.

Gastric Carcinoma: Does Lymph Node Dissection Alter Survival?

Wanebo HJ, Kennedy BJ, Winchester DP, et al (Brown Univ, Providence, RI; Univ of Minnesota, Minneapolis; Northwestern Univ, Chicago; et al)

J Am Coll Surg 183:616–624, 1996 7–34

Objective.—Whether extensive regional lymph node dissection improves survival in patients with gastric cancer is controversial. A prospective review of records of 18,346 patients from a gastric cancer study conducted by the American College of Surgeons examined survival in the 10% who had extragastric node dissection.

Methods.—From the 3,804 patients having curative resection and a follow-up of 5 years or longer, outcome in patients having extragastric lymph node dissection was compared with outcome in patients who did not.

Results.—There were 695 patients having dissection of the N2 nodes (hepatic, celiac axis, or splenic nodes), 1,529 having dissection of the N1 nodes (perigastric, gastric, or both), and 677 having no dissection. Whether the remaining 903 patients had nodes removed is not known. Five-year survival rates were 55.3% for stage I disease, 34.3% for stage II, 16.6% for stage III, and 4.3% for stage IV. Five-year survival rates were 26.3% for patients having N2 node dissection, 30% for those having N1 node dissection, and 35.6% for those having no nodal dissection. Patients with stage I disease having N1 or N2 node dissection had improved survival compared with patients having no nodal dissection. There was no significant survival difference between groups for patients with higher stage disease (Table 3). Of patients receiving radiation therapy, those with N1 dissection or no nodal dissection lived longer than those having N2 dissection. Disease-free survival rates at 5 years were 35.5% for N2 dissection, 40.4% for N1 dissection, and 50.6 for no nodal dissection.

Conclusion.—Gastric node dissection appears to have conferred no survival benefit in patients with gastric cancer.

TABLE 3.—Gastrectomy With Curative Intent: Survival by Lymph Node Dissection and Stage

	Lymph node dissection		
Stage	*Perigastric and gastric*	*Hepatic, celiac, and splenic*	*None*
All stages			
Patients, n	1,500	683	666
5-Year survival, percent	30.0	26.3	35.6
Median survival time, mo	24.8	19.7	29.5
p=.001			
Stage I			
Patients, n	326	117	224
5-Year survival, percent	61.1	62.5	47.8
Median survival time, mo	86.4	96	54.1
p=.002			
Stage II			
Patients, n	363	101	141
5-Year survival, percent	37.2	33.5	31.6
Median survival time, mo	34.3	30.3	25.6
p=.075			
Stage III			
Patients, n	552	270	134
5-Year survival, percent	15.8	18.2	20.9
Median survival time, mo	19.8	17.9	17.9
p=.844			
Stage IV			
Patients, n	183	155	56
5-Year survival, percent	3.0	7.0	10.0
Median survival time, mo	8.5	10.5	10.1
p=.849			

Abbreviations: n, number; *mo,* months.
(Courtesy of Wanebo HJ, Kennedy BJ, Winchester DP, et al: Gastric carcinoma: Does lymph node dissection alter survival? *J Am Coll Surg* 183:616–624, 1996. By permission of the *Journal of the American College of Surgeons.*)

Survival Benefit of Extended D2 Resection for Proximal Gastric Cancer

Volpe CM, Driscoll DL, Miloro SM, et al (State Univ of New York, Buffalo)
J Surg Oncol 64:231–236, 1997 7–35

Objective.—The frequency of proximal gastric cancer has increased significantly. It affects 4 times as many men as women. Because it has a poor prognosis, the optimal surgical strategy is still being sought. A retrospective analysis and comparison of the outcomes of patients treated with a standard D1 gastrectomy vs. those treated by en bloc removal of the primary tumor and extended lymph node dissection (D2 gastrectomy) were presented.

Methods.—The records of 62 patients (5 females), aged 33 to 85 years, with gastric cancer were divided into the extended resection group (D2, D2.5) and the limited resection group (D1, D1.5). Kaplan-Meier survival curves were generated for both groups. Prognostic factors were determined using multivariate analysis.

Results.—There were 54 adenocarcinomas. Lymph node metastases were found in 73% of patients. Overall and disease-free survival were

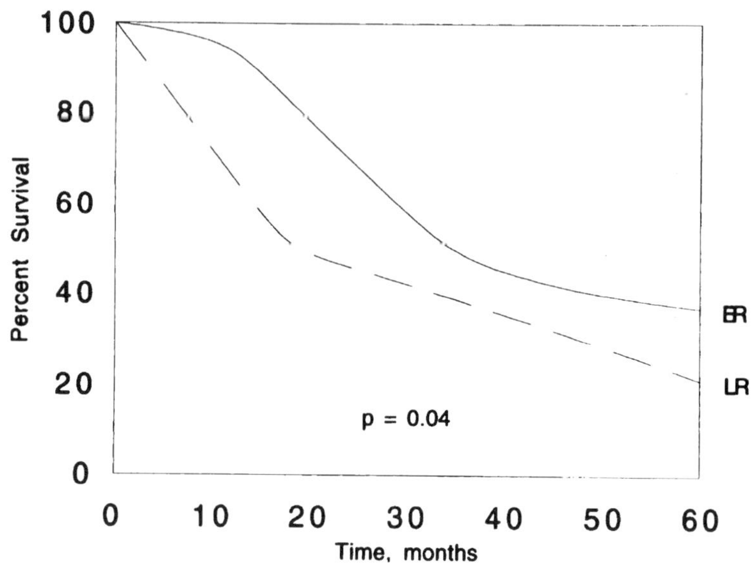

FIGURE 1.—Overall survival rates for the 2 resection groups. The difference in survival between the 2 curves is statistically significant. *Abbreviations: ER*, extended resection; *LR*, limited resection. (Courtesy of Volpe CM, Driscoll DL, Miloro SM, et al: Survival benefit of extended resection for proximal gastric cancer. *J Surg Oncol* 64:231–236, copyright 1997. Reprinted by permission of Wiley-Liss, Inc., a subsidiary of John Wiley & Sons, Inc.)

higher for the extended resection group (Figs 1 and 2). Lymph node status, disease stage, and extent of resection were significant predictors of overall and disease-free survival. After multivariate analysis, only the latter 2 remained as significant predictors of overall and disease-free survival.

Conclusion.—Extended resection appears to be superior as the treatment of choice for proximal gastric cancer.

▶ The extent of the lymphadenectomy performed for operable gastric adenocarcinoma remains an area of controversy. Published reports from areas of the world where gastric cancer is both endemic and epidemic support a radical lymphadenectomy over and above what is normally performed in the United States. The majority of these reports consist of retrospective reviews indicating subsets of patients who will benefit from this approach.

The article by Volpe et al. (Abstract 7–35) suggests a benefit from extended lymph node dissection (D2) for patients with proximal gastric adenocarcinoma. This benefit is manifested in both recurrence-free and overall survival when compared with a group of similar patients undergoing less than a D2 nodal dissection. One must temper an enthusiastic support for this approach, however, as this report represents a retrospective analysis in a nonrandomized patient population and cannot be a reference source for specifically justifing a more radical operative procedure.

The article from the patient care evaluation study conducted by the American College of Surgeons and authored by Wanebo et al. (Abstract 7–34) also

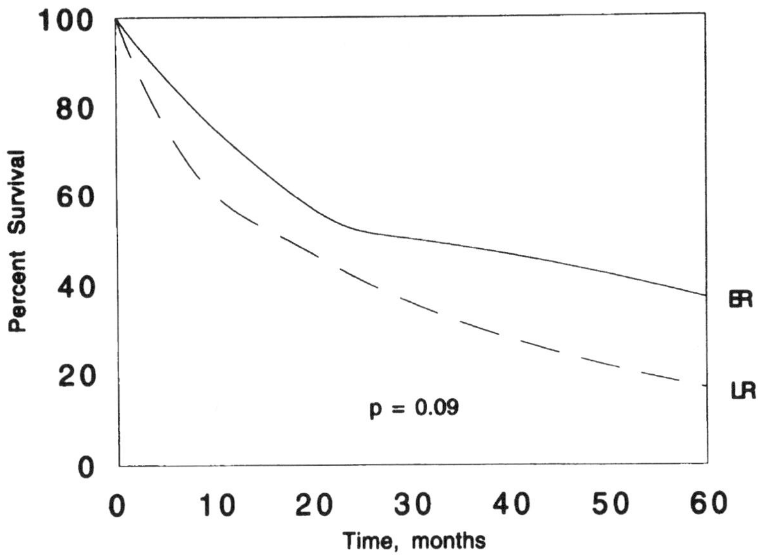

FIGURE 2.—Comparison of disease-free survival between the extended resection (*ER*) group, and the limited resection (*LR*) group. (Courtesy of Volpe CM, Driscoll DL, Miloro SM, et al: Survival benefit of extended resection for proximal gastric cancer. *J Surg Oncol* 64:231–236, copyright 1997. Reprinted by permission of Wiley-Liss, Inc., a subsidiary of John Wiley & Sons, Inc.)

suggests that a subgroup of patients—namely, those with stage I gastric cancer—may benefit from an extended lymphatic dissection. Again, it is clear from reviewing this article that this is a conclusion based on a large patient care study and certainly does not represent a prospective database.

There are several ongoing large, multi-institutional, randomized studies[1, 2] that have not, to date, shown any benefit for a radical lymphadenectomy (D2) as opposed to the standard lymphatic dissection (D1 or even D0). Additional information on this topic may be forthcoming. Until then, no standards of surgical care can be established in this regard.

B.L. Eisenberg, M.D.

References

1. Dent DM, Madden MV, Price SK: Randomized comparison of R1 and R2 gastrectomy for gastric carcinoma. *Br J Surg* 75:110–112, 1988.
2. Bonenkamp JJ, Songun I, Hermans J, et al: Randomised comparison of morbidity after D1 and D2 dissection for gastric cancer in 996 Dutch patients. *Lancet* 345:745–748, 1995.

Recommendations for Follow-up Care of Individuals With an Inherited Predisposition to Cancer: I. Hereditary Nonpolyposis Colon Cancer

Burke W, for the Cancer Genetics Studies Consortium (Univ of Washington, Seattle; Johns Hopkins Univ, Baltimore, Md; Univ of Texas, Houston; et al)

JAMA 277:915–919, 1997 7–36

Introduction.—Many individuals who are genetically susceptible to hereditary nonpolyposis colorectal cancer can now be identified by genetic testing, and they need appropriate counseling about cancer surveillance and follow-up options. A task force of experts in medical genetics, oncology, primary care, gastroenterology, and epidemiology was convened by the Cancer Genetics Studies Consortium, organized by the National Human Genome Research Institute. A search of MEDLINE was conducted, and studies of evaluation of cancer risk, surveillance, and risk reduction in individuals genetically susceptible to colon cancer were identified. Recommendations were developed during a 14-month period.

Recommendations.—The efficacy of cancer surveillance to lower the risk of cancer in genetically susceptible individuals is unknown. It is recommended that individuals with hereditary nonpolyposis colorectal cancer-associated mutations have a colonoscopy every 1–3 years, beginning at age 25 years. Screening for endometrial cancer also is recommended. No recommendations were made regarding prophylactic surgery because of a lack of evidence of clinical benefit. Individuals interested in genetic testing should be advised that the effectiveness of risk reduction measures is unknown. Whenever possible, individuals with cancer-predisposing mutations should receive care within the context of research designed to measure clinical outcome.

Discussion.—Early screening for cancer may reduce access to health insurance and compromise long-term health care. These recommendations are preliminary and controversial, and they do not apply to most individuals with a family history of colon cancer. Such families do not have the characteristics of an autosomal dominant inheritance of cancer predisposition. Members of such families have significantly lower cancer risks than individuals with hereditary nonpolyposis colorectal cancer-associated mutations.

► This article reviews the present information and subsequent recommendations from the National Human Genome Research Institute concerning issues regarding patients with hereditary nonpolyposis colon cancer (HNPCC). It is important to realize that we are at the beginning of the new era in medicine as we define genetic molecular markers of risk for individual patients and inherited familial traits that may predispose to a heightened incidence of malignancy. In this article, it is emphasized that, although patients may fit the strict definition of HNPCC by the Amsterdam Criteria, there is no consensus because of a lack of clinical data that close follow-up screening or prophylactic surgery will prevent the onset of colon cancer. It is logical, however, in identified high-risk patients and particularly in those individuals that carry a specific and documented gene mutation that screening colonoscopy every 1–3 years beginning at an early age, preferably in context with informed consent and counseling, may prevent or decrease the severity of the disease. It is also important to recognize that family members may be predisposed to other cancers such as endometrial carcinoma in the case of HNPCC. The medical community needs to become more aware of the latest information with regard to genetic testing and susceptibility and become a resource to concerned patients seeking advice for treatment and follow-up recommendations.

B.L. Eisenberg, M.D.

Long-term Results of Preoperative Radiation Therapy Alone for Stage T_3 and T_4 Rectal Cancer

Ahmad NR, Nagle D (Thomas Jefferson Univ, Philadelphia)

Br J Surg 84:1445–1448, 1997 7–37

Introduction.—Little information is available regarding the long-term results of preoperative radiotherapy followed by surgery for locally advanced rectal carcinomas. The time course and pattern of failure were assessed for 74 patients with clinical stage T3 or T4 (cT3–4) rectal cancer treated with preoperative radiotherapy for whom long-term follow-up was available.

Methods.—All 74 patients received a median of 45.0 Gy of radiation alone and then surgery 4–8 weeks later. Patients were followed up every 3 months during the first 2 years, every 6 months for the next 3 years, and annually thereafter. The median follow-up was 90 months. Local control, freedom from distant metastasis, and disease-free survival were determined.

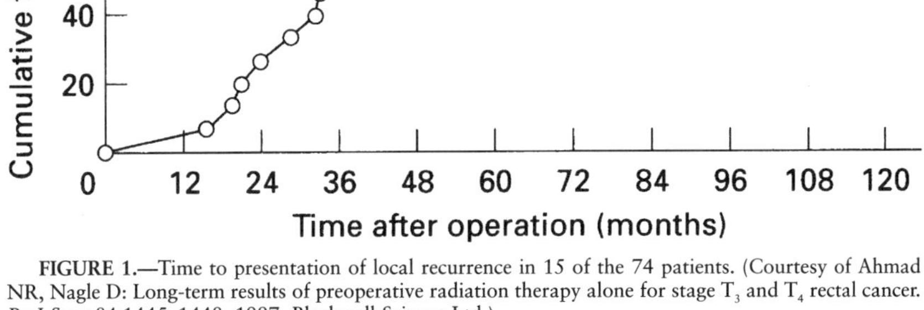

FIGURE 1.—Time to presentation of local recurrence in 15 of the 74 patients. (Courtesy of Ahmad NR, Nagle D: Long-term results of preoperative radiation therapy alone for stage T_3 and T_4 rectal cancer. *Br J Surg* 84:1445–1448, 1997. Blackwell Science Ltd.)

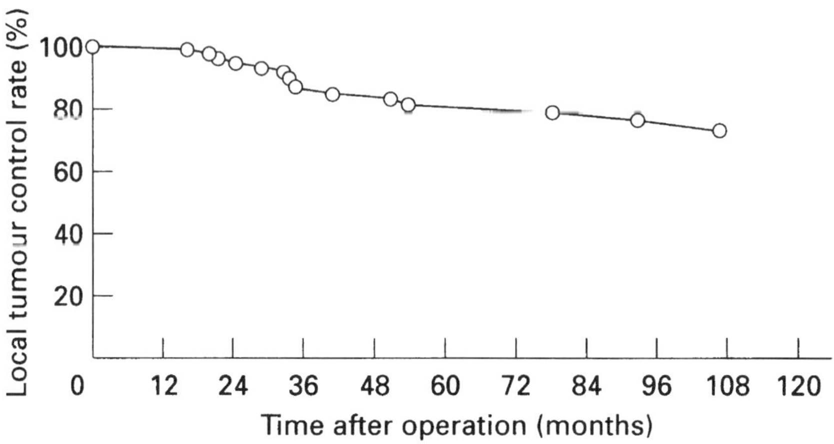

FIGURE 2.—Overall actuarial rate of local tumor control. (Courtesy of Ahmad NR, Nagle D: Long-term results of preoperative radiation therapy alone for stage T_3 and T_4 rectal cancer. *Br J Surg* 84:1445–1448, 1997. Blackwell Science Ltd.)

Results.—Of 74 patients, 3 tumors (4%) were pathologic stage T0 (pT0), 19 (26%) were pT1–2, and 52 (70%) were pT3–4. Involved lymph nodes were detected in 32% of patients. The crude local failure rate was 20% (15 patients), and the median time to local recurrence was 34 months. Eighty percent of local failures were observed within 54 months (Fig 1). The overall 5-year local control rate was 80%; the 10-year rate was 73% (Fig 2). The crude distant failure rate was 42% (31 patients), and the median time to distant metastases was 24 months. Eighty percent of distant metastases were observed within 57 months (Fig 3). The overall actuarial rates for freedom from distant metastases were 64% for 5 years

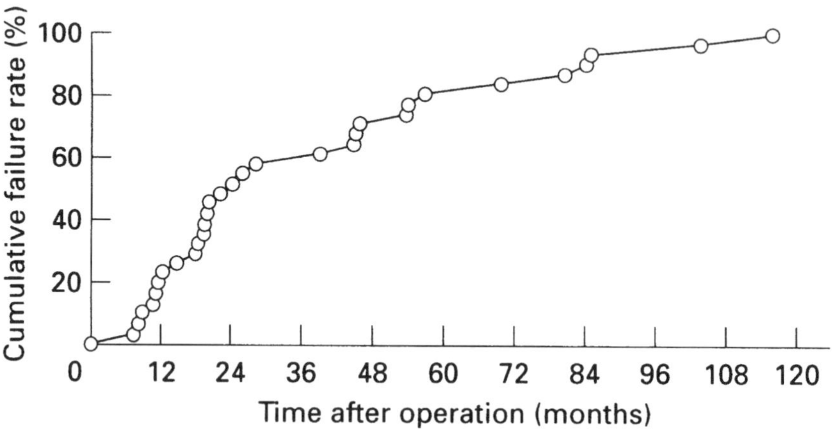

FIGURE 3.—Time to presentation of distant metastases in 31 of the 74 patients. (Courtesy of Ahmad NR, Nagle D: Long-term results of preoperative radiation therapy alone for stage T_3 and T_4 rectal cancer. *Br J Surg* 84:1445–1448, 1997. Blackwell Science Ltd.)

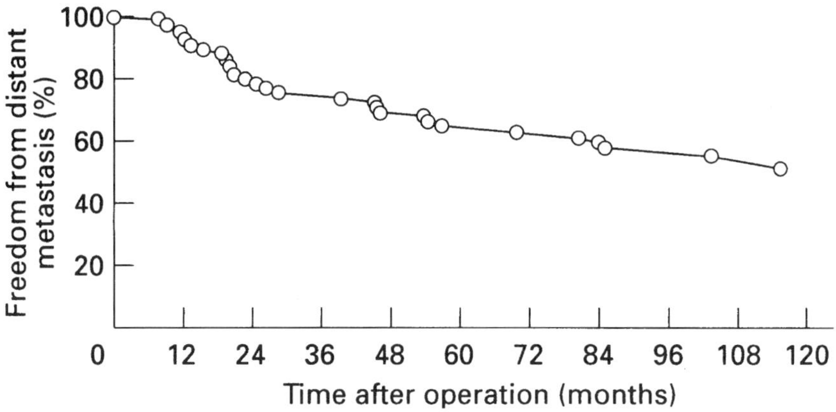

FIGURE 4.—Overall actuarial rate of freedom from distant metastases. (Courtesy of Ahmad NR, Nagle D: Long-term results of preoperative radiation therapy alone for stage T_3 and T_4 rectal cancer. *Br J Surg* 84:1445–1448, 1997. Blackwell Science Ltd.)

and 51% for 10 years (Fig 4). There were no significant differences in the rate of freedom from distant metastases when clinical stage or pathologic N stage were compared (Table 3). There was a trend toward a lower rate of freedom from distant metastases in patients with high pathologic T stage carcinomas.

Conclusion.—The interval to local and distant disease recurrence was prolonged in patients who received preoperative radiotherapy for locally advanced rectal cancer. The high distant failure rate with radiation alone indicates that adjuvant systemic therapy may be worthwhile.

► Clinically advanced rectal cancer is still a major problem. This is a review of 74 locally advanced lesions of the rectum treated with preoperative

TABLE 3.—Actuarial Rates of Freedom From Distant Metastasis

	No. of patients	Rate of freedom from distant metastasis (%) 5 years	10 years
Overall	74	64	51
Clinical tumour stage			
cT_3	44	70	55
cT_4	30	55	42
Pathological tumour stage			
pT_{0-2}	22	85	67
pT_{3-4}	52	55	43*
Pathological node stage			
pN_0	46	70	57
pN^+	24	54	42

**P* < 0.07 (pT3–4 vs. pT0–2, log rank test.

(Courtesy of Ahmad NR, Nagle D: Long-term results of preoperative radiation therapy alone for stage T_3 and T_4 rectal cancer. *Br J Surg* 84:1445–1448, 1997. Blackwell Science Ltd.)

radiotherapy. These patients all received 4,500 rad followed by surgery 1–2 months later.

The 5- and 10-year figures on local control, freedom from metastases, and disease-specific survival are really excellent.

E. Glatstein, M.D.

Mutated *p53* Gene Is an Independent Adverse Predictor of Survival in Colon Carcinoma

Pricolo VE, Finkelstein SD, Hansen K, et al (Rhode Island Hosp, Providence; Brown Univ, Providence, RI)
Arch Surg 132:371–375, 1997 7–38

Introduction.—A complex multistep process occurring through a series of gene mutations is involved in large-bowel tumorigenesis. Varying degrees of biological aggressiveness to colorectal carcinomas may be conferred by the presence of certain genetic alterations. There has been intense investigation into determining a correlation between genetic damage and cancer prognosis. The applicability of a method for genetic mutational analysis—topographic genotyping—was applied to the study of colorectal cancer behavior, which was assessed in terms of stage at diagnosis, pattern of metastatic dissemination, and survival figures. The impact of *p53* gene mutations on long-term survival of patients with colorectal cancer was determined.

Methods.—There were 71 patients with stage II colon carcinoma and 70 with stage III colon carcinoma involved in the mutational analysis. Using amplification and direct sequencing by polymerase chain reaction, archival pathology specimens were analyzed for point mutations of exons from the *p53* gene. The impact of patient survival was assessed by examining *p53* mutations and adverse histopathologic features, such as poor differentiation, lymphovascular invasion, and mucin production.

Results.—For patients with stage II colon carcinoma, the median overall survival was 64 months and for those with stage III disease, it was 34 months. Throughout the follow-up period, the single most important risk factor associated with poorer survival both in patients with stage II and stage III colon carcinoma was the presence of a *p53* mutation. In patients with stage II colon carcinoma, a *p53* mutation increased the risk of death by 2.82 times and in stage III patients, the risk was increased by 2.39 times. An additive effect on the cumulative risk of death between adverse histopathologic variables and *p53* mutations was observed.

Conclusion.—An independent adverse prognostic value in colon cancer is carried by the presence of *p53* mutations. In the future, therapeutic choices are likely to be affected by the applicability of mutational analysis in clinical practice.

► Oncogene mutational events may play an important role in the initiation and clinical activation of gastrointestinal malignancies. Certainly, *p53* mutation and the subsequent effect on cell cycle dynamics and clonal expansion have been studied in colorectal cancer. This paper provides a large series of patients with documented clinical follow-up demonstrating the usefulness of evaluating this molecular marker as an independent prognostic factor. The study is particularly important because it not only evaluates immunohistochemical expression of mutated protein but correlates that finding with direct sequencing for "hot spot" mutations incorporating polymerase chain reaction analysis. These techniques may have wide applicability to solid-tumor genetic risk–profiling for adjuvant trials as well as the development of future interventional therapy.

B.L. Eisenberg, M.D.

8 Adult Leukemia

Case/Control Study of the Role of Splenectomy in Chronic Lymphocytic Leukemia

Seymour JF, Cusack JD, Lerner SA, et al (Royal Melbourne Hosp, Australia; Univ of Texas, Houston)

J Clin Oncol 15:52–60, 1997 8–1

Objective.—Whereas splenectomy is the treatment of choice for patients with advanced chronic lymphocytic leukemia with cytopenia and splenomegaly, definitive evidence of improved survival is lacking or difficult to interpret. Results were presented of a retrospective analysis evaluating the morbidity and mortality of splenectomy in patients with chronic lymphocytic leukemia to determine the probability of hematologic response, the patients most likely to benefit, and the influence of splenectomy on survival.

Methods.—In a study with a case-control format, 55 patients with chronic lymphocytic leukemia underwent splenectomy between October 1971 and September 1993. Factors predictive of survival, age, serum albumin level, sex, hemoglobin level—and, where available, markers of disease severity, number of therapies, and time from diagnosis—were included in the multivariate analysis. Survival was calculated by the Kaplan-Meier method. Survivals were compared using the log-rank test.

Results.—Blood loss and blood product use during splenectomy were modest. Enlarged spleens were found in 96% of patients. Postoperative hospital stays ranged from 6 to 39 days. Perioperative complications included minor wound or urinary tract infections in 10 patients, pneumonia or basal atelectasis in 14, septicemia in 3, and intestinal perforation in 2. All 5 patients who died of septic complications had a perioperative performance status of 2 or greater. Spleen weight was a significant predictor of low hemoglobin and neutrophil levels. The 30-day mortality rate was similar for patients and controls. There was no significant difference in duration of survival of patients and controls. There was a trend toward increased survival in splenectomized patients with Rai stage IV disease.

Conclusion.—Morbidity and mortality are modest after splenectomy in patients with advanced chronic lymphocytic leukemia. Whereas splenectomized patients experience significant improvements in hemoglobin and neutrophil levels, survival is not increased compared with that of control patients. Splenectomized patients with Rai stage IV disease tend to have increased survival.

▶ This retrospective analysis is of importance because the role of splenectomy in patients with chronic lymphocytic leukemia has not been recently revisited. Furthermore, this study represents a relatively large cohort of patients (55) and compares the results with those achieved with fludarabine-treated patients. This study shows that splenectomy can be performed with only minimal morbidity, mortality, and resource utilization in patients with advanced chronic lymphocytic leukemia and significant pancytopenia. Most patients had significant hematologic benefits, and the degree of improvement correlated with spleen weight. Importantly, splenectomy done for symptomatic management had no detrimental impact on survival compared with the control population. Although many physicians do not often consider splenectomy anymore for chronic lymphocytic leukemia, this report revisits that approach.

M.S. Tallman, M.D.

International Scoring System for Evaluating Prognosis in Myelodysplastic Syndromes

Greenberg P, Cox C, LeBeau MM, et al (Stanford Univ, Calif; Rochester Med Ctr, NY; Univ of Chicago; et al)

Blood 89:2079–2088, 1997 8–2

Introduction.—Many different scoring systems have been used to evaluate prognosis in patients with myelodysplastic syndrome (MDS). However, these systems continue to be imprecise, with variable sensitivity and specificity. The International MDS Risk Analysis Workshop was held in an attempt to develop a consensus prognostic risk-based analysis system. The development of the International Prognostic Scoring System (IPSS) for MDS was reported.

Methods.—Cytogenetic, morphologic, and clinical data were analyzed from 7 large, risk-based studies that had previously been used to generate prognostic systems for MDS. The study included data on 816 patients with primary MDS, including 759 who were analyzed for acute myeloid leukemia (AML) evolution. The critical prognostic variables from these patients were analyzed to develop a consensus prognostic system, one that used a more refined bone marrow cytogenetic classification. The performance of the IPSS was compared with that of previous classification methods.

Results.—On univariate analysis, the main factors affecting evolution to AML were cytogenetic abnormalities, percentage of myoblasts in bone marrow, and number of cytopenias. In addition to these, age and sex also had a significant impact on survival. In terms of cytogenetic abnormalities, outcomes were good for patients with normal, −Y alone, del(5q) alone, and del(20q) alone patterns; poor for those with 3 or more abnormalities or anomalies of chromosome 7; and intermediate for those with other abnormalities.

The IPSS model was generated by combining these genetic subgroups with percentage of bone marrow blasts and number of cytopenias by multivariate analysis. Weighted by statistical power, the variables were able to identify distinct risk subgroups, defined by the time needed for 25% of patients to undergo evolution to AML: low risk, 31% of patients, 9.4 years; intermediate-1 (INT-1) risk, 39% of patients, 3.3 years; intermediate-2 (INT-2) risk, 22% of patients, 1.1 years; and high risk, 8% of patients, 0.2 year. Median survival was 5.7 years for the low-risk group, 3.5 years for the INT-1 group, 1.2 years for the INT-2 group, and 0.4 years for the high-risk group. Survival analysis was further improved by stratification for age.

Conclusions.—The IPSS system identifies key prognostic features, emphasizes the importance of stratification by age, and improves the ability to evaluate prognosis in MDS, compared with previously reported risk-based classifications. Use of the IPSS will aid in the design and interpretation of treatment trials for MDS.

► The IPSS collates a large amount of data from a large group of patients with primary MDS. It is important because of the large number of patients studied. Patients with refractory anemia and refractory anemia with ringed sideroblasts clearly have a significantly more favorable survival and significantly decreased risk for evolution to AML. This scoring system emphasizes the importance of cytogenetic subtypes with respect to both overall survival and risk of evolution to AML. These issues will only continue to become more important as new agents, including amifostine and topotecan, are available for the treatment of patients with MDS.

M.S. Tallman, M.D.

Major Activity of Cladribine in Patients With De Novo B-Cell Prolymphocytic Leukemia

Saven A, Lee T, Schlutz M, et al (Scripps Clinic and Research Found, La Jolla, Calif; Hoag Cancer Ctr, Newport Beach, Calif; Virginia Mason Med Ctr, Seattle)

J Clin Oncol 15:37–43, 1997 8–3

Introduction.—De novo B-cell prolymphocytic leukemia (B-PLL) is a distinct clinicopathologic entity distinguished by marked lymphocytosis, massive splenomegaly, an aggressive course, and a poor prognosis. Cladribine (2-chlorodeoxyadenosine [2–CdA]) is a new purine analogue that exhibits potent activity in the treatment of indolent lymphoproliferative diseases. The response to cladribine is reported in 8 patients with de novo B-PLL.

Methods.—Patients were treated with 0.1 mg/kg/day cladribine for 7 days by continuous infusion or with 0.14 mg/kg/day infused over 2 hours for 5 days. A median of 3 courses was administered every 28–35 days until the maximum response or prohibitive toxicity occurred. Peripheral blood and bone marrow aspirates were evaluated before and after treatment to determine the toxicity and the response.

Results.—Five patients achieved a complete response (CR). The median duration of a CR was 14 months. Two of 4 patients with a CR in whom peripheral blood immunophenotypic analysis was performed had no circulating B-PLL cells, and 1 had no residual disease on Southern blot analysis. Three patients had grade 3 or 4 myelosuppression, 4 patients had bacterial infections, and 2 had herpes zoster infections.

Conclusion.—Cladribine was highly effective and had a favorable toxicity profile in this small series of patients with de novo B-PLL. Larger investigations are needed to determine the efficacy, toxicity, and potential beneficial effects on survival.

▶ Although the number of patients in this study is small, the authors report an excellent response rate for a particularly aggressive lymphoproliferative disorder, prolymphocytic leukemia. These observations are particularly important because the disease does not respond well to chemotherapy with conventional alkylating agents. The major toxic effects were the same as those seen with alkylating agents and other purine analogues and included myelosuppression and infection. Nevertheless, 5 of 8 patients achieved a CR, and the median response rate was 14 months; these are remarkable observations that will need confirmation in larger studies.

M.S. Tallman, M.D.

Hepatosplenic Candidiasis in Patients With Acute Leukemia: Incidence and Prognostic Implications

Anttila V-J, Elonen E, Nordling S, et al (Helsinki Univ Central Hosp; Univ of Helsinki)

Clin Infect Dis 24:375–380, 1997 8–4

Introduction.—Hepatosplenic candidiasis, a distinct form of invasive candidiasis seen in patients with acute leukemia, appears to be increasing in incidence. Questions remain about the incidence of hepatosplenic candidiasis and its associated mortality. The incidence among, risk factors for, and survival of adult patients with acute leukemia and hepatosplenic candidiasis during a 14-year period were reviewed.

Patients.—A total of 562 adult patients with leukemia treated at a tertiary care hospital between 1980 and 1993 were studied. The incidence of hepatosplenic candidiasis was approximately 7%. The affected patients were 20 males and 18 females, with a mean age of 46 years. Patients with acute myeloid leukemia were less likely to be affected than those with acute lymphatic leukemia (5% vs. 11%). The annual incidence of infection increased fivefold during the experience. The patients survived for a median of 9.5 months. Twenty-six percent were alive at the end of follow-up.

Findings.—Survival was better for patients whose leukemia was in remission before receiving their last cytotoxic treatment before the development of hepatosplenic candidiasis than for those with newly diagnosed, refractory, or relapsed leukemia. Of 11 patients who died within 3 months after the diagnosis of infection, all were found to have infection at autopsy.

Conclusions.—A significant increase in the incidence of leukemia-associated hepatosplenic candidiasis has occurred since this entity was first recognized in the early 1980s. The outcome of hepatosplenic candidiasis is linked to the stage of the patient's leukemia. Mortality is lower for patients whose leukemia is in remission when the infection develops. More effective preventive and therapeutic antifungal treatments for hepatosplenic candidiasis are needed.

▶ Patients receiving antileukemic chemotherapy are at significant risk for the development of fungal infections, including hepatosplenic candidiasis. This paper is useful because a large number of patients were studied. Several interesting observations were made during the study, including the fact that almost 7% of patients had hepatosplenic candidiasis develop, and that its incidence was twice as high among patients with acute lymphoid leukemia than among those with acute myeloid leukemia. Not unexpectedly, patients whose last cytotoxic chemotherapy preceded the development of hepatosplenic candidiasis faired better with respect to overall survival than did patients with newly diagnosed, refractory, or relapsed leukemia. Unfortunately, the fatality rate from hepatosplenic candidiasis remains relatively high. It can be helped with new and improved antifungal medications including, perhaps, liposomal amphotericin.

M.S. Tallman, M.D.

A Pilot Study of All-*Trans* Retinoic Acid in Patients With Philadelphia Chromosome-Positive Chronic Myelogenous Leukemia

Cortes J, Kantarjian H, O'Brien S, et al (Univ of Texas, Houston)
Leukemia 11:929–932, 1997 8–5

Background.—Retinoids have been shown to inhibit clonal growth in acute myeloid leukemia. This clinical study investigates the effect of single-agent therapy retinoids on Ph-positive chronic myelogenous leukemia (CML).

Method.—The 13 patients studied exhibited chronic phase CML diagnosed more than 1 year before the study began. These patients were resistant to IFN-alpha therapy. Patients were in the chronic, accelerated, and blastic phases of the disease (N = 7, 5, 1 respectively). Patients were required to stop other forms of therapy 2 weeks before beginning retinoid therapy. All patients had been treated extensively before participating in this study. Patients were treated with 175mg/m^2 of all-*trans* retinoic acid (ATRA) divided into 2 doses per day. This treatment continued until drug toxicity or disease progression became evident. Therapy continued for a median of 56 days (11 to 190).

Results.—All but 1 late chronic patient showed no response to therapy. This patient showed a decrease in white blood cell count. But, the effect was transient. One patient was removed from therapy because of toxicity. Eighty percent (n = 4) of accelerated phase patients showed some antileukemic effect. They had a decrease in blasts in the bone marrow and blood and showed favorable basophil or promyelocyte ratios. This response was transient. The blastic phase patient did not show any improvement.

Conclusion.—ATRA as a single-agent therapy is not an adequate treatment for advanced stage Ph-positive CML. Even so, the antileukemic effect recorded by other studies deserves further investigation and might be used in combination with other therapies for advanced CML.

▶ Given the remarkable advance in the treatment of patients with acute promyelocytic leukemia with all-*trans* retinoic acid, it is of considerable interest to determine if this differentiating agent has effects in patients with other hematologic malignancies. Therefore, this study of 13 patients with Philadelphia chromosome-positive chronic myeloid leukemia warrants attention, because 4 of the 5 patients in accelerated phase had some evidence of antileukemic effect, as indicated by a decrease in the number of bone marrow or peripheral blood blasts, promyelocyte, and basophil percentages. The dose of all-*trans* retinoic acid was quite high at 175 mg/m^2 given daily, and it is of interest that this was relatively well tolerated. Therefore, it may be worth pursuing this differentiating agent, perhaps in combination with other differentiating agents, chemotherapy, or biological response modifiers.

M.S. Tallman, M.D.

Intensive Postremission Chemotherapy Without Maintenance Therapy in Adults With Acute Lymphoblastic Leukemia

Dekker AW, for the Dutch Hemato-Oncology Research Group (Univ Hosp Utrecht, The Netherlands; Dr Daniel den Hoed Cancer Ctr, Rotterdam, The Netherlands; Leyenburg Hosp, The Hague; et al)

J Clin Oncol 15:476–482, 1997 8–6

Objective.—Recent years have seen no improvement in the results of treatment for adult acute lymphoblastic leukemia (ALL). It has been suggested that intensive consolidation or intensification therapy may be beneficial, but the best approach to treatment for patients who go into remission is unclear. The results of intensive consolidation therapy without maintenance therapy were examined in adults with ALL.

Methods.—The phase II, Dutch Hemato-Oncology Group trial included 130 adult patients with ALL, aged 16–60 years. All received standard induction therapy. This was followed by postinduction chemotherapy, consisting of 3 courses of high-dose cytarabine, 2,000 mg/m^2 every 12

hours for 4 doses, combined with amsacrine in course 1, mitoxantrone in course 2, and etoposide in course 3. For CNS prophylaxis, the patients received 10 injections of intrathecal methotrexate. Allogeneic bone marrow transplantation was considered for patients younger than 50 years who had an HLA-identical sibling. However, no maintenance therapy was given.

Results.—The complete remission rate was 73% overall, 82% in patients younger than 50 years and 41% in those older than 50 years. Chemotherapy resistance was encountered in 13% of patients, and mortality during induction therapy was 14%. The only factors significantly associated with response to induction chemotherapy were age and performance status. Four patients died while receiving consolidation therapy. Overall survival at 5 years was estimated at 22% overall and 26% for patients younger than 35 years. Five-year disease-free survival was 28% for patients younger than 35 years, 25% for those aged 35–50 years, and 0% for those older than 50 years. Older age and CD34 expression were adverse prognostic factors. The rate of isolated CNS relapse was just 3%.

Conclusions.—The outcomes of intensive consolidation therapy without maintenance therapy for adult patients with ALL do not compare favorably with those of studies using long-term maintenance therapy. The use of high-dose cytarabine, combined with intrathecal methotrexate, does appear effective in preventing CNS relapse. However, high-dose cytarabine is not an adequate substitute for prolonged postremission maintenance therapy.

▶ The treatment of adults with ALL remains problematic. The current therapeutic approach involves several phases of treatment including the maintenance phase, modeled after a successful approach for children with this disease. The disappointing results suggest what others have found, namely that maintenance therapy appears to be important in the treatment of adults with ALL. Although high-dose cytarabine may contribute to the prevention of CNS disease, it does not appear to be an acceptable substitute for prolonged maintenance therapy.

M.S. Tallman, M.D.

Extramedullary Leukemia Adversely Affects Hematologic Complete Remission Rate and Overall Survival in Patients With t(8;21) (q22;q22): Results From Cancer and Leukemia Group B 8461

Byrd JC, Weiss RB, Arthur DC, et al (Cancer and Leukemia Group B, Chicago; Roswell Park Cancer Inst, Buffalo, NY; Walter Reed Army Med Ctr, Washington, DC)

J Clin Oncol 15:466–475, 1997 8–7

Objective.—Some patients with acute myeloid leukemia (AML) have extramedullary involvement (EML). The t(8;21)(q22;q22) translocation is a major cytogenetic risk factor for EML. There are conflicting reports about the prognostic significance of this translocation. The outcomes of patients with the t(8;21)(q22;q22) karyotype and EML at presentation were studied.

Methods.—The analysis included 1,454 consecutive patients entered into Cancer and Leukemia Group B trials of therapy for de novo AML. Of these, 84 patients were found to have the t(8;21)(q22;q22) karyotype. These patients were examined for evidence of EML, including granulocytic sarcomas, subcutaneous nodules, leukemia cutis, and meningeal leukemia. The investigators analyzed the clinical characteristics and outcomes of those patients with t(8;21)(q22;q22) who did and did not have EML.

Results.—Eight of 84 patients with t(8;21)(q22;q22) had EML. The manifestation of EML occurred as granulocytic sarcomas (mainly paraspinal) in 7 patients and symptomatic meningeal leukemia in 1. There was no difference in baseline variables for patients with and without EML. Fifty percent of patients with t(8;21)(q22;q22) and EML achieved complete hematologic remission (CR) compared with 92% of patients without EML. The median duration of CR was 15 months for patients with EML vs. 38 months for those without. The median survival time was 5 months for those with EML vs. 60 months for those without EML. The short survival time of patients with EML may have been related to inadequate local therapy (i.e., radiotherapy or intrathecal therapy). This lack led to residual or recurrent EML after induction chemotherapy or at relapse in 3 patients and to irreversible neurologic deficits in 4. There was 1 patient with EML who received high-dose cytarabine intensification, and this was the only patient with EML who was alive and in CR.

Conclusions.—The remission and survival rates are reduced for patients with AML with the t(8;21)(q22;q22) translocation and EML. These patients should be considered for aggressive local and induction chemotherapy. Additional research is needed to determine the efficacy of cytarabine intensification in this patient subgroup.

► Patients with AML (French-American-British classification M2) with an associated t(8;21) translocation are thought to have a relatively favorable prognosis. However, a subgroup of such patients appears to have a proclivity for granulocytic sarcomas. This retrospective study confirms that patients with this subtype of AML with EML have inferior outcomes, that is, poor effective CR and overall survival rates. The mechanisms by which EML develops in these patients and the optimal therapeutic approach will require further study.

M.S. Tallman, M.D.

Long-term Survival and Development of Secondary Malignancies in Patients With Acute Myeloid Leukemia Treated With Aclarubicin or Daunorubicin Plus Cytosine Arabinoside Followed by Intensive Consolidation Chemotherapy in a Danish National Phase III Trial

de Nully Brown P, for the Danish Society of Haematology Study Group on AML (Univ Hosp Rigshopitalet, Copenhagen; Aarhus Univ Hosp, Denmark; Odense Univ Hosp, Denmark; et al)

Leukemia 11:37–41, 1997 8–8

Background.—Anthracycline and cytosine arabinoside (ara-C) induction therapy produces a high rate of complete remission in adults with acute myeloid leukemia (AML). However, even with intensive consolidation therapy, the relapse rate is high. The authors previously reported the results of a randomized, phase 3 trial of a new treatment approach for *de novo* AML: ara-C combined with daunorubicin (DNR) or aclarubicin (ACR) in a 3 + 7 regimen as induction therapy, followed by early intensive consolidation therapy with 2 alternating cycles of high-dose ara-C and 2 cycles of amsacrine plus etoposide, and then 3 days of daunomycin plus 7 days of ara-C. Long-term follow-up data on this approach were reported.

Methods.—A total of 174 patients, aged 17–65 years, with *de novo* AML were studied. All surviving patients were followed up for a minimum of 7 years. The results were evaluated in terms of long-term survival and risk of secondary neoplasms.

Results.—Overall survival was 23% at 5 years and 19% at 10 years, with no significant survival difference between the DNR or ACR regimens. Ninety-nine patients went into complete remission after 1 or 2 courses of induction chemotherapy, with survival of 35% at 5 years and 31% at 10 years. Five-year survival was 57% for patients younger than 40 years vs. 27% for those aged 40–60 years. The standardized incidence ratio of secondary neoplasms was 3.41. Four of these 7 neoplasms were diagnosed at the same time as AML or shortly thereafter, and thus were unrelated to the AML chemotherapy. The remaining 3 secondary neoplasms were not significantly more than expected, with a standardized incidence ratio of 1.46.

Conclusions.—At 5 years, more than 20% of patients with AML treated with ara-C–based induction chemotherapy followed by early, intensive consolidation chemotherapy are alive and in complete remission; such patients have a very good chance of surviving for the next 5 years as well. This intensive chemotherapy regimen does not appear to cause any increased risk of solid tumors; however, patients with AML do seem to be at increased risk of simultaneously diagnosed solid tumors.

► As more patients survive after intensive chemotherapy for a variety of malignant diseases, the risks of secondary malignancy are important to identify. In this report of 174 patients with previously untreated AML, 7 secondary neoplasms were identified. Four of these cases were diagnosed simultaneously at or shortly after diagnosis of AML and were clearly unrelated. The 3 malignancies that developed after AML was diagnosed were not more than would be expected based on the patient population. Therefore, it appears that there is no significant risk for second malignancies with antileukemic chemotherapy that includes an anthracycline and cytarabine.

M.S. Tallman, M.D.

9 Adult Lymphoma

CHOP Is the Standard Regimen in Patients $\geq$ 70 Years of Age With Intermediate-grade and High-grade Non-Hodgkin's Lymphoma: Results of a Randomized Study of the European Organization for Research and Treatment of Cancer Lymphoma Cooperative Study Group

Tirelli U, Errante D, Van Glabbeke M, et al (Division of Med Oncology and AIDS, Aviano, Italy; Aviano Cancer Ctr, Italy; Gen Hosp, Ravenna, Italy, et al)

J Clin Oncol 16:27–34, 1998 9–1

Introduction.—Age is the most significant prognostic factor independently related to poor survival in patients with intermediate- and high-grade non-Hodgkin's lymphoma (NHL). There is a significantly higher incidence of severe and moderate toxicity in elderly patients who receive intensive chemotherapy regimens at standard doses used in younger patients. Treatment-related deaths occur in 37% of older adults undergoing the cyclophosphamide, doxorubicin, vincristine, and prednisone (CHOP) regimen. Reported were results of a randomized trial in which the general clinical condition and performance status of elderly patients was used to devise a chemotherapy regimen.

Methods.—Patients 70 years of age or older with stage II, III, or IV intermediate- and high-grade NHL with Eastern Cooperative Oncology Group performance status less than 4 and acceptable cardiac, renal, and liver status were randomized to receive 6 courses of either mitoxantrone, etoposide, and prednisone (VMP) or CHOP. Doses were adjusted according to performance status and the general condition of each patient. Patients were followed for response and survival.

Results.—The median patient age was 75 years. The overall response rate for CHOP was significantly better than for VMP (50% vs. 77%). The complete response rates were borderline significant: CHOP, 45% and VMP, 27%. Progression-free survival rates at 2 years were 55% and 25%, respectively, for CHOP and VMP. Patients receiving the CHOP regimen had significantly more alopecia and neurologic and gastrointestinal toxicities than patients receiving VMP.

Conclusion.—Even with decreased dosage, CHOP is the treatment of choice in patients older than 70 years with stages II to IV intermediate- and high-grade NHL. Using a careful and patient-oriented approach in elderly patients can yield a good complete response rate and acceptable toxicity.

► The treatment of older adults with intermediate-grade and high-grade NHL remains controversial. This is generally attributable to reduced tolerance to intensive chemotherapy. The results of this study are important because they continue to support the general principle that CHOP chemotherapy is the standard approach for patients 70 years of age and older with advanced intermediate- or high-grade lymphoma. An additional important observation in this study is the fact that the more favorable outcome of patients treated with CHOP held to patients with good, as well as poor, performance status. Therefore, even in the latter patient population, CHOP remains the gold standard with which new approaches should be compared.

M.S. Tallman, M.D.

Mantle Cell Lymphoma: A Clinicopathologic Study of 80 Cases

Argatoff LH, Connors JM, Klasa RJ, et al (Univ of British Columbia, Vancouver)

Blood 89:2067–2078, 1997 9–2

Introduction.—Mantle cell lymphoma (MCL) accounts for approximately 5% of cases of malignant lymphomas. Although it is recognized as a distinct entity, there are limited data on the clinical and pathologic characteristics of this tumor. A 7-year clinicopathologic review of MCL is presented.

Methods.—The retrospective study included 80 cases of MCL seen at 1 Canadian cancer referral center. The clinical and histologic findings were reviewed to identify prognostically significant factors.

Findings.—Seventy percent of patients were men, and 88% had advanced disease; the mean age was 63 years. The patients survived for a median of 43 months. The only clinical factor with a significant effect on prognosis was performance status.

On histologic examination, none of the tumors showed proliferative centers. A few cases with diffuse architecture had occasional compressed germinal centers, but these lacked a normal mantle zone (MZ). The architecture was classified as diffuse in 78% of cases, "nodular" in 16%, and MZ zone in 6%. The nodular cases were those with well-defined nodularity but no significant MZ pattern. If the pattern was mixed, the case was assigned to the pattern occupying more than 50% of the cross-sectional area of all sections available for review. Five cases had so many blastic cells that it was difficult to distinguish MCL from lymphoblastic lymphoma. The survival rate was not significantly different for cases that had some degree of transformation but that were not truly blastic. However, outcome was poor for patients with more than 20 mitotic figures per high-powered field. Twenty-seven of 69 cases analyzed had peripheral blood (PB) involvement by lymphoma cells. The typical pattern was a polymorphous mixture of small, medium, and large lymphocytes. The major cell type had a slightly irregular nucleus with fine chromatin, a small nucleolus, and a thin rim of gray-blue cytoplasm. There were also some cells with a morphological picture similar to that of small cleaved cells or chronic lymphocytic leukemia cells and some immature cells with L1 and L2 lymphoblast-like morphological characteristics. Some patients with PB involvement did not have an elevated lymphocyte count. Patients with a leukemic presentation had a significantly reduced survival rate.

On bone marrow biopsy, lymphomatous infiltration was found mainly in an interstitial or intertrabecular location. This infiltrate could be arranged in nodular aggregates and/or diffuse infiltrates. The cellular morphological findings were very close to those of MCL in lymph nodes, without large transformed cells and proliferative centers. Bone marrow involvement was positive in 50 cases, not evident in 25 cases, and unknown in 5. There were no significant differences in outcome between these groups. The overall survival rate tended to be shorter for patients with heavy MCL involvement. Immunophenotyping by flow cytometry disclosed a characteristic pattern.

Conclusions.—In this clinicopathologic review of MCL, factors associated with a poor prognosis include increased mitotic activity, blastic morphological features, and PB involvement at presentation. The criteria for a true MZ pattern in this tumor are undefined and variable between observers. This study permits no conclusions about the effectiveness of different treatments because none of the treatment groups did well.

▶ This paper is important because it describes the characteristics of a relatively uncommon but aggressive form of MCL. Prognostically important factors include increased mitotic activity, blastic morphologic characteristics, and PB involvement in the diagnosis. Unlike the diagnosis of diffuse large cell lymphoma, the diagnosis of MCL was not significantly influenced by age, stage, lactate dehydrogenase level, or extranodal involvement. This study emphasizes the importance of recognizing this histologic subtype of lymphoma because the standard clinical indicators of prognosis have little influence on outcome and the general outlook is unfavorable. Novel approaches to this disease are needed.

M.S. Tallman, M.D.

Marginal Zone B Cell Lymphoma of the Parotid Glands: Results of a Randomised Trial Comparing Radiotherapy to Combined Therapy

Avilés A, Delgado S, Huerta-Guzmán J (Natl Med Ctr, México City)

Eur J Cancer 32B:420–422, 1996 9–3

Background.—Monocytoid B-cell lymphoma, a well-recognized clinicopathologic entity characterized by monocytoid B cells, has recently been allocated to the low-grade malignant lymphoma group as marginal zone B-cell lymphoma (MZBCL). Reported were the findings of a prospective

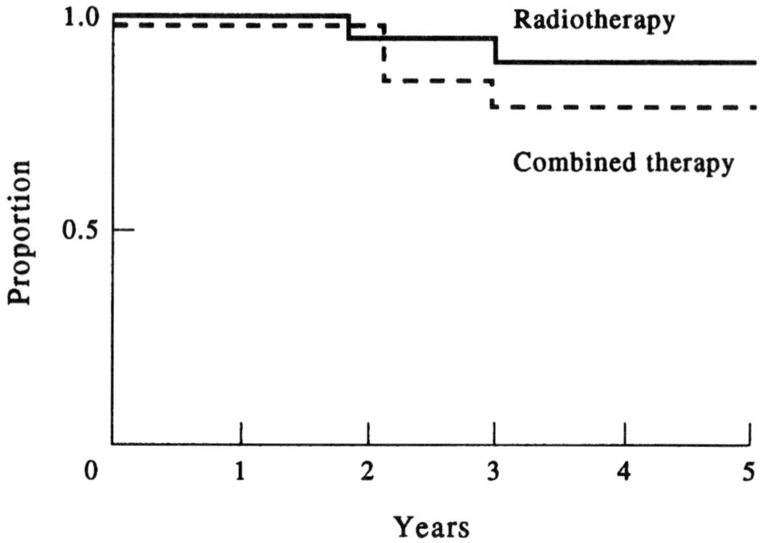

FIGURE 1.—Actuarial duration of time to treatment failure. (Reprinted from *Eur J Cancer* 32B, courtesy of Avilés A, Delgado S, Huerta-Guzmán J: Marginal zone B cell lymphoma of the parotid glands: Results of a randomised trial comparing radiotherapy to combined therapy, pp 420–422, copyright 1996, with kind permission from Elsevier Science Ltd, The Boulevard, Langford Lane, Kidlington 0X5 1GB, UK.)

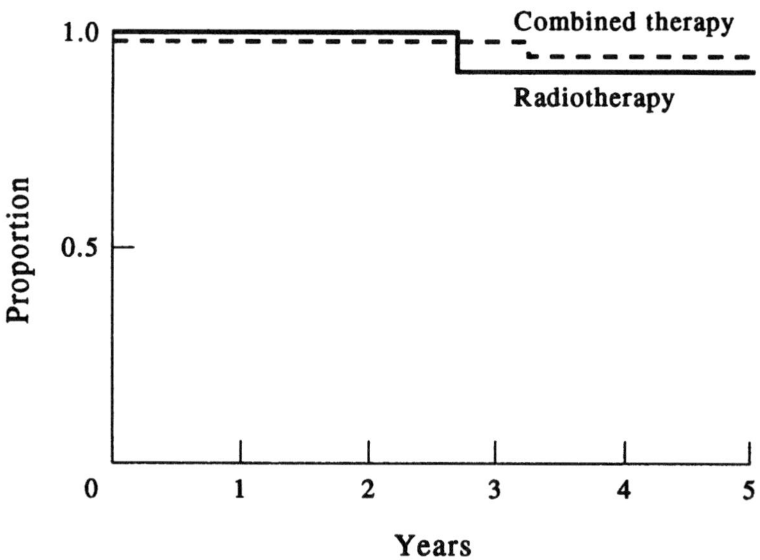

FIGURE 2.—Overall survival. (Reprinted from *Eur J Cancer* 32B, courtesy of Avilés A, Delgado S, Huerta-Guzmán J: Marginal zone B cell lymphoma of the parotid glands: Results of a randomised trial comparing radiotherapy to combined therapy, pp 420–422, copyright 1996, with kind permission from Elsevier Science Ltd, The Boulevard, Langford Lane, Kidlington 0X5 1GB, UK.)

clinical trial involving a small group of patients with MZBCL localized to the parotid glands (stage I) or adjacent lymph nodes (stage II) treated with radiotherapy alone or with combined therapy.

Methods.—Thirty-nine patients were assigned randomly to radiotherapy with extended fields, 4,500 Gy, alone or combined with a chemotherapeutic regimen of cyclophosphamide, vincristine, and prednisone.

Findings.—The complete remission rate was 100% in both groups. Time to treatment failure was 90% and 80% respectively at 5 years in patients given radiotherapy alone and in those given combined treatment. Overall 5-year survival rates were 90% and 95%, respectively. None of these differences were significant (Figs 1 and 2).

Conclusion.—Although these patients tolerated adjuvant chemotherapy well, its use in the initial treatment of early-stage MZBCL offered no advantages over radiotherapy alone. Radiotherapy continues to be the best strategy for treating such patients.

► This paper evaluates 39 patients who had MZBCL of the parotid gland(s). Patients received either radiation therapy alone or radiation therapy plus adjuvant chemotherapy with cyclophosphamide, vincristine, and prednisone. The treatment was randomized. The survival and time to relapse were excellent in both arms of the study. It is said in this paper that patients with MZBCL have better outcomes than patients with mucosa-associated lymphoid tissue (MALT) lymphomas. If the MALT lymphomas are really restricted to small lymphocytic lesions, the type that used to be categorized as "pseudolymphomas," I am not sure I agree with that at all. The authors have identified the syndrome of lymphoma with indolent B-cell characteristics for which chemotherapy has added nothing of a curative nature as yet.

E. Glatstein, M.D.

Cutaneous Histopathology of Sézary Syndrome: A Study of 41 Cases With a Proven Circulating T-Cell Clone

Trotter MJ, Whittaker SJ, Orchard GE, et al (Univ of British Columbia, Vancouver; St John's Inst, London; St Thomas' Hosp, London)

J Cutan Pathol 24:286–291, 1997 9–4

Introduction.—Sézary syndrome is an uncommon variant of cutaneous T-cell lymphoma (CTCL) that is typified by erythroderma, pruritis, adenopathy, and circulating atypical T lymphocytes with cerebriform nuclei. There is a need for numerous skin biopsy specimens because variable cutaneous histopathology makes differentiation from benign forms of erythroderma difficult. Sézary syndrome may be further refined by including only patients with a circulating peripheral blood population of clonal T cells. Seventy-nine skin biopsies from 41 patients were examined to define the spectrum of cutaneous histopathology in Sézary syndrome in patients with clinical and molecular evidence of CTCL.

TABLE 2.—Skin Biopsy Patterns in Patients With Sézary Syndrome

	Patients with at least one skin biopsy diagnostic of CTCL (n=30)	Patients without a skin biopsy diagnostic of CTCL (n=11)
Non-specific changes	7	19
Lymphocytic band, no atypia	1	4
Lymphocytic band, with atypia	18	—
MF-like	30	—

(Courtesy of Trotter MJ, Whittaker SJ, Orchard GE: Cutaneous histopathology of Sézary syndrome: A study of 41 cases with proven circulating T-cell clone. *J Cutan Pathol* 24:286–291, 1997. Copyright 1997 Munksgaard International Publishers Ltd., Copenhagen, Denmark.)

Methods.—Skin biopsy samples underwent cutaneous histopathology examination. Peripheral blood samples were collected for genotypic studies.

Results.—All 41 patients with Sézary syndrome had a TCR-β gene rearrangement in peripheral blood. Histopathologic examination revealed features consistent with chronic dermatitis in 26 of 79 (33%) skin biopsy specimens. Biopsy of erythrodermic skin revealed lack of evidence of CTCL in 11 of 41 patients (Tables 2 and 3). Survival of these 11 patients did not differ from the remaining 30 patients with evidence of CTCL on skin biopsy. In the 30 patients with changes diagnostic of CTCL, 23% had dermal lymphocytic band with atypical lymphocytes, and 38% had mycosis fungoides–like infiltrate.

Conclusion.—Skin biopsies are useful in the diagnostic evaluation of patients with suspected Sézary syndrome. Of 79 biopsies, 48 had evidence diagnostic of CTCL. Multiple biopsies and analysis of peripheral blood for clonal T-cell population is highly recommended when considering a diagnosis of Sézary syndrome.

► Sézary syndrome is an uncommon variant of the rare condition, mycosis fungoides. Personally I do not like the term *cutaneous T-cell lymphoma*

TABLE 3.—Skin Biopsy Results in Patients With Sézary Syndrome: Biopsy Patterns Observed Before and After Identification of Circulating T-cell Clone

	Skin biopsies obtained prior to identification of circulating T-cell clone	Skin biopsies obtained coincident with or after identification of circulating T-cell clone
Non-specific changes	13	13
Lymphocytic band, no atypia	3	2
Lymphocytic band, with atypia	11	7
MF-like	10	20
	16/37 (43%) not diagnostic of CTCL	15/42 (36%) not diagnostic of CTCL

(Courtesy of Trotter MJ, Whittaker SJ, Orchard GE: Cutaneous histopathology of Sézary syndrome: A study of 41 cases with proven circulating T-cell clone. *J Cutan Pathol* 24:286–291, 1997. Copyright 1997 Munksgaard International Publishers Ltd., Copenhagen, Denmark.)

because it implies we know a great deal more about this disease than we do. In addition, I have seen many a lymphoma, B cell, or T cell involved in the skin, and I do not honestly believe that labeling it as CTCL is helpful. Patients who have Sézary syndrome are characterized largely by erythroderma, pruritus, adenopathy, and the circulating T cells with cerebriform nuclei originally described by Sézary. They do not really have plaques, although I consider the whole skin to be one big plaque.

The authors have a good number of patients in this unusual setting and their conclusions are very reasonable, considering their data. Because there is a circulating cell component, we desperately need effective systemic treatment for this condition. At the moment, what that treatment is really is not clear.

There is a component of the biology of this disease that is clearly molecular, and these approaches will be more common in the future.

E. Glatstein, M.D.

Primary Anaplastic Large-cell Lymphoma in Adults: Clinical Presentation, Immunophenotype, and Outcome

Tilly H, for the Groupe d'Etudes des Lymphomes de l'Adulte (Centre Henri Becquerel, Rouen, France; Hôpital Henri Mondor, Créteil, France; Centre Hospitalier Lyon-Sud, Pierre Bénite, France; et al)

Blood 90:3727–3734, 1997 9–5

Objective.—As many as 8% of lymphomas are anaplastic, CD30+, large-cell lymphomas. Recent studies have clarified the biological characteristics of these tumors, which include proliferation of pleomorphic large neoplastic lymphoid cells that strongly express the CD30 antigen. However, the differences in clinical behavior from other large-cell lymphomas remain uncertain. The presentation, immunophenotypic findings, and clinical outcomes of anaplastic large-cell lymphoma (ALCL) were compared with those of nonanaplastic diffuse large-cell lymphoma (non-ALCL).

Methods.—The study was based on a large multicenter trial of treatment for aggressive lymphoma. Morphologic and CD30 expression studies identified 146 cases of ALCL. Their characteristics and outcomes were compared with those of 1,695 cases of non-ALCL.

Findings.—Patients with ALCL were more likely to be male and of younger age than those with non-ALCL. The ALCL patients were also more likely to have B symptoms. Although the ALCL patients were more likely to have skin and lung involvement, there was no difference in the frequency of bone marrow involvement. In the ALCL group, 38% of patients had a B-cell tumor phenotype, 34% had a T phenotype, and 22% had a null phenotype. The ALCL group had a better response to chemotherapy, better event-free survival, and better overall survival. On multivariate analysis, anaplastic tumors were independently associated with longer survival, though not with event-free or overall survival.

Conclusions.—Anaplastic large-cell lymphoma is a tumor with heterogeneous phenotypic and genotypic characteristics. However, it affects a homogeneous patient population and carries a better prognosis than other diffuse large-cell lymphomas. Among patients with ALCL, prognosis is unaffected by phenotype, although survival is predicted by the clinical variables of the International Prognostic Index. It remains to be seen whether ALCL requires a specific treatment approach.

▶ This paper is useful because it reports presenting features, immunophenotyping, and clinical outcome of a large number of patients with a relatively uncommon, fairly recently recognized lymphoma, ALCL. Interestingly, overall survival was better for the cohort of patients with ALCL than for those with non-ALCL. It is important to recognize that patients with ALCL have a distinct entity which overall has a more favorable outcome than that seen in patients with other diffuse large-cell lymphomas. It is important to establish a diagnosis.

M.S. Tallman, M.D.

Incidence, Predictive Factors, and Outcome of Lymphoma Transformation in Follicular Lymphoma Patients

Bastion Y, Sebban C, Berger F, et al (Hospitalier Lyon-Sud, Pierre-Benite, France; Hôpital E Herriot, Lyon, France)

J Clin Oncol 15:1587–1594, 1997 9–6

Background.—Follicular lymphoma (FL) has a relatively indolent course, but is not curable, with survival after diagnosis ranging from 7 to 9 years. The conversion of low-grade lymphoma to more aggressive disease over this period is associated with poor outcome. No predictive factors for this transformation have been identified. This retrospective study of FL patients was performed to analyze the incidence, risk factors, and outcome of transformation.

Study Design.—From 1975 to 1990, 220 FL patients, with a median age at diagnosis of 53, participated in this study. Transformation was defined as progression to a more aggressive diffuse lymphoma. At disease progression or transformation, patients were restaged by clinical examination, CT scan, bone marrow aspirate and biopsy, lactate dehydrogenase level and presence of B symptoms. The median duration of follow-up was 9 years.

Findings.—The overall incidence of transformation was 24% in this group. The probability of transformation was 22% at 5 years and 31% at 10 years, with a tendency to plateau after 6 years. The risk factors for transformation were no complete remission after initial therapy, low serum albumin level, and b_2-microglobulin level greater than 3 mg/l at diagnosis. Multivariate analysis indicated that only b_2-microglobulin was an independent prognostic factor for freedom-from-transformation survival. Transformation was involved in 44% of the deaths in the study group and was associated with poor outcome. After transformation, there was a median survival duration of only 7 months.

Conclusions.—This large retrospective study of patients with FL demonstrated that transformation is an early event in the course of this disease and is associated with poor outcome. Transformation is usually observed in patients with adverse prognostic factors and those who do not achieve complete remission after initial treatment. These findings may be useful in the selection of appropriate treatment for FL patients with varying prognostic factors.

▶ Predictive factors for transformation included failure to achieve complete remission after initial therapy, low serum albumin level, and elevated β_2-microglobulin level at diagnosis. These observations are important since once transformation occurred, it accounted for 44% of all deaths, and was associated with a poor outcome, with a median survival of only 7 months. This information is useful because such patients may be selected for alternative strategies.

M.S. Tallman, M.D.

Stanford-Kaiser Permanente G1 Study for Clinical Stage I to IIA Hodgkin's Disease: Subtotal Lymphoid Irradiation Versus Vinblastine, Methotrexate, and Bleomycin Chemotherapy and Regional Irradiation

Horning SJ, Hoppe RT, Mason J, et al (Stanford Univ, Calif; Kaiser-Permanente Med Care Program, Oakland, Calif)

J Clin Oncol 15:1736–1744, 1997 9–7

Background.—An earlier study by these authors indicated that chemotherapy with vincristine, methotrexate, and bleomycin (VBM) plus regional irradiation was as effective as subtotal lymphoid irradiation (STLI) in asymptomatic patients with pathologic stage I and II Hodgkin's disease. In this study, patients' disease was staged clinically and the outcomes with VBM plus regional irradiation were compared with STLI alone in patients with clinical stage I or IIA Hodgkin's disease.

Methods.—Previously untreated patients with clinical stage I or II disease were randomly assigned to receive either STLI (n = 43) or VBM + regional irradiation (n = 35). The groups were stratified to maintain similar patient characteristics of age, sex, number of Ann Arbor disease sites, histologic stage (nodular sclerosing or mixed cellularity), and treating institution between groups. In the STLI arm of the study, the total dose to involved regions was 40 to 44 Gy and to uninvolved regions was 30 to 40 Gy. Patients in the VBM + regional irradiation arm received 2 cycles of intravenous vinblastine (6 mg/m^2), bleomycin (10 U/m^2), and methotrexate (30 mg/m^2) on days 1 and 8 every 28 days. Regional irradiation began about 2 weeks after the second VBM cycle and involved 35 to 36 Gy to involved regions and 30 to 35 Gy to uninvolved regions. Then, about 2 weeks after irradiation, another 4 courses of VBM were used.

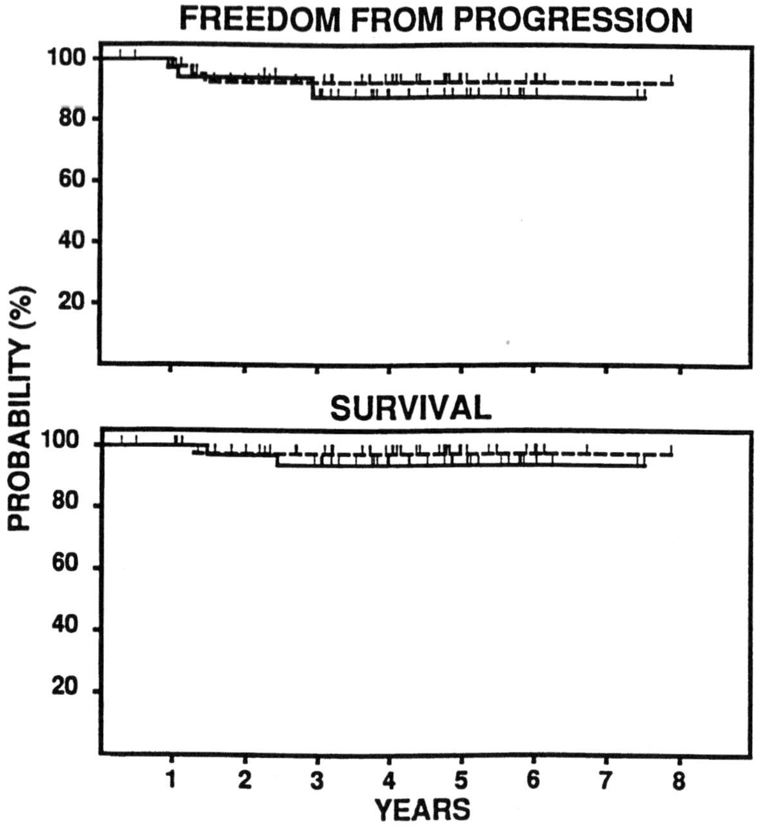

FIGURE 1.—Freedom from progression and overall survival in 78 favorable clinical stage I to II patients treated from 1988 to 1995 with STLI (n = 43, *dashed line*) or VBM + regional irradiation (n = 35, *solid line*). (Courtesy of Horning SJ, Hoppe RT, Mason J, et al: Stanford-Kaiser Permanente G1 study for clinical stage I to IIA Hodgkin's disease: Subtotal lymphoid irradiation versus vinblastine, methotrexate, and bleomycin chemotherapy and regional irradiation. *J Clin Oncol* 15:1736–1744, 1997.)

Findings.—The median follow-up has been 4 years. At 5 years, 92% of patients treated with STLI and 87% of patients treated with VBM + regional irradiation are free of disease (Fig 1). A total of 7 patients experienced relapse. In all 3 patients who had a relapse after STLI disease developed in the untreated pelvis that extended to the paraaortic lymph nodes. Relapses in the 4 patients in the VBM + regional irradiation group occurred at the previously irradiated mediastinum, at the margin of the irradiated field, or in the bone marrow. Second-line therapy was begun for these 7 patients, and 6 are currently alive and their disease is in remission. Nine patients in both groups had toxic side effects related to the regimen, although the side effects were milder for those in the VBM + regional irradiation group.

Conclusions.—After 4 years of follow-up, results of STLI are comparable with those of VBM + regional irradiation in the disease-free progression and survival of patients with clinical stage I and IIA Hodgkin's disease. Furthermore, VBM + regional irradiation is a potentially less toxic regimen than STLI for these patients with favorable disease. Further research is needed to determine the utility of this regimen, particularly the reduction of toxicity.

► This is certainly an exciting article on combined modality treatment of Hodgkin's disease. These Stanford investigators randomly assigned 78 patients with clinical stage I or II Hodgkin's disease, to receive either subtotal lymphoid radiation or VBM chemotherapy plus regional radiotherapy. All patients had laparotomy to confirm their favorable presentation. The results are truly superb, with the 4-year freedom from relapse rate at 92% and 87%, respectively, and even better survival rates. At the investigational level, their point clearly has been made that modest chemotherapy and localized radiation are equivalent to more aggressive radiation in these patients.

I believe one of the more serious problems in Hodgkin's disease today is that many practicing physicians are essentially experimenting with patients who have Hodgkin's disease. They are taking chemotherapy regimens that are established to be curative with 6 or more cycles, and giving fewer than that either with or without radiation therapy. When the data are lacking for *confirming* curability by a new regimen, it seems to me very dangerous to cut back on the extent of that treatment. The Stanford studies are unique because of the method of patient follow-up and randomization to 1 of 2 different treatments. One of the treatments is usually the state-of-the-art and the other is the combined modality investigational treatment, which in this series has proved to be quite good.

Some practicing physicians need to be reminded that, when they read about a new treatment (of any type), there is a learning curve associated with implementing that new treatment. This is research, but very unglamorous "confirmatory" in type. Nonetheless, it is research. One wonders what kind of consent form such physicians in practice are having patients sign. I believe the medicolegal implications are major.

E. Glatstein, M.D.

Is Combined Modality Therapy Necessary for Advanced Hodgkin's Disease?

Mendenhall NP, Bennett CJ Jr, Lynch JW Jr (Univ of Florida, Gainesville)
Int J Radiat Oncol Biol Phys 38:583–592, 1997 9–8

Objective.—Whether single or combined modality therapy is optimal management for patients with advanced Hodgkin's disease was the subject of a retrospective analysis.

Methods.—The 141 patients (30 female), aged 5 to 73 years, with clinical or pathologic stage III or IV Hodgkin's disease treated at the University of Florida between October 1964 through December 1989 were followed for a median of 13.5 years. There were 55 patients who received combined modality therapy (CMT), 50 who received chemotherapy only (CX), and 36 who received only radiotherapy (RT). Freedom from relapse, probability of overall survival, and probability of cause-specific survival were determined. Poor prognostic factors were tabulated, and fatal and nonfatal complications were recorded.

Results.—Ten-year survival rates varied with the disease stage and type of therapy received (Table 2). According to multivariate analysis, freedom from relapse was related to tumor diameter, number of sites, stage, age, presence of B symptoms, splenic involvement, and the number of cycles of chemotherapy, and use of doxorubicin-based chemotherapy. The majority of patients with nonbulky Stage IIIA disease were in the RT group, and freedom from relapse in this group was related to splenic involvement and age. Ten-year freedom from relapse and overall survival rates at 10 years for patients with tumors 6 cm or smaller were 53% and 58% for the RT group, 60% and 56% for the CX group, and 83% and 71% for the CMT group. Freedom from relapse was significantly higher for the CMT group than for the CX group. Overall survival rates were not significantly different between groups.

TABLE 2.—Ten-Year Results in Advanced Stage Hodgkin's Disease

		Stage						
Treatment		IIIA (%)	IIIB (%)	All III (%)	IVA (%)	IVB (%)	All IV (%)	All patients (%)
RT	FFR	50	60	52	0	50	33	50
		n = 26	*n* = 7	*n* = 33	*n* = 1	*n* = 2	*n* = 3	*n* = 36
	OS	64	14	53	0	100	67	55
		n = 26	*n* = 7	*n* = 33	*n* = 1	*n* = 2	*n* = 3	*n* = 36
	CSS	72	26	64	0	100	67	64
		n = 26	*n* = 7	*n* = 33	*n* = 1	*n* = 2	*n* = 3	*n* = 36
CMT	FFR	91	60	85	50	56	53	77
		n = 23	*n* = 19	*n* = 42	*n* = 4	*n* = 9	*n* = 13	*n* = 55
	OS	80	40	65	75	56	64	65
		n = 23	*n* = 19	*n* = 42	*n* = 4	*n* = 9	*n* = 13	*n* = 55
	CSS	88	43	71	75	56	64	69
		n = 23	*n* = 19	*n* = 42	*n* = 4	*n* = 9	*n* = 13	*n* = 55
CX	FFR	67	52	56	0	28	27	43
		n = 6	*n* = 21	*n* = 27	*n* = 1	*n* = 22	*n* = 23	*n* = 50
	OS	42	66	60	0	19	17	39
		n = 6	*n* = 21	*n* = 27	*n* = 1	*n* = 22	*n* = 23	*n* = 50
	CSS	83	70	73	0	23	21	49
		n = 6	*n* = 21	*n* = 27	*n* = 1	*n* = 22	*n* = 23	*n* = 50
All patients	FFR	68	63	66	33	37	36	57
		n = 55	*n* = 47	*n* = 102	*n* = 6	*n* = 33	*n* = 39	*n* = 141
	OS	68	47	59	44	33	35	53
		n = 55	*n* = 47	*n* = 102	*n* = 6	*n* = 33	*n* = 39	*n* = 141
	CSS	79	54	69	44	38	39	61
		n = 55	*n* = 47	*n* = 102	*n* = 6	*n* = 33	*n* = 39	*n* = 141

Abbreviations: FFR, freedom from relapse; *OS*, overall survival; *CSS*, cause-specific survival; *RT*, radiotherapy alone; *CMT*, combined modality therapy; *CX*, chemotherapy alone.

(Reprinted by permission of the publisher from Mendenhall NP, Bennett CJ Jr, Lynch JW Jr: Is combined modality therapy necessary for advanced Hodgkin's disease? *Int J Radiat Oncol Biol Phys* 38:583–592, copyright 1997 by Elsevier Science Inc.)

Ten-year freedom from relapse and overall survival rates at 10 years for patients with tumors smaller than 6 cm were 44% and 45% for the RT group, 9% and 0% for the CX group, and 72% and 58% for the CMT group. Both freedom from relapse and overall survival rates were significantly higher for the CMT group than for the CX group. Patterns of relapse involved sites of initial disease in 14 of 91 patients treated with radiotherapy (RT and CMT patients) and in 20 of 50 CX patients. Fatal blood disorders developed in 10 patients. Of the 68 deaths, 31 were from Hodgkin's disease.

Conclusion.—Patients receiving combined modality therapy did better than patients receiving single modality therapy. Patients with bulky disease so treated had increased survival and freedom from relapse, and patients without bulky disease had increased freedom from relapse. Most complications were dose related.

► This is a report on the experience at the University of Florida in treating stages III and IV Hodgkin's disease by a variety of techniques. The data appear to suggest that there is a benefit of combined modality treatment for most patients with advanced disease. Of course, there are prospectively randomized studies that demonstrate quite convincingly that in patients who receive chemotherapy and achieve a complete remission, no benefit is derived.

This gets me to the point of frustration with what is happening in Hodgkin's disease treatment today. Many people want to modify the chemotherapy that is shown to be curative or the radiation that is shown to be curative and put together some form of hybrid, without a formal investigation or investigational consent. Even when an investigator is trying to repeat what has been reported by another investigator, the second investigator is, in fact, doing confirmatory research without acknowledging it.

Personally, I am interested in combined modality treatment and am more than anxious to cooperate in almost any kind of combined modality protocol. On the other hand, I do not see a reason for *routinely* trying to cure the patient twice, thereby subjecting the patient to the risks of both modalities. If the modalities have to be modified into 1 package, as they have attempted to do at Stanford University, that is a noble goal. The Stanford approach (Abstract 9–7) condenses the chemotherapy into something like 16 weeks, with the Stanford 5 regimen, plus an additional few weeks of involved field treatment. This makes some sense.

On the other hand, what I see happening in practice is that physicians treat patients with 2 or 3 planned cycles of chemotherapy but then see that there is residual disease and want to push for a full course of doxorubicin, bleomycin, vinblastine, and dacarbazine, and still want to use radiation—although now the patient has been put into complete remission. I can understand the frustrations and difficulties of dealing with some of these problems, but that is what investigation is about. It seems to me that some physicians have to learn the difference between being a private practitioner and being an investigator.

As far as the Florida results are concerned, stage IIIB disease appears to be a reasonable candidate for combined modality studies. This might also be true of stage IV disease, but I think that takes some real defining of what stage IV disease is, when picking appropriate patients for combined modality treatment. Age is also an important factor, both from the standpoint of outcome, and the use of additional modalities.

E. Glatstein, M.D.

Is Comprehensive Lymphatic Irradiation for Low-grade Non-Hodgkin's Lymphoma Curative Therapy? Long-term Experience at a Single Institution

De Los Santos JF, Mendenhall NP, Lynch JW Jr (Univ of Florida, Gainesville)

Int J Radiat Oncol Biol Phys 38:3–8, 1997 9–9

Objective.—Only radiotherapy has been proven to alter the course of indolent non-Hodgkin's lymphoma (NHL). There has been insufficient follow-up to determine whether this alteration constitutes a "cure." An update of the University of Florida's 10-year experience regarding relapse-free and absolute survival rates for patients with stage I–III low-grade NHL given comprehensive lymphatic irradiation (CLI) was presented.

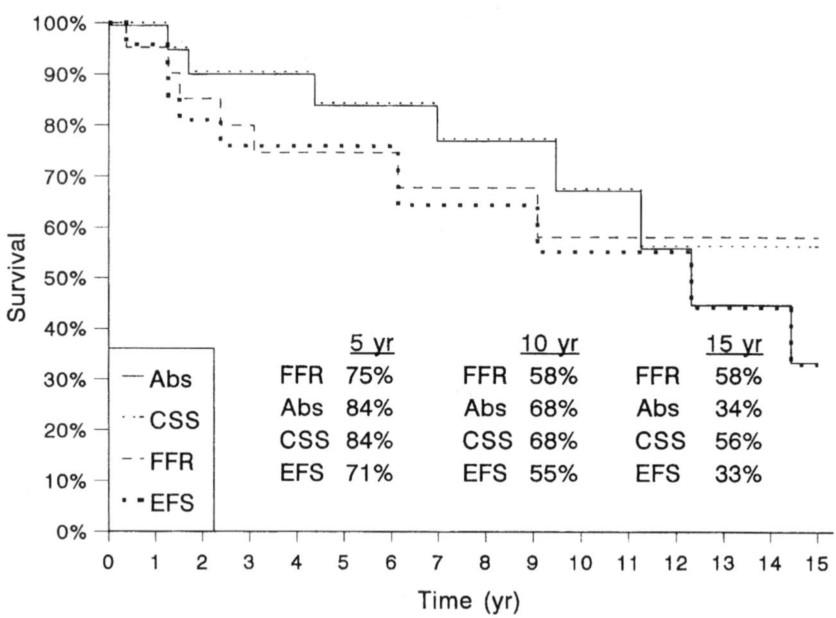

FIGURE 1.—Survival rates at 5, 10, and 15 years for 21 patients with non-Hodgkin's lymphoma treated with comprehensive lymphatic irradiation. (Reprinted by permission of the publisher from De Los Santos JF, Mendenhall NP, Lynch JW Jr: Is comprehensive lymphatic irradiation for low-grade non-Hodgkin's lymphoma curative therapy? Long-term experience at a single institution. *Int J Radiat Oncol Biol Phys* 38:3–8, copyright 1997 by Elsevier Science Inc.)

TABLE 2.—Patterns of Relapse

Pattern of relapse	No. of pts. with low-grade recurrence* (n = 4)	No. of pts. with high-grade transformation† (n = 3)
Outside treatment field	1	1
Generalized disease	1	0
Marginal recurrence	1	0
In treatment field‡	1	2

*Time to recurrence: 17 months, 21 months, 29 months, and 6 years.
†Time to recurrence: 5 months, 38 months, and 9 years.
‡Doses of 20, 23, and 30 Gy.
Abbreviation: pts., patients.
(Reprinted by permission of the publisher from De Los Santos JF, Mendenhall NP, Lynch JW Jr: Is comprehensive lymphatic irradiation for low-grade non-Hodgkin's lymphoma curative therapy? Long-term experience at a single institution. *Int J Radiat Oncol Biol Phys* 38:3–8, copyright 1997 by Elsevier Science Inc.)

Methods.—Between 1966 and 1992, 21 patients (10 women), aged 31 to 76 years, treated with CLI, were followed for an average of 14 years (24.5 years in the case of stage III patients). Most clinically involved sites received 30 Gy and most clinically uninvolved sites received 25 Gy or more. Kaplan-Meier survival curves were constructed.

Results.—At the time of analysis, 10 patients had died (Fig 1). No Stage I or II patients died of NHL. One stage III patient had disease progression. Seven patients had a relapse (Table 2). Three of 4 patients treated after

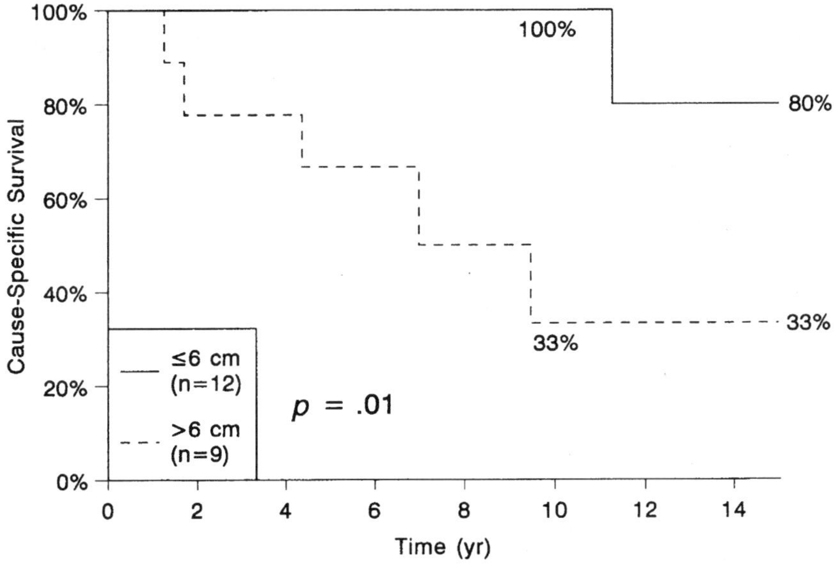

FIGURE 2.—Cause-specific survival according to disease bulk (6 cm or less vs. more than 6 cm) for 21 patients with non-Hodgkin's lymphoma treated with comprehensive lymphatic irradiation. (Reprinted by permission of the publisher from De Los Santos JF, Mendenhall NP, Lynch JW Jr: Is comprehensive lymphatic irradiation for low-grade non-Hodgkin's lymphoma curative therapy? Long-term experience at a single institution. *Int J Radiat Oncol Biol Phys* 38:3–8, copyright 1997 by Elsevier Science Inc.)

relapse with chemotherapy, including 1 patient who received additional radiotherapy, survived from 28 months to 11 years after salvage. Bulky disease was prognostic of cause-specific survival (Fig 2). Treatment was generally well-tolerated, although 3 patients were unable to complete the therapy. Five patients had additional malignancies, but only 1 was possibly radiation induced. Treatment times varied from 1.1 to 11.1 months.

Conclusion.—Comprehensive lymphatic irradiation can be curative for low-grade non-Hodgkin's lymphoma. The treatment, ranging from 1.1 to 11.1 months, was generally well tolerated.

► This paper from Florida suggests that CLI is potentially curable for patients with stages I, II, and "limited" stage III indolent histology lymphoma. The authors had only 21 cases, so it is a little hard to make a lot out of this study. In addition, the follow-up was only about 15 years, at least according to the graphs which are difficult to interpret.

I think, at the moment, the standard of practice for stage I and II disease is to treat a mantle or inverted Y or some variation of that, but not to treat on both sides of the diaphragm. I believe that is still investigational. As for stage III disease, I believe the standard of practice is "watch-and-wait" treatment or combined modality treatment, but not radiation alone. I do not think the data are sufficient to convince anyone that those practices are better than others, but the results seem to be reasonable in terms of side effects, efficacy, time of treatment, and overall costs.

E. Glatstein, M.D.

Long-term Outcome of Treatment for Ann Arbor Stage I Hodgkin's Disease: Prognostic Factors for Survival and Freedom From Progression

Vlachaki MT, Hagemeister FB, Fuller LM, et al (Univ of Texas MD Anderson Cancer Ctr, Houston)

Int J Radiat Oncol Biol Phys 38:593–599, 1997 9–10

Introduction.—For patients with very early Hodgkin's disease, radiation therapy offers excellent short-term survival. There is debate over the pretreatment evaluation, extent of irradiation, role of chemotherapy, and importance of prognostic factors in this situation. Several adverse clinical prognostic factors in patients treated with radiation only have been suggested. The long-term results of radiotherapy for stage I Hodgkin's disease were studied retrospectively.

Patients.—A total of 145 patients treated for stage I Hodgkin's disease during a 20-year period were studied. The patients were 93 men and 52 women, with a median age of 31 years. Before treatment, all patients underwent lymphangiography and bone marrow aspiration with biopsy. Seventy percent had laparotomy. One hundred thirty-three patients had subdiaphragmatic disease, whereas 12 had infradiaphragmatic adenopathy. Only 5 patients had B symptoms present. Disease subtype was lymphocyte predominance in 18% of patients, nodular sclerosis in 41%,

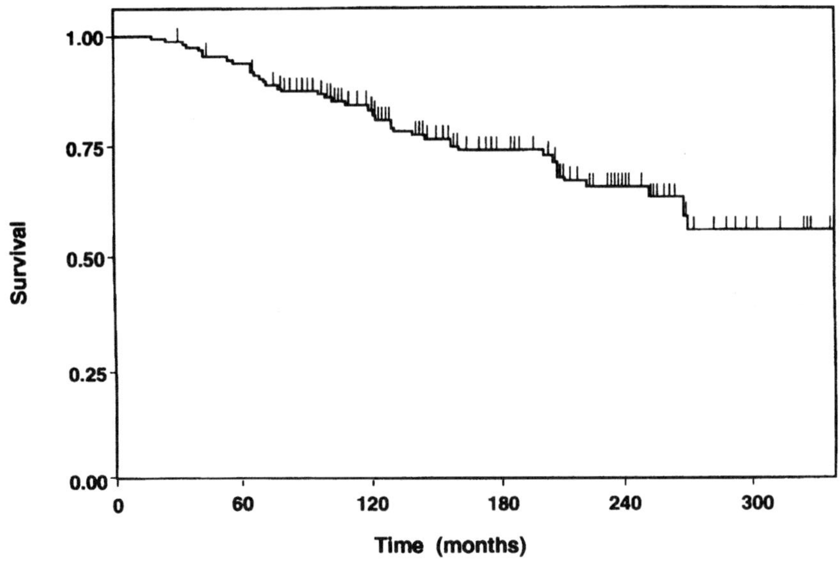

FIGURE 1.—Survival. (Courtesy of Vlachaki MT, Hagemeister FB, Fuller LM, et al: Long-term outcome of treatment for Ann Arbor stage I Hodgkin's disease: Prognostic factors for survival and freedom from progression. *Int J Radiat Oncol Biol Phys* 38:593–599. Copyright 1997, Elsevier Science Inc. Reprinted by permission.)

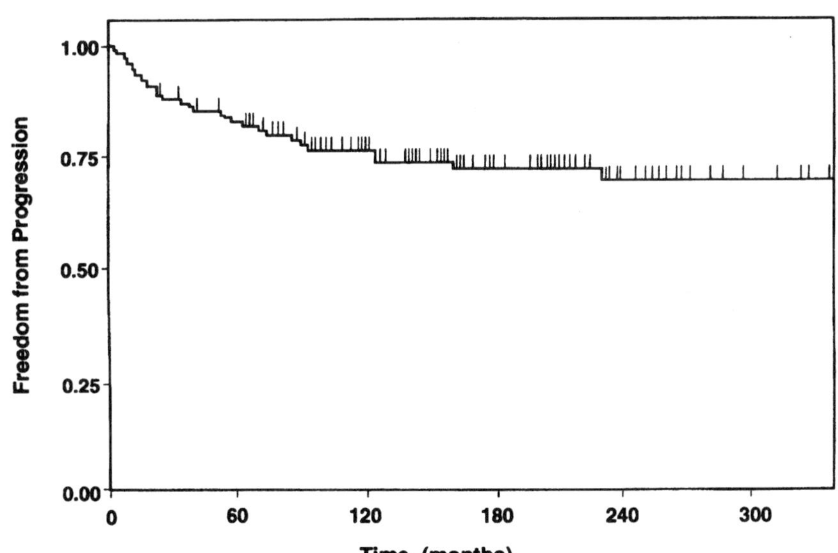

FIGURE 2.—Freedom from progression. (Courtesy of Vlachaki MT, Hagemeister FB, Fuller LM, et al: Long-term outcome of treatment for Ann Arbor stage I Hodgkin's disease: Prognostic factors for survival and freedom from progression. *Int J Radiat Oncol Biol Phys* 38:593–599. Copyright 1997, Elsevier Science Inc. Reprinted by permission.)

mixed cellularity in 41%, and unclassified with primary splenic involvement in 1 patient.

Treatment.—All patients received radiotherapy. In addition, 11% received combination chemotherapy. Forty-nine percent of patients had radiation to involved and regional field, 43% had mantle or inverted-Y extended-field radiation, and 8% had subnodal total irradiation.

Outcomes.—Median follow-up was 16.5 years and median survival was 14 years. Ten-year survival was 83% and 20-year survival was 66% (Fig 1). Age greater than 40 years at diagnosis was the only factor significantly related to decreased survival. Eleven of 43 deaths were caused by Hodgkin's disease; the rest were from intercurrent causes, including treatment-related causes. Median progression-free interval was 10.5 years. Freedom from progression was 76% at 10 years and 69% at 20 years (Fig 2). Thirteen percent of relapses occurred after 10 years. Freedom from progression was better for women than for men; age, histologic subtype, disease bulkiness, site of involvement, and chemotherapy had no effect. Just 12 patients received subtotal nodal irradiation. This group had a 10-year freedom from progression of 92%, compared with 65% for patients receiving less extensive treatment.

Conclusions.—The results of radiation therapy for stage I Hodgkin's disease are very good. However, the possibility of late relapse mandates long-term follow-up. Of all factors analyzed, age is the only factor to affect survival; freedom from progression is somewhat affected by sex. Excellent freedom from progression was demonstrated in patients receiving subtotal nodal irradiation, suggesting the need for further study of this treatment.

► The outcome for patients who have been treated for stage I Hodgkin's disease is obviously excellent. Moreover, that is a reflection of a variety of different treatments. This is a study from M.D. Anderson that shows excellent freedom from progression, about 75% at 10 years and about 66% survival at 20 years. Even in stage I disease, they show that over the age of 40 was a poor prognostic factor. In their experience at Houston, additional chemotherapy after radiation did not influence the freedom of progression. The differences in freedom from progression according to the laparotomy group appears statistically very strongly positive in significance, in favor of patients who were surgically explored compared to those who were not explored. On the other hand, survival showed only a trend but not a statistical significance.

E. Glatstein, M.D.

10 Pediatric Solid Tumors

Potential Role of Proton Therapy in the Treatment of Pediatric Medulloblastoma/Primitive Neuro-Ectodermal Tumors: Spinal Theca Irradiation

Miralbell R, Lomax A, Russo M (Univ Hosp, Geneva; Paul Scherrer Inst, Villigen, Switzerland)

Int J Radiat Oncol Biol Phys 38:805–811, 1997 10–1

Introduction.—In children with medulloblastoma or other primitive neuroectodermal tumors, irradiation of the spina theca is considered an indispensable part of any strategy aiming to reduce the chances of spinal failure. Standard megavoltage photon beam radiation therapy, however, can result in bone marrow suppression, thyroid hypofunction, gonadal damage, and vertebral growth arrest. Research is underway to reduce the morbidity of spinal theca irradiation in medulloblastoma. A posterior, variably modulated proton beam was compared with a standard posterior 6-MV x-ray beam to determine the dose distribution achievable.

Methods.—A standard set of posterior 6-MV x-ray fields was compared with a posterior modulated 100 MeV proton beam (spot scanning method) to determine the dose distribution that could be achieved in this comparative dosimetric study. The potential improvements with proton therapy were evaluated by using dose-volume histograms to examine the coverage of the target, as well as to determine the dose to the vertebral bodies (growth plates), lungs, heart, and liver.

Results.—In both treatment plans, the target, which was the spinal dural sac, received the full prescribed dose. Both methods delivered the prescribed dose of 30 Gy to the target volume. With 6-MV x-rays, the proportion of the vertebral body volume receiving 50% or more of the prescribed dose was 100%, and with the proton beam, the proportion receiving 50% or more was 20%. The proton beam was able to completely avoid the heart, the liver, and in all likelihood the thyroid and gonads; however, for 6-MV x-rays, more than 60% of the dose prescribed to the target was delivered to 44% of the heart volume.

Conclusions.—Proton therapy may have a potential role in decreasing the dose and toxicity to the critical structures in the irradiation of the spinal neuraxis in medulloblastoma/primitive neuroectodermal tumors. This approach is especially attractive for intensive chemotherapy protocols and for very young children because of the potential reductions in bone marrow toxicity and growth retardation. Additional advantages of proton therapy that may ensure a long-term posttreatment morbidity-free survival are its potential for sparing the thyroid gland, the posterior heart wall, and the gonads.

► This paper addresses the potential advantage of a proton beam in the treatment of pediatric medulloblastoma. The potential advantage is simply the absence of an exit dose, giving a remarkably limited exposure to radiation. On the other hand, the big question is whether proton therapy is sufficiently better in terms of outcome to justify the enormous expense that will be involved in this kind of treatment. That remains to be seen.

E. Glatstein, M.D.

11 Brain Tumors

Dose Estimation to Critical Organs From Vertex Field Treatment of Brain Tumors

Das IJ, Cheng C-W, Fein DA, et al (Fox Chase Cancer Ctr, Philadelphia; Univ of Arizona, Tucson; Thomas Jefferson Univ, Philadelphia)

Int J Radiat Oncol Biol Phys 37:1023–1029, 1997 11–1

Introduction.—Patients with brain tumors undergoing radiation therapy sometimes need a noncoplanar vertex field that irradiates the entire length of the body. Although this field has important advantages in sparing normal brain tissues and increasing the dose to the target tumor, it may

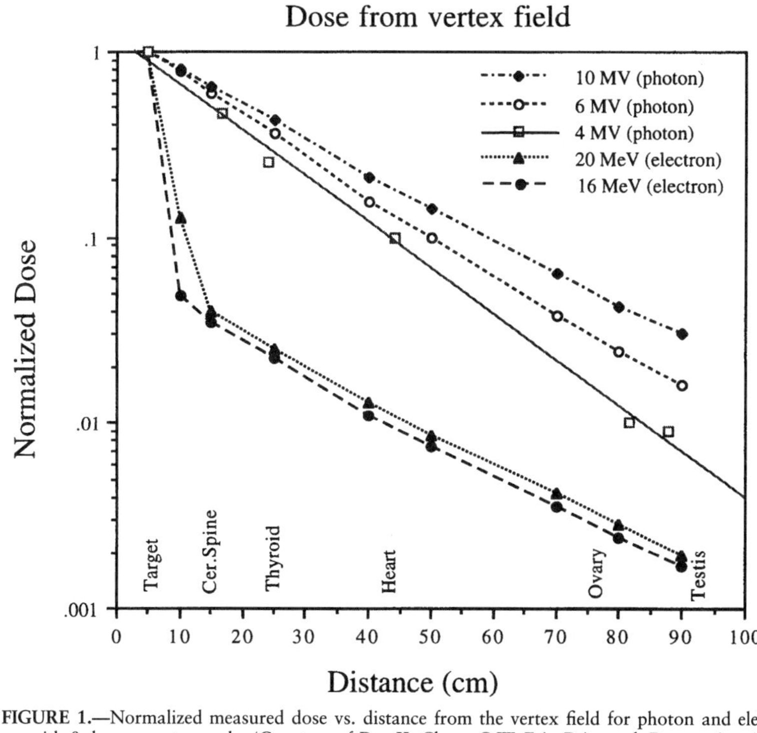

FIGURE 1.—Normalized measured dose vs. distance from the vertex field for photon and electron beams with 0-degree gantry angle. (Courtesy of Das IJ, Cheng C-W, Fein DA, et al: Dose estimation to critical organs from vertex field treatment of brain tumors. *Int J Radiat Oncol Biol Phys* 37:1023–1029, 1997. Copyright 1997 with permission from Elsevier Science.)

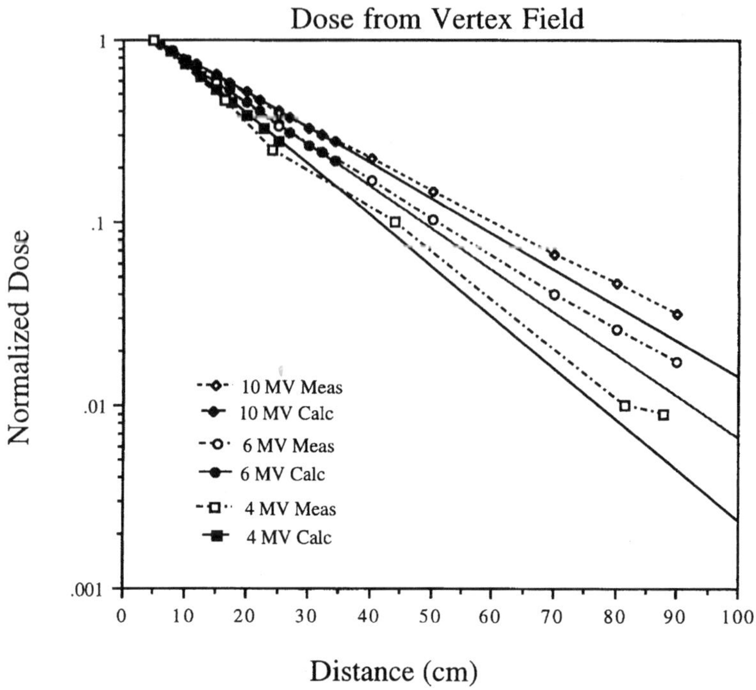

FIGURE 3.—Comparison of the measured and calculated normalized dose vs. distance from the vertex for the photon beams. (Courtesy of Das IJ, Cheng C-W, Fein DA, et al: Dose estimation to critical organs from vertex field treatment of brain tumors. *Int J Radiat Oncol Biol Phys* 37:1023–1029, 1997. Copyright 1997 with permission from Elsevier Science.)

expose various critical structures. The radiation doses to normal tissues—including the thyroid, spinal cord, heart, and genitals—with the vertex field were estimated.

Methods.—A clinically used vertex field was applied to an anthropomorphic Rando phantom. The field included 4-, 6-, and 10-MV photon beams and 16- and 20-MeV electron beams. An ion chamber appropriately positioned within the phantom was used for dosimetry. The radiation doses were normalized to the target dose at a depth of 5 cm. Head flexion and extension were mimicked by rotating the gantry angle up to 20 degrees. The measured radiation doses were compared with the doses estimated using an exponential best fit to the depth dose table.

Findings.—As an example, a 6-MV photon beam was associated with a measured normalized dose of 60% to the cervical spinal cord, 36% to the thyroid, 16% to the heart, 2.5% to the ovaries, and 1.6% to the testicles. For electron beams, organ doses were 4–10 times lower than with photon beams (Fig 1). With all energies used, the primary beam dose to the gonads was less than 5% of the target dose, although the actual dose depended on the body structure, length, and posture. Flexing the head by 5 degrees had little effect on the radiation dose elsewhere in the body. However, head rotation of greater than 10 degrees lowered doses by a factor of 10^{-2} to organs located farther than 40 cm from the prescription point. The measured doses were as much as 35% higher than the doses estimated from the fitted curves (Fig 3).

Conclusions.—A significant dose to the gonads could occur if the entire prescribed treatment were delivered using a vertex field. The data provide an empirical equation for measuring the critical organ doses at known distances for children and smaller patients. The risks may be accepted for patients with malignant tumors; however, the long-term complications must be assessed in younger patients and those with curable tumors. The results suggest that the radiation dose to critical organs could be reduced by using a 3-dimensional planning system to arrange beams in other nonaxial planes, and by using electron beams for the vertex field.

► One of the reasons that radiation therapy for brain tumors has not often included a vertex field is that it has been difficult to image the vertex field for purposes of verification of the treatment fields as part of a quality assurance program. That problem has now been solved by a number of different techniques. This paper demonstrates some important physical characteristics of the vertex field that put some restrictions on what one can do. The major point the authors are emphasizing is that a vertex field goes the longitudinal length of the patient's torso and as such, the vertex field may potentially affect extracranial organs. Ultimately, it comes down to exactly what dose of radiation is delivered to what point and by what means.

E. Glatstein, M.D.

12 Lung Cancer

Extrapulmonary Small Cell Carcinoma

Galanis E, Frytak S, Lloyd RV (Mayo Clinic and Mayo Found, Rochester, Minn)

Cancer 79:1729–1736, 1997 12–1

Background.—Extrapulmonary small-cell carcinoma (EPSCCA), an entity distinct from small-cell lung carcinoma, is underrecognized. One experience with this tumor was reviewed.

Methods.—The tumor registry database at 1 center was used to identify the records of all patients with EPSCCA treated between 1974 and 1994. Eligibility criteria included normal chest radiograph results, a CT scan of the chest, sputum cytology, and/or negative bronchoscopy results.

TABLE 1.—EPSCCA: Primary Disease Site and Smoking History

Disease site	No. (%)	Gender (M/F)	Smoking history	Location
GI	29(36%)	15/14	14/29 (48%)	Colorectal 13 Esophagus 8 Pancreas 7 Gallbladder 1
HEENT	14 (17%)	11/3	8/14 (57%)	Salivary glands 6 Sinuses 7 Thyroid 1
GU	12 (15%)	10/2	8/12 (67%)	Bladder 7 Prostate 4 Penis 1
GYN	10 (12%)	0/10	7/10 (70%)	Cervix 7 Ovary 2 Endometrium 1
Upper resp	5 (6%)	4/1	5/5 (100%)	Larynx 4 Trachea 1
UP-lymph nodes	5 (6%)	4/1	4/5 (80%)	Submandibular 3 Inguinal 1 Retroperitoneal 1
Thymus	3 (4%)	0/3	3/3 (100%)	
UP-other	2 (2%)	2/0	2/2 (100%)	Brain 1 Liver 1
Peritoneum	1(1%)	0/1	0 (0%)	Pelvic Peritoneum

Abbreviations: GI, gastrointestinal system; *HEENT*, ear, nose, and throat; *GU*, genitourinary system; *GYN*, internal genitalia; *Upper resp*, upper respiratory system; *UP*, unknown primary.

(Courtesy of Galanis E, Frytak S, Lloyd RV: Extrapulmonary small cell carcinoma. *Cancer* 79:1729–1736, © 1997 American Cancer Society. Reprinted by permission of Wiley-Liss, Inc., a subsidiary of John Wiley & Sons, Inc.)

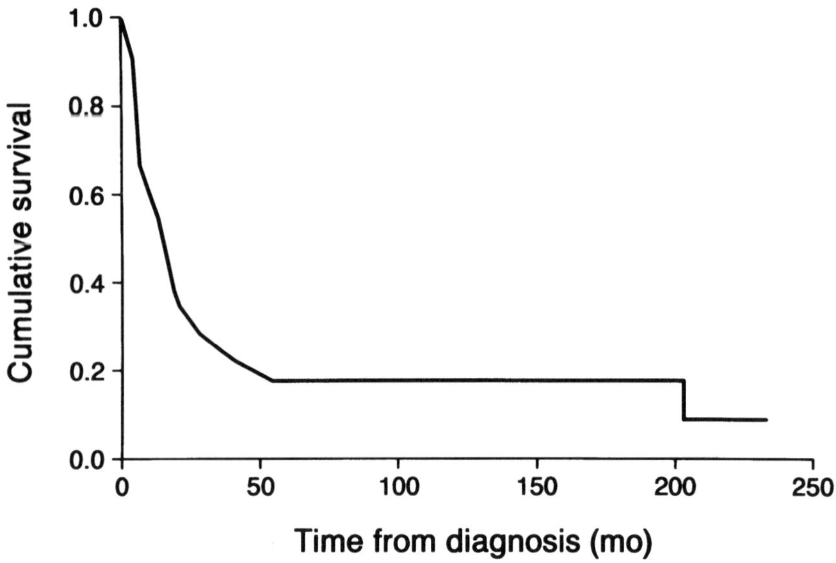

FIGURE 4.—Survival curve for all patients with extrapulmonary small-cell carcinoma. (Courtesy of Galanis E, Frytak S, Lloyd RV: Extrapulmonary small cell carcinoma. *Cancer* 79:1729–1736, ©1997 American Cancer Society. Reprinted by permission of Wiley-Liss, Inc., a subsidiary of John Wiley & Sons, Inc.)

Findings.—The primary sites of EPSCCA were the gastrointestinal system in 29 patients; the ear, nose, and throat in 14; the genitourinary system in 12; internal genitalia in 10; the upper respiratory system in 5; unknown primary lymph nodes in 5; other unknown primary in 2; the thymus in 3; and the peritoneum in 1. Seventy-one of these 81 patients attended follow-up examinations. Fifty-four had limited disease. This group included 40 patients undergoing surgery. Twenty-five percent were alive and disease free at least 3 years postoperatively; the rest relapsed, with a median disease-free survival of 6 months. Six of 54 patients with limited disease underwent chemotherapy and radiation therapy; 5 of them relapsed at a median of 11.5 months. Another 8 patients received radiation therapy only; all had recurrences at a median of 5 months. Platinum-based chemotherapy was used in 22 patients with extensive or recurrent disease. The response rate to this treatment was 72%, with a median duration of 8.5 months. Of the 7 patients given doxorubicin-based chemotherapy, 57% responded, with a median duration of 4.5 months. Overall disease-free survival and overall survival rates were 26% and 38%, respectively, at 3 years, and 13% each at 5 years (Table 1; Fig 4).

Conclusions.—Extrapulmonary small-cell carcinoma is usually fatal, with a 5-year survival rate of only 13%. Surgery can be curative in a small percentage of patients with small tumors confined to the organ of origin. Adjuvant chemotherapy should be considered in certain patients undergoing surgery. Combined chemotherapy and radiation therapy may be as effective as surgery for the primary treatment. Disease extent at diagnosis is the best predictor of survival.

► This is one of those papers that only a place like the Mayo Clinic can turn out—a large series of EPSCCAs over a 20-year period. The authors had 81 such patients with primary sites including 29 gastrointestinal; 14 ear, nose, and throat; 12 genitourinary; and a mixture of others. They point out the poor prognosis and the need for systemic treatment.

E. Glatstein, M.D.

Utility of Screening Procedures for Detecting Recurrence of Disease After Complete Response in Patients With Small Cell Lung Carcinoma

Perez EA, Loprinzi CL, Sloan JA, et al (Mayo Clinic and Found, Rochester, Minn; Cedar Rapids Oncology Project CCOP, Iowa)

Cancer 80:676–680, 1997 12–2

Introduction.—In patients who were curatively treated for various malignancies, there has been renewed interest in evaluating routine follow-up procedures. Little evidence exists that follow-up testing of patients who achieve a complete response after chemotherapy for small-cell lung carcinoma impacts the natural history of the disease. The usefulness of follow-up testing for patients whose disease was considered to be in complete remission after systemic chemotherapy for small-cell lung carcinoma, was studied.

Methods.—There were 115 patients with small-cell lung carcinoma who had achieved a complete response after chemotherapy-radiotherapy and who later had disease progression. There were 57 patients with extensive-stage disease and 58 patients with limited-stage disease. Patients were examined every 4 months in the first year and every 6 months thereafter. Follow-up included examination of clinical history, chest radiography, chemistry group, hematology group, and physical examinations. To determine the first test to identify disease recurrence, whether the recurrence was diagnosed at the time of routine follow-up or between scheduled follow-up evaluations, the sites of recurrence, and patient outcome, patients' records were evaluated.

Results.—In the first follow-up year, 56 patients (49%) had recurrences. In the second year, 51 (44%) had recurrences. After 2 years, 8 patients (7%) had recurrences. Clinical histories signaled recurrences in 71% of patients, physical examination signaled recurrences in 10% of patients, chest radiographs signaled recurrences in 12%, and, abnormal results of chemistry testing signaled recurrences in 6% of patients. Symptoms that prompted visits between scheduled appointments signaled recurrences in 59% of patients, and 41% of recurrences were detected at scheduled clinical visits. All of the patients in this study had died at last follow-up with a median survival of 115 days after diagnosis of recurrences. For patients with recurrent small-cell lung carcinoma, there is a lack of curative therapy.

Conclusion.—Clinical histories and physical examinations are the most fruitful means of detecting evidence of recurrent lung carcinoma. This is consistent with data regarding the follow-up of other curatively treated cancers, such as melanoma and breast carcinoma. Routine blood tests appear to be of little value and chest radiography in asymptomatic patients detects recurrences in a small proportion of patients.

► Sometime during this generation, physicians developed the compulsion to order tests on most patients seen for routine visits. Whether it is a result of defensive medicine, consumer demand, or lack of confidence in the modern day physical examination, it is more common than not that patients leaving our offices have a chest radiograph or blood tests or both measures. This article should give some heart to the old-fashioned physician who takes a history and performs physical examinations. I'm sure if Hippocrates were alive today, a corollary of one of his aphorisms would be *primun non iubere* ("first, do not order").

P.J. Loehrer, Sr., M.D.

The Impact of Surgical Adjuvant Thoracic Radiation Therapy for Patients With Nonsmall Cell Lung Carcinoma With Ipsilateral Mediastinal Lymph Node Involvement

Sawyer TE, Bonner JA, Gould PM, et al (Mayo Clinic and Mayo Found, Rochester, Minn)

Cancer 80:1399–1408, 1997 12–3

Background.—Recurrence rates and survival in nonsmall cell lung carcinoma are generally worse for patients with ipsilateral mediastinal (American Joint Committee on Cancer [AJCC] class N2) lymph node involvement than in those with less nodal involvement (N0 or N1). Perhaps this poorer outcome is the result of retained subclinical local disease; if so, then adjuvant thoracic radiotherapy (TRT) to treat sites of retained disease may help improve outcomes in such patients. These authors put this hypothesis to the test.

Methods.—Complete surgical resection for lung carcinoma was performed for 224 patients (143 men and 81 women) with squamous cell, adenosquamous, or large cell carcinoma or adenocarcinoma. All patients had at least 1 involved N2 lymph node station. No patient had metastatic disease before the thoracotomy, nor had any patient received prior radiation or chemotherapy. Adjuvant TRT was used in 88 patients (39%) at a median dose of 50.4 Gy.

Results.—At a median follow-up of 3.5 years, 158 of 224 patients (71%) had died, for an overall survival rate of 29%. Local recurrence rates at 4 years were significantly better in the group treated with surgery and TRT (17%) than in the group treated by surgery alone (60%) (Fig 1).

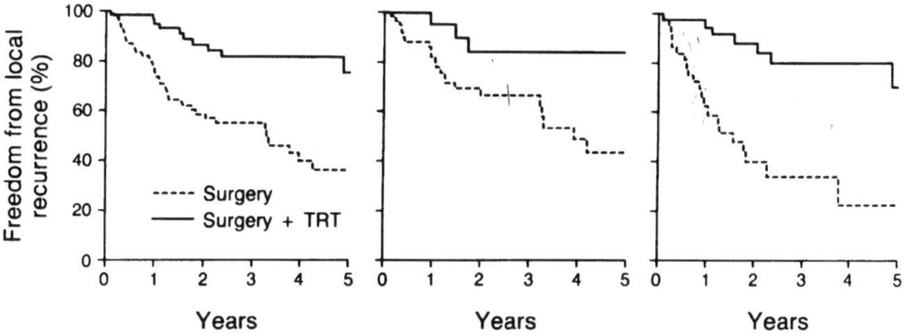

FIGURE 1.—The addition of postoperative thoracic radiotherapy (*TRT*) was associated with a significantly higher rate of freedom from local recurrence (compared with surgery alone) for (*left*) the entire group of patients ($P < 0.0001$), (*middle*), patients with 1 involved N2 lymph node ($P = 0.02$), and (*right*) patients with >1 involved N2 lymph node ($P < 0.0001$). (Courtesy of Sawyer TE, Bonner JA, Gould PM, et al: The impact of surgical adjuvant thoracic radiation therapy for patients with nonsmall cell lung carcinoma with ipsilateral mediastinal lymph node involvement. *Cancer* 80:1399–1408, 1997.)

Local recurrences were the first site of failure in 50% of the patients who had surgery alone, yet local disease recurrence happened in only 16% of patients who also received TRT (statistically significant difference) (Table 4). Overall survival at 4 years was also significantly better in the group treated with surgery and TRT (43%) than in the group treated by surgery alone (22%) (Fig 2). Multivariate analysis indicated that TRT, the absence of superior mediastinal lymph node involvement, and less N1 lymph node involvement were significant independent predictors of outcome in these patients.

TABLE 4.—Failure Patterns and Sequencing of Failure (224 Patients)

Endpoint	TRT	No. of patients	No. of events	4-yr actuarial rate, %	95% CI at 4 yrs	*P** value
Freedom from local	Yes	73	10	83	73–94	
recurrence†	No	124	43	40	28–57	<0.0001
Freedom from local	Yes‡	73	9	84	74–95	
recurrence as first site of recurrence†	No	124	36	50	38–66	0.0001
Freedom from distant	Yes	88	35	55	44–69	
recurrence	No	136	77	32	23–43	0.0002
Freedom from distant	Yes‡	88	32	59	48–72	
recurrence as first site of recurrence	No	136	64	35	26–47	0.002
Freedom from any	Yes	73	34	51	40–66	
recurrence	No	124	82	19	13–30	<0.0001

TRT, Thoracic radiotherapy; *95% CI*, 95% confidence interval.
*Log rank test.
†Total of 197 patients in the local recurrence analysis; the other 27 were immediately censored because they never underwent a documented study to assess local disease status.
‡Includes patients with simultaneous local and distant recurrence at the time of first recurrence.
(Courtesy of Sawyer TE, Bonner JA, Gould PM, et al: The impact of surgical adjuvant thoracic radiation therapy for patients with nonsmall cell lung carcinoma with ipsilateral mediastinal lymph node involvement. *Cancer* 80:1399–1408, 1997.

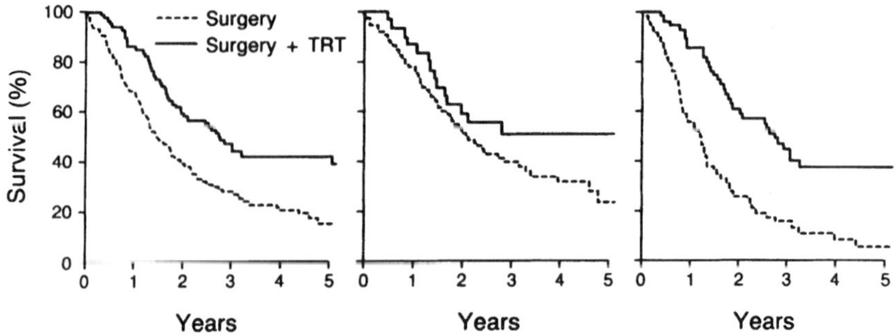

FIGURE 2.—The addition of postoperative thoracic radiotherapy (*TRT*) was associated with a significantly higher survival rate (compared with surgery alone) for (*left*) the entire group of patients (P = 0.0005), (*middle*), patients with 1 involved N2 lymph node (P = 0.17, not statistically significant), and (*right*) patients with >1 involved N2 lymph node (P < 0.0001). (Courtesy of Sawyer TE, Bonner JA, Gould PM, et al. The impact of surgical adjuvant thoracic radiation therapy for patients with nonsmall cell lung carcinoma with ipsilateral mediastinal lymph node involvement. *Cancer* 80:1399–1408, 1997. Copyright © 1997 American Cancer Society. Reprinted by permission of Wiley-Liss, Inc., a subsidiary of John Wiley & Sons, Inc.)

Conclusions.—Resection plus adjuvant TRT improved not only local recurrence rates, but also overall survival more so than resection alone in these patients with N2 lymph node involvement. The recurrences that did develop with TRT were more often at a site distant from the primary site, further supporting the role of TRT in improving local disease control. Further research is needed to define the role of TRT in prolonging disease-free control and survival in patients with non–small-cell lung cancer with N2 lymph node involvement.

▶ Following the Lung Cancer Study Group's investigation with postoperative radiation after a complete mediastinal "cleanout" for non–small-cell lung cancer, it has been difficult to know quite what to recommend. Typically, patients with lung cancer do not have a mediastinal cleanout procedure but just simply some sampling at the time of the surgical resection. The question remains: just how much can be accomplished with postoperative radiation in a setting of limited metastatic disease? The Lung Cancer Study Group involved patients after mediastinal cleanout procedure and resection with no gross residual disease and randomly assigned them to postoperative radiation or no radiation. They showed a statistically significant improvement in local control with radiation therapy, but no enhancement of survival. The highly selected nature of these patients is evident from the fact that the surgical resection alone was associated with a 30% long-term survival. That was obviously not typical for advanced lung cancer.

In the Lung Cancer Study Group experience, only 20% of their patients had N2 disease, which is probably an indication of why the patients did so well with surgery alone. In this retrospective analysis, all patients had N2 disease, which is a sharp distinction. Approximately 40% of patients received postoperative radiation therapy but were not in the randomized group. Postoperative radiation markedly reduced the local recurrence rate, which was 60% with surgery alone, and effectively doubled the actuarial

4-year survival rate. Despite its retrospective nature, this study strongly suggests that postoperative radiation therapy is beneficial for both local control and survival when mediastinal nodes are involved.

The Lung Cancer Study Group's investigation was flawed not only by a minority of their patients with N2 disease, but also by the fact that they evaluated only squamous cell carcinoma, neglected the other histologic findings, and that the uppermost nodes of resection had to be negative (benign) in order for patients to be included in their randomization. This retrospective study from the Mayo Clinic does not have such restrictions. In addition, it should be pointed out that the typical procedure performed in this country is not a mediastinal cleanout at all, but simple removal of the lobe or lung and the taking of some adjacent lymph nodes. Right or wrong, that is the procedure typically done. The case for postoperative radiation therapy remains a strong one.

E. Glatstein, M.D.

Wedge Resection Versus Lobectomy for Stage I (T1 N0 M0) Non-Small-Cell Lung Cancer

Landreneau RJ, Sugarbaker DJ, Mack MJ, et al (Allegheny Univ, Pittsburgh, Pa; University of Pittsburgh, Pa; Harvard Univ, Boston; et al)
J Thorac Cardiovasc Surg 113:691–700, 1997 12–4

Background.—The value of nonanatomic wedge resection in the treatment of stage I non–small-cell lung cancer relative to the current gold standard, anatomic lobectomy, has not been established definitively. The efficacy of the video-assisted thoracic surgical (VATS) approach to wedge resection of peripheral lung cancers also has not been studied directly.

Methods.—The outcomes of 219 consecutive patients with pathologic stage I (T1 N0 M0) non–small-cell lung cancer were analyzed. Resection was performed in 42 patients, VATS wedge resection in 60, and lobectomy in 117.

Findings.—Operative mortality rate was 3% in patients undergoing lobectomy and 0% in those having wedge resection. Five-year survival was

TABLE 2.—Wedge Resection Versus Lobectomy for Stage I (T1 N0 M0) Lung Cancer

	Open WR	*VATS WR*	*vs*	*Lobectomy*	*p Value*
Operative mortality (%)	0	0	vs	3.3	0.20
Postop. stay (days)	7.7	6.3	vs	10.6	0.0002
Local recurrence (%)	24	16	vs	9	0.07
Local/systemic recurrence (%)	30	26	vs	19	0.22

Abbreviation: ER, wedge resection.

(Courtesy of Landreneau RJ, Sugarbaker DJ, Mack MJ, et al: Wedge resection versus lobectomy for stage I (T1 N0 M0) non-small-cell lung cancer. *J Thorac Cardiovasc Surg* 113:691–700, 1997.)

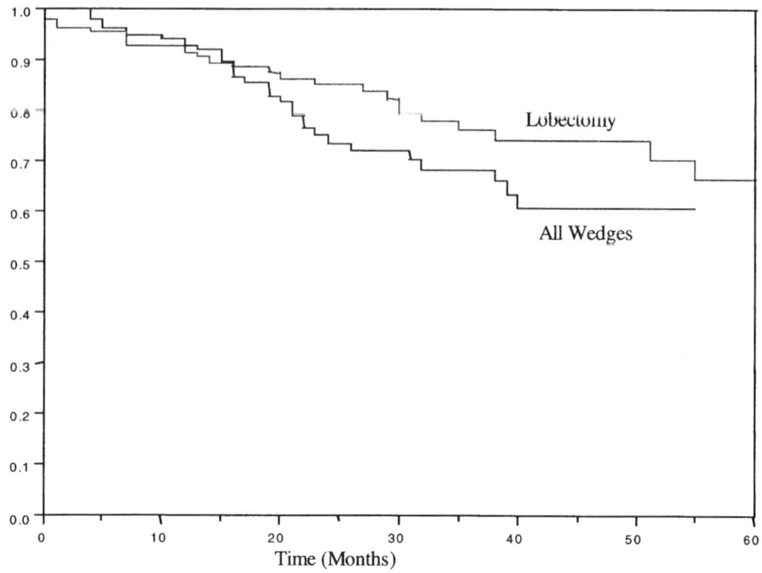

FIGURE 2.—Five-year actual survival differences noted between all patients having wedge resection and all those having lobectomy. (Courtesy of Landreneau RJ, Sugarbaker DJ, Mack MJ, et al: Wedge resection versus lobectomy for stage I (T1 N0 M0) non-small-cell lung cancer. *J Thorac Cardiovasc Surg* 113:691–700, 1997.)

58% for patients who underwent open wedge resection, 65% for those with VATS wedge resection, and 70% for those who underwent lobectomy (Table 2). In log rank testing, significant differences were noted among survival curves during the 5-year study, a result of a significantly greater non–cancer-related death rate by 5 years among patients undergoing wedge resection (Fig 2).

Conclusion.—In patients with cardiopulmonary physiologic impairment, wedge resection by open thoracotomy or VATS approaches appears to be a viable "compromise" treatment for stage I T1 N0 M0 non–small-cell lung cancer. Because the risk for local recurrence is increased, anatomical lobectomy continues to be the surgical treatment of choice for such cancer in patients with adequate physiologic reserve.

▶ This article is a retrospective review of 219 patients with pathologic Stage I non–small-cell lung cancer who underwent open wedge resection, video-assisted wedge resection, or lobectomy. More than half of the patients had the lobectomy. There were no significant differences with regard to histology. Patients who underwent wedge resections tended to be older and had poor pulmonary function. There were no operative deaths among patients who had a wedge resection, but there was a 3% operative mortality among those who had a lobectomy. Within the first year, survival curves were similar. However, by 5 years patients who had an open wedge resection had a 58% survival rate, whereas those who had a video-assisted wedge resection had a 65% survival rate, and those with a lobectomy had a 70% survival rate.

It is important to recall that these data are not based on any randomization and that there are undoubtedly subtle differences among the patients themselves under each heading. The data seem reasonably clear that, all things being equal (which they are usually not), a lobectomy would seem to be the procedure of choice for this kind of problem.

E. Glatstein, M.D.

Factors Influencing Long-term Survival After Lung Metastasectomy

Robert JH, Ambrogi V, Mermillod B, et al (Geneva Univ Hosp; Royal Brompton Natl Heart and Lung Hosp, London)

Ann Thorac Surg 63:777–784, 1997 12–5

Introduction.—Reported survivals for patients undergoing resection of lung metastases are sometimes even better than those reported after surgery for primary lung cancer. However, the available data are insufficient to draw conclusions about how metastasectomy works and in whom it should be done. A 14-year experience with lung metastasectomy was reviewed to identify those patients most likely to benefit.

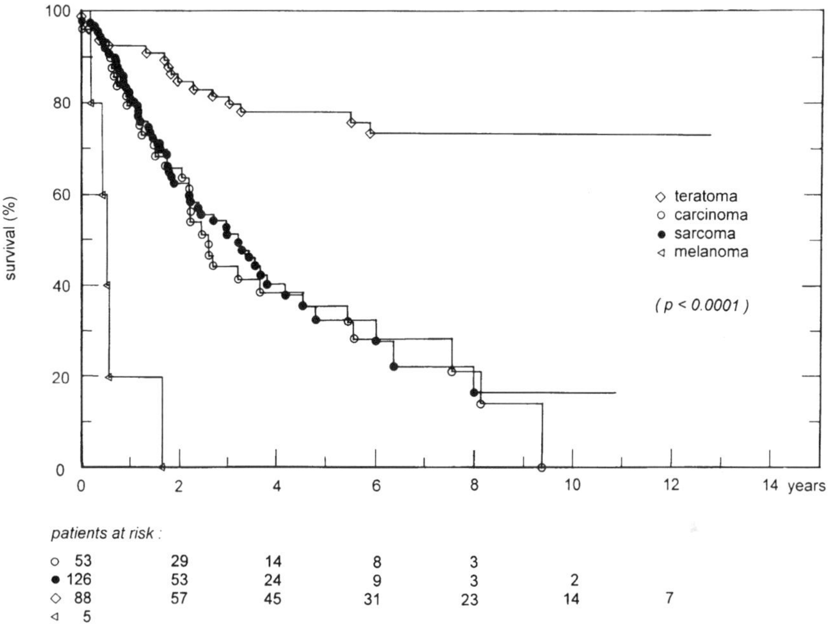

FIGURE 2.—Survival in relation to histology. (Courtesy of Robert JH, Ambrogi V, Mermillod B, et al: Factors influencing long-term survival after lung metastasectomy. *Ann Thorac Surg* 63:777–784, 1997. Reprinted with permission from the Society of Thoracic Surgery.)

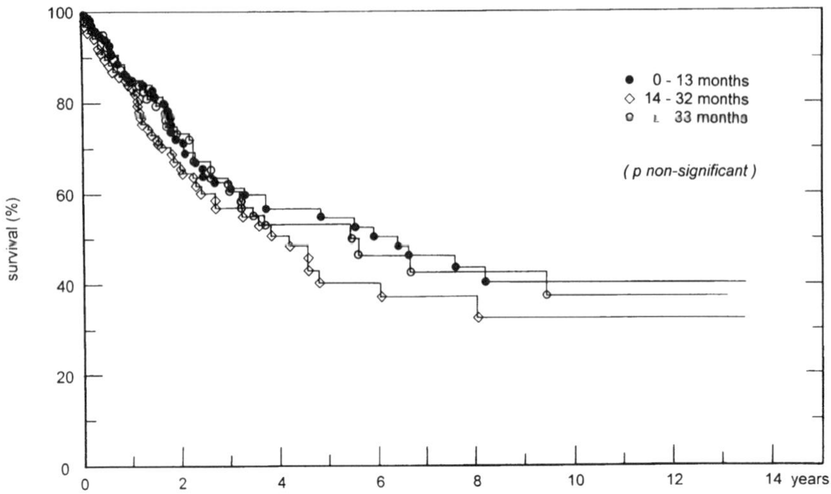

patients at risk :

● 89	53	36	24	15	8	5
◇ 95	40	23	13	7	2	1
○ 92	48	26	12	8	6	1

FIGURE 4.—Survival in relation to disease-free interval from primary treatment to (first) metastasectomy. (Courtesy of Robert JH, Ambrogi V, Mermillod B, et al: Factors influencing long-term survival after lung metastasectomy. *Ann Thorac Surg* 63:777–784, 1997. Reprinted with permission from the Society of Thoracic Surgery.)

Methods.—From 1980 to 1993, 276 patients underwent one or more lung metastasectomies. The patients were 193 males and 83 females, with a mean age of 38 years. In each patient, complete excision of all intrathoracic disease was considered feasible, and reliable control of primary disease had been achieved. Sixty-three patients subsequently required a second-stage metastasectomy, 12 had 3 stages, and 2 had 4 stages. On univariate and multivariate analyses, disease-free interval, size, and number of resected metastases were assessed for predictive value.

Results.—Forty-six percent of patients had primary sarcoma, 32% had teratoma, and 53% had carcinoma. Two-year actuarial survival was 69%, with a 95% confidence interval (CI) of 62% to 74%. Survival decreased to 48% at 5 years (95% CI 40% to 55%) and 35% at 10 years (95% CI 23% to 44%). On multivariate analysis, almost all useful predictive information was obtained from histologic examination (Fig 2). The median disease-free interval was 21 months; this parameter had no effect on survival (Fig 4). Number of metastases had some predictive value (Fig 5).

Conclusions.—Some patients undergoing lung metastasectomy achieve long-term survival. The major determinant of survival appears to be histologic tumor type. Metastasectomy may be considered even for patients with a short disease-free interval, numerous metastatic lesions, or even recurrent tumor deposits after a first or second metastasectomy.

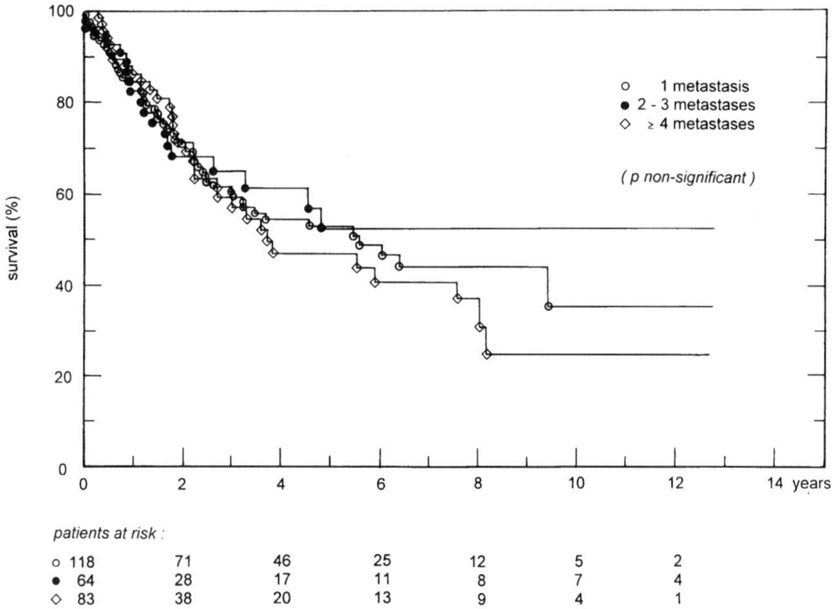

FIGURE 5.—Survival according to the number of metastases excised at first metastasectomy. (Courtesy of Robert JH, Ambrogi V, Mermillod B, et al: Factors influencing long-term survival after lung metastasectomy. *Ann Thorac Surg* 63:777–784, 1997. Reprinted with permission from the Society of Thoracic Surgery.)

▶ The role of metastasectomy for metastases seems to go through cycles of acceptability. This retrospective study would suggest that it has a major role to play. When one looks at the survival in relationship to histology, one sees that the role to play is related predominantly to teratomas, and to a lesser degree sarcoma. For melanoma there is not even a hint of benefit, and for carcinomas it is obviously a question of selection.

It is unfortunate that the data on relationship to disease-free interval from primary treatment to the first metastasectomy and the data on the survival by number of metastases excised are not broken down by the histology. Particularly for the carcinomas I suspect that would be helpful for a proper interpretation.

I think it is important to note there is no other clinically curative alternative to metastasectomy and that there is a realistic cure rate for teratomas and sarcomas, at least measured at 5 years, after aggressive surgery. The key is in the patient selection because it appears that there is a subpopulation of patients with metastatic disease confined to pulmonary tissue.

E. Glatstein, M.D.

13 Head and Neck Cancer

Comparison of Cost and Function in Reconstruction of the Posterior Oral Cavity and Oropharynx: Free vs Pedicled Soft Tissue Transfer
Tsue TT, Desyatnikova SS, Deleyiannis F W-B, et al (Univ of Kansas, Kansas City; Univ of Washington, Seattle; Virginia Mason Med Clinic, Seattle)
Arch Otolaryngol Head Neck Surg 123:731–737, 1997 13–1

Introduction.—Technological advances have diminished the differences between the benefits and drawbacks of free flaps (FF) and pedicled pectoralis major myocutaneous flaps (PMMF) in the treatment of patients undergoing reconstruction of the posterior oral cavity and oropharynx. The cost and intangible functional results of FF and PMMF reconstruction were compared in patients undergoing surgery for posterior or oropharyngeal lesions.

Methods.—Medical and accounting records of 53 consecutive patients undergoing FF (29 patients) or pedicled PMMF (24 patients) for extirpation of neoplastic or osteoradionecrotic lesions were reviewed from January 1991 to December 1995. Median patient follow-up time was 298 days.

Results.—The operative time was significantly longer for patients who underwent FF reconstruction than it was for those who underwent PMMF reconstruction. Intensive care unit and hospital stays were similar for patients in both groups. The cost of treatment for patients who underwent FF reconstructions was $41,122. For patients with PMMF reconstructions, the cost was $37,160. This significant difference in treatment cost was the result of increased professional fees required for microsurgical FF reconstruction. These expenses were offset by intangible cost differences. Patients in the PMMF group had an increased rate of flap-related complications, compared with patients in the FF group. At final follow-up, 4 (15%) patients in the FF group and 3 (15%) patients in the PMMF group had a tracheotomy. In the PMMF group, 17 (85%) patients required enteral tube feedings, and 6 (30%) patients were eating a soft diet, compared with 11 (39%) and 18 (64%) in the FF group (both differences were significant).

Conclusion.—When direct costs are compared, there is only a modest difference in the reconstruction costs of FF and PMMF. The intangible costs of PMMF reconstruction outweighed the direct costs of FF. The functional benefits of FF reconstruction seem to justify the slightly increased expense of its use.

▶ This is a cost comparison and also a comparison of functional results following free flap vs. pedicled soft tissue reconstruction in the management of posterior oral cavity and oropharyngeal lesions. Certainly the cost for these procedures is significant. The difference between them seems relatively modest.

Personally, I am not enthusiastic about cost comparison studies. I am anxious to see who has developed better ways of treating cancer. In this era of bean counters, cost considerations are not trivial. I only hope they are not ultimately used as the sole basis for deciding *how* patients should be treated. In the meantime, whether I like it or not, we will see more of these types of analyses.

E. Glatstein, M.D.

Resection and Immediate Microvascular Reconstruction in the Management of Osteoradionecrosis of the Mandible

Shaha AR, Cordeiro PG, Hidalgo DA, et al (Mem Sloan-Kettering Cancer Ctr, New York)

Head Neck 19:406–411, 1997 13–2

Background.—Patients with advanced cancers of the head and neck are often treated with high doses of radiation. This treatment can lead to the development of osteoradionecrosis (ORN) of the mandible, and advanced ORN of the mandible can be difficult to treat. Six patients with advanced ORN of the mandible were treated with surgical resection of the affected portion of the mandible with immediate mandibular reconstruction and microvascular free-tissue transfer.

Methods.—All 6 patients had head or neck cancer and were exposed to postoperative radiotherapy, ranging in dosage from 6,000 to 7,900 cGy. From 5 months to 17 years later, these patients had ORN. Initial treatment was conservative and included local débridement, oral irrigation, and antibiotics. In 3 cases, hyperbaric oxygen was employed. Despite this treatment, the necrosis was not responsive and progressed to mucosal ulceration and bone exposure. These patients were treated with mandibular resection, followed by an osteotomized, contoured fibular graft. The cutaneous surface was utilized to resurface the soft-tissue defect.

Results.—The surgery was well tolerated with no significant postoperative complications. Hospitalization duration was for a median of 15 days. Two patients had minor wound sepsis that required removal of some hardware. Cosmetic and functional results were satisfactory. All patients are now capable of eating at least a soft diet.

Conclusions.—The management of advanced ORN remains controversial. For these patients, radical resection of the involved portion of the mandible, followed by free microvascular reconstruction appears to be a good option. Once the wound has healed, osseointegrated implants should be considered to improve the functional results. This was achieved for 1 patient in this series.

▶ Osteoradionecrosis of the mandible has been a major challenge in the management of head and neck cancer for some time. These investigators from Memorial Sloan-Kettering have used a radical resection of the mandible with immediate microvascular reconstruction to deal with ORN. They treated 6 patients this way, all of whom had failed initial conservative management, which included hyperbaric oxygen in 3.

This operative procedure appears to have been effective in dealing with this problem, and those who are interested should read the article carefully and look at exactly what the procedure is and how it has been carried out.

E. Glatstein, M.D.

Pterygopalatine Fossa and Maxillary Nerve Infiltration in Nasopharyngeal Carcinoma

Chong VFH, Fan Y-F (Singapore Gen Hosp)

Head Neck 19:121–125, 1997 13–3

Background.—Although rare in Western countries, nasopharyngeal carcinoma occurs in up to 30/100,000 Chinese each year. As a rare complication, it can extend through the pterygopalatine fossa (PPF) to affect the maxillary and infraorbital nerves. These authors examined the frequency of PPF and maxillary nerve involvement in a series of patients with nasopharyngeal carcinoma.

Methods.—The overall series consisted of 114 patients with nasopharyngeal carcinoma proven by histologic examination. All patients underwent MRI and CT to define the extent of tumor invasion, including infraorbital involvement. In particular, T1-weighted MRI best shows the replacement of fat that characterizes the PPF, and contrast-enhanced coronal MRI best shows involvement of the maxillary nerve in the foramen rotundum (Fig 1E, F).

Findings.—Fifteen percent of the patients (17 of 114) had tumor extending anteriorly into the PPF. Whereas perineural infiltration of the maxillary nerve was uncommon in the series as a whole (4 of 114 patients), it was seen in one fourth of patients with PPF involvement. All patients whose MR images showed maxillary nerve enhancement also had hypoesthesia of the cheek; hypoesthesia was ipsilateral in almost half of these patients (8 of 17, or 47%).

Conclusion.—In this series, 15% of patients with nasopharyngeal carcinoma had tumor infiltration into the PPF. Maxillary nerve involvement was common in such cases, and could be identified clinically by hypoes-

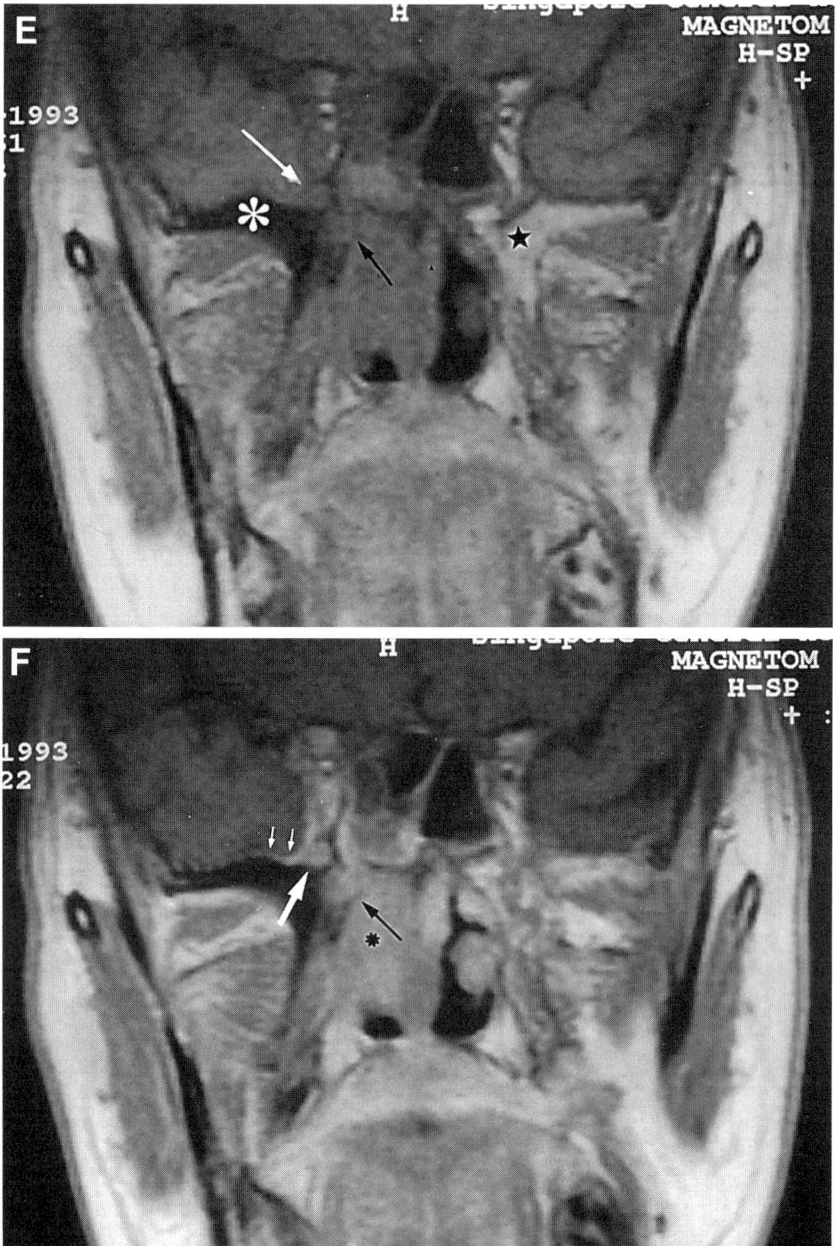

FIGURE 1.—**E**, coronal T1-weighted MRI shows enlargement of the right maxillary nerve (*white arrow*). The right sphenoid bone shows low signal intensity (*asterisk*). The signal intensity of the left sphenoid bone is normal (*star*). Note the enlarged right Vidian canal (*black arrow*). **F**, contrast-enhanced coronal MRI shows enhancement of the right maxillary nerve (*white arrow*). Note the dural enhancement (*small arrows*) and mass in the right nasal fossa (*asterisk*). There is also perineural infiltration of the Vidian nerve (*black arrow*). (Courtesy of Chong VFH, Fan Y-F: Pterygopalatine fossa and maxillary nerve infiltration in nasopharyngeal carcinoma. *Head Neck* 19:121–125, 1997. Reprinted by permission of John Wiley & Sons, Inc.)

thesia over the cheek. Perineural infiltration occurred in 1 of 4 of these patients, and its presence affected both the planning of the treatment and the patient's prognosis.

▶ This paper evaluates involvement of the maxillary nerve and PPF in patients with nasal pharyngeal carcinoma. I include this article because I think the MR pictures are really quite spectacular and of use in helping us assess this area in the future.

E. Glatstein, M.D.

Timing of Edentulation and Extraction in the Management of Oral Cavity and Oropharyngeal Malignancies

Doerr TD, Marunick MT (Wayne State Univ, Detroit; Harper Hosp, Detroit)

Head Neck 19:426–430, 1997 13–4

Objective.—An oral evaluation before surgery and radiotherapy for head and neck cancer is important for the timing of extractions. Providing a sufficient healing period after extraction minimizes the risk of osteoradionecrosis. A retrospective review of the safety and efficacy of concurrent extractions and surgery vs. delayed postsurgical extractions compared the postoperative courses and addressed management of patients with head and neck cancer.

Methods.—There were 32 patients (4 women), with an average age of 52 years, who had concurrent extractions and surgery and 23 patients (4 women), with an average age of 52 years, who had postsurgical extractions.

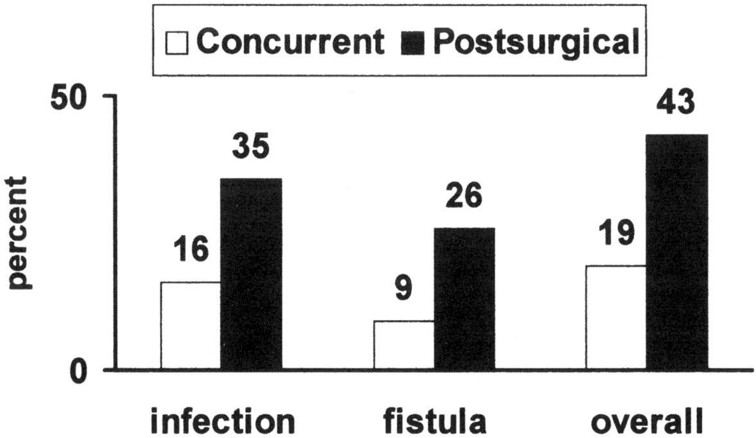

FIGURE 1.—Postoperative wound complications. (Courtesy of Doerr TD, Marunick MT: Timing of edentulation and extraction in the management of oral cavity and oropharyngeal malignancies. *Head Neck* 19:426–430, 1997. Reprinted by permission of John Wiley & Sons, Inc.)

Results.—Five patients in the concurrent group had wound infections and 3 had orocutaneous fistulas, whereas in the postsurgical group, the numbers were nonsignificantly higher (8 and 6, respectively) (Fig 1). Average postoperative stays were significantly longer in the postsurgical group (27 days) than in the concurrent group (15 days). Average stays with and without complications were also shorter in the concurrent group.

Conclusion.—Patients with head and neck cancer who have extractions concurrent with surgery have fewer complications and shorter hospitalizations than patients having postsurgical extractions.

▶ In radiation therapy, there is a constant struggle regarding the subject of retaining teeth in the management of patients who have head and neck cancer. This particular study from Detroit looks at patients who were not randomized but who underwent dental extractions either at the time of the surgical procedure or postoperatively. The data show that patients do best who have their teeth removed at the time of surgery.

It is unfortunate that the authors did not investigate patients who had their teeth removed before the surgery. If we think the teeth cannot be salvaged and have to be removed, our usual policy is to take the teeth out before the surgical procedure, even if it delays surgery and/or radiation for a couple of weeks. Unfortunately, the authors have no data on that type of management.

E. Glatstein, M.D.

Carcinoma of the Nasopharynx Treated by Radiotherapy Alone: Determinants of Local and Regional Control

Sanguineti G, Geara FB, Garden AS, et al (Univ of Texas, Houston)

Int J Radiat Oncol Biol Phys 37:985–996, 1997 13–5

Background.—Nasopharyngeal carcinoma is rare (less than 0.5/100,000 in the United States), but regional or local recurrences are common (up to 60% of patients). This large, retrospective article examined almost 400 cases of carcinoma of the nasopharynx treated by radiotherapy, to determine specific prognostic factors for regional and local recurrences.

Methods.—From 1954 to 1992, 378 patients (286 men and 92 women; median age, 52 years) with nasopharyngeal carcinoma were treated. Treatment methods evolved over the years, although radiotherapy remained the cornerstone of treatment. The total radiation dose was based on tumor stage and ranged from 60.2 to 72.0 Gy. Most patients (three quarters) were seen with advanced disease, including squamous cell carcinoma in 51% of patients and lymphoepithelioma in 41%. Also, most (three quarters) had positive neck nodes. Cranial nerve involvement (typically cranial nerves VI and V) occurred in 8% of patients.

Findings.—Almost half of the patients (49%) have died, with 5-, 10-, and 20-year actuarial survival rates of 48%, 34%, and 18%, respectively.

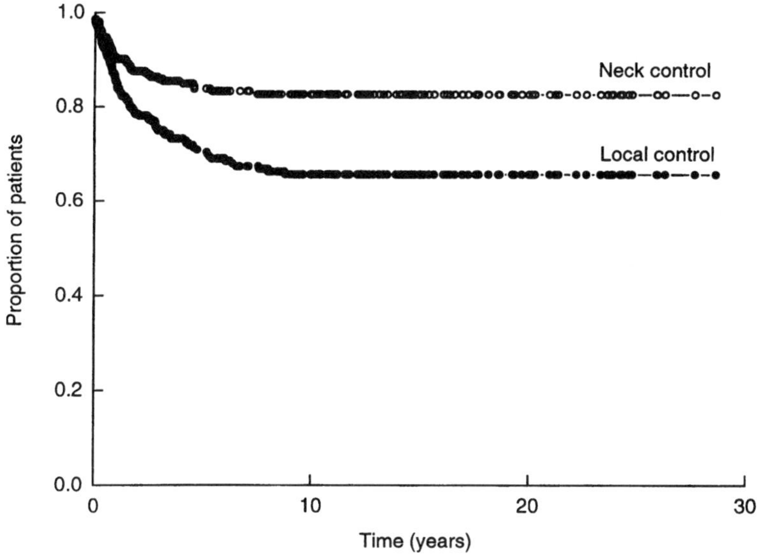

FIGURE 1.—Overall actuarial control rates at the primary site and the neck. (Reprinted by permission of the publisher from Sanguineti G, Geara FB, Garden AS, et al. Carcinoma of the nasopharynx treated by radiotherapy alone: Determinants of local and regional control. *Int J Radiat Oncol Biol Phys* 37:985–996, copyright 1997 by Elsevier Science Inc.)

However, local and regional control rates have been better, with local control rates at 5, 10, and 20 years of 71%, 66%, and 66%, respectively, and regional control rates of 84%, 83%, and 83%, respectively (Fig 1). Local recurrence was experienced by 26% of patients at a median of 13 months after treatment. The stage of the tumor (greater stages had worse prognosis), the type of tumor (worse prognosis for squamous cell carcinoma), the presence of skull base erosion, and the presence of cranial nerve deficits were significantly associated with poorer local control rates. In fact, patients with both skull base erosion and cranial nerve deficits had higher local failure rates than patients with only 1 of these features (Fig 4). Regional recurrence was experienced by 13% of patients at a median of 8.2 months after treatment. The nodal stage (nodal involvement had worse prognosis) and the type of squamous cell tumor (worse prognosis for moderately or well-differentiated tumors) were significantly associated with poorer regional control rates. Grade 3 to 5 complication rates at 5, 10, and 20 years were 16%, 19%, and 19%, respectively. Treatment-related complications were responsible for 12 deaths (3%) (all had grade 5 complications), and all these occurred before 1976.

Conclusion.—This article establishes benchmarks in the evaluation of local and regional recurrences after treatment of nasopharyngeal carcinoma. Local recurrences were more likely in patients with advanced squamous cell carcinoma with skull base erosion and/or cranial nerve deficits. Regional recurrences were more likely in patients with moderately or well-differentiated squamous cell cancer with nodal involvement. These

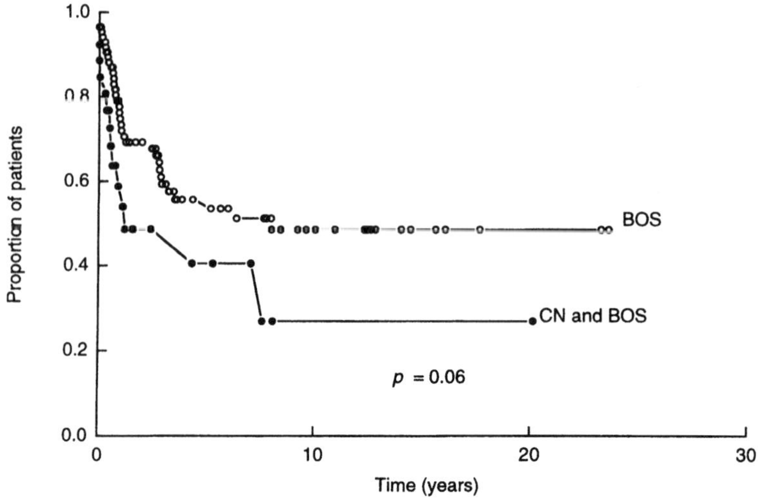

FIGURE 4.—Local control as a function of the presence of base of skull erosion (*BOS*) and cranial nerve (*CN*) deficit. Local control rates were lower for patients who had both features ($P = 0.06$). (Reprinted by permission of the publisher from Sanguineti G, Geara FB, Garden AS, et al. Carcinoma of the nasopharynx treated by radiotherapy alone: Determinants of local and regional control. *Int J Radiat Oncol Biol Phys* 37:985–996, copyright 1997 by Elsevier Science Inc.)

patients are candidates for other treatments such as dose escalation or adjunctive chemotherapy.

▶ This is a large retrospective paper from the M.D. Anderson Cancer Center at the University of Texas dealing with a nearly 40-year experience and just under 400 patients with nasopharyngeal carcinoma treated by radiation therapy alone. Their 5-, 10-, and 20-year actuarial survival rates were 48%, 34%, and 18%, respectively. Local control figures were considerably better. Because of the size of the patient group and the fact that it comes from the M.D. Anderson Hospital, it is likely that this will be the standard reference on outcome for nasopharyngeal carcinoma for the next several years.

E. Glatstein, M.D.

Definitive Radiotherapy for T3 Squamous Cell Carcinoma of the Glottic Larynx

Mendenhall WM, Parsons JT, Mancuso AA, et al (Univ of Florida, Gainesville)
J Clin Oncol 15:2394–2402, 1997 13–6

Purpose.—There is ongoing debate about the treatment of T3 squamous cell carcinoma of the glottic larynx. Whereas most American patients are treated surgically, patients in Canada may be treated by radiation therapy alone, with surgery reserved for salvage treatment. The results of radiotherapy alone for patients with T3 cancer of the true vocal cords were reported.

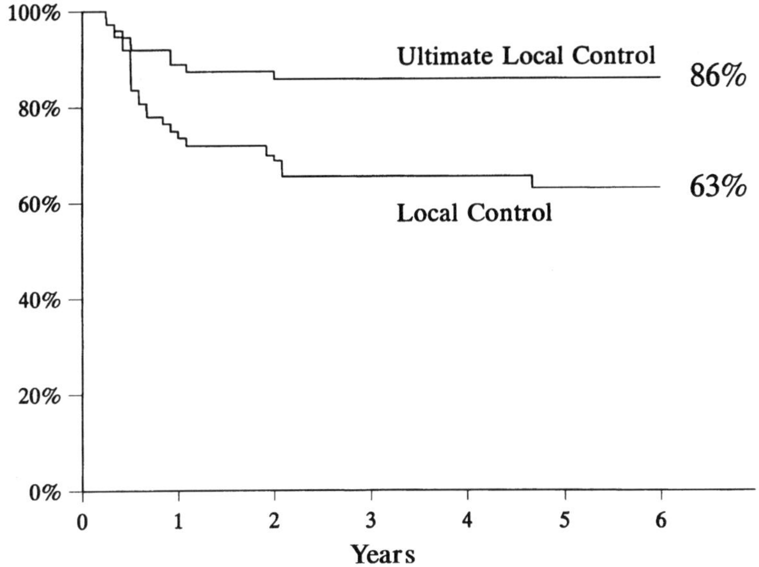

FIGURE 1.—Local control (after radiotherapy alone) and ultimate local control (after salvage therapy). (Courtesy of Mendenhall WM, Parsons JT, Mancuso AA, et al: Definitive radiotherapy for T3 squamous cell carcinoma of the glottic larynx. *J Clin Oncol* 15:2394–2402, 1997.)

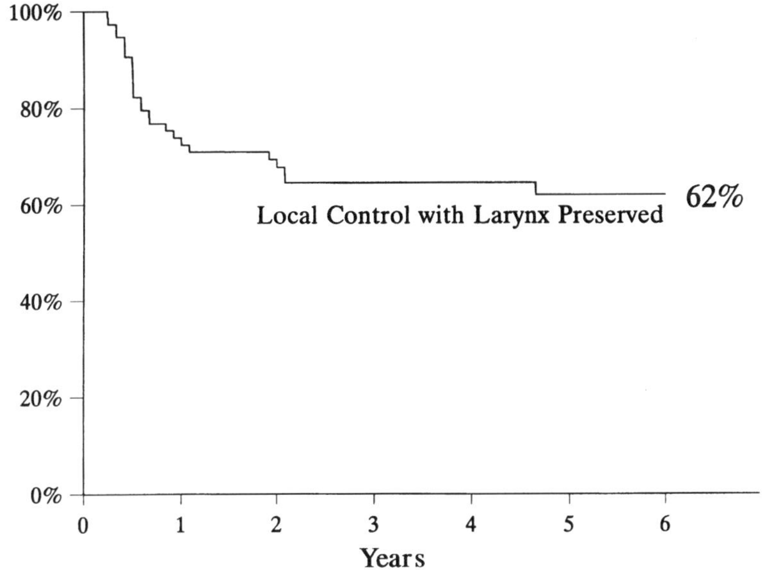

FIGURE 3.—Local control with laryngeal voice preservation. (Courtesy of Mendenhall WM, Parsons JT, Mancuso AA, et al: Definitive radiotherapy for T3 squamous cell carcinoma of the glottic larynx. *J Clin Oncol* 15:2394–2402, 1997.)

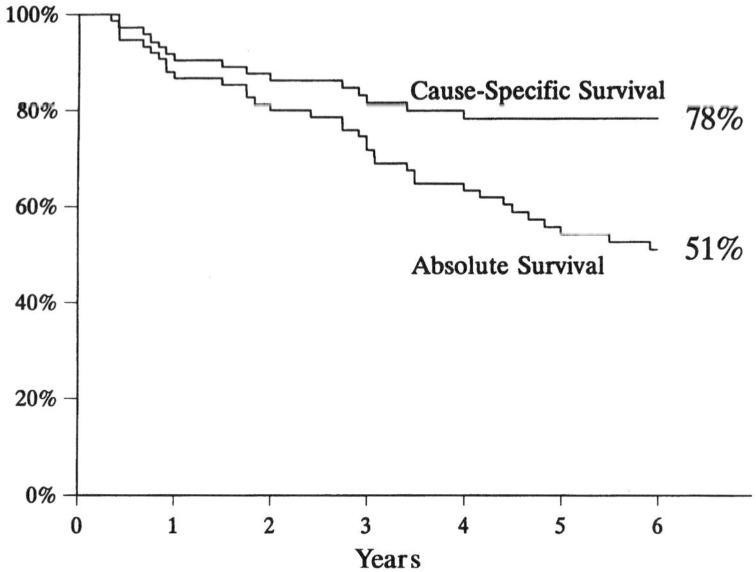

FIGURE 5.—Absolute survival and cause-specific survival. (Courtesy of Mendenhall WM, Parsons JT, Mancuso AA, et al: Definitive radiotherapy for T3 squamous cell carcinoma of the glottic larynx. *J Clin Oncol* 15:2394–2402, 1997.)

Methods.—A total of 75 patients with previously untreated T3 squamous cell carcinoma of the glottic larynx were studied. All patients received radiotherapy, 73 with curative intent. The other 2 patients underwent a planned neck dissection after radiotherapy. None was given adjuvant chemotherapy. Follow-up was at least 2 years for all patients, and 85% were followed up for at least 5 years. Follow-up was complete. Primary tumor volume was calculated from pretreatment CT scans in 38 patients.

Results.—Local control rate was 63% at 5 years and 86% after salvage therapy (Fig 1). Sixty-two percent of patients had local control with laryngeal voice preservation (Fig 3). This outcome was achieved in 87% of patients with a pretreatment tumor volume of 3.5 cm^3 or less vs. 29% in those with larger tumor volumes. Local control was unrelated to whether the vocal cord regained mobility or remained fixed after radiation therapy. Five-year absolute survival was 54%, whereas cause-specific survival at the same time was 78% (Fig 5). On multivariate analysis, cause-specific survival was significantly associated with pretreatment tracheostomy.

Conclusions.—Long-term locoregional control and survival with radiotherapy alone are similar to those achievable with surgery in patients with T3 squamous cell carcinoma of the true vocal cords. Primary tumor volume appears to affect the chances of local control after radiotherapy. It remains to be seen whether induction chemotherapy followed by radiation therapy could offer still better results.

▶ Advanced carcinoma of the glottis tends to be treated with both surgery and radiation. Exactly why is not clear to me because this series, as well as others, show excellent results with radiation therapy alone, coupled with a surgical salvage. Despite the bias of many surgeons, these data from University of Florida show excellent results with radiation alone and raise the question of a controlled clinical trial.

E. Glatstein, M.D.

14 Skin Cancer

Optimal Selective Sentinel Lymph Node Dissection in Primary Malignant Melanoma

Leong SPL, Steinmetz I, Habib FA, et al (Univ of California, San Francisco)

Arch Surg 132:666–673, 1997 14–1

Objective.—Whether there is a benefit from sentinel lymph node dissection in patients with melanoma is controversial. Sentinel lymph node (SLN) mapping using lymphoscintigraphy may help distinguish those patients who would benefit from lymph node dissection. Results of 163 consecutive patients with stage I melanoma who had undergone immediate preoperative lymphoscintigraphy followed by intraoperative SLN mapping were evaluated.

Methods.—Technetium-99m sulfur colloid was injected intradermally around the biopsy sites. Isosulfan blue was injected intradermally around the melanoma site before surgery. Most patients preferred general anesthesia for the mapping process. Sentinel lymph nodes were defined as radiolabeled lymph nodes or nodes detected with blue dye.

Results.—Sentinel lymph nodes were detected in 160 patients. The 3 failures involved the head. A total of 303 SLNs and 144 adjacent nodes were removed, and 11.6% were positive for micrometastases. Thirty (18.4%) patients had micrometastases. Complete lymph node dissection was performed in 22 patients, and 1.01% were positive compared to 46.3% of lymph nodes detected by lymphoscintigraphy. Significantly more SLNs than non-SLNs had micrometastases. During an average follow-up period of 463 days, 7 recurrences were reported, 5 (3.8%) from the SLN group and 2 (6%) from the non-SLN group. Second melanomas developed in 2 patients.

Conclusion.—Immediate preoperative lymphoscintigraphy followed by intraoperative mapping is an effective technique for identifying and locating SLNs. The incidence of SLN micrometastases was 18.4%.

► The standard of care for the management of melanomas has undergone a rather drastic change in the last few years. This was precipitated by the proven benefit of alpha-interferon[1] in the adjuvant therapy of patients with high-risk melanoma and the routine use of lymphatic mapping and SLN biopsy in the staging of melanoma. This article from the group at the University of California at San Francisco utilizes a double-mapping technique of vital dye and gamma probe detection with a yield of approximately 20% microscopic positive nodal disease. In addition, approximately 20% of patients will have additional nodal metastases noted after complete nodal dissection. This is substantially in agreement with other institutional series of SLN biopsy. Although the majority of patients in this series had general anesthesia, it has become routine in our institution as well as others to do lymphatic mapping and SLN biopsy and wide local excision of the primary site using local anesthesia with IV-assist sedation. This makes the procedure a cost-effective, simple outpatient surgery. Clinical trials are presently underway to evaluate whether a complete nodal dissection or adjuvant therapy is actually necessary for all patients with microscopic SLN positivity detected by either immunohistochemistry or reverse transcription-polymerase chain reaction technology. When available, this information will help crystallize therapeutic paradigms for patients with cutaneous malignant melanoma.

B.L. Eisenberg, M.D.

Reference

1. Kirkwood JM, Strawderman MH, Ernstoff MS: Interferon-alpha 2b adjuvant therapy of high-risk resected cutaneous melanoma: the Eastern Cooperative Oncology Group Trial EST 1684. *J Clin Oncol* 14:7–17, 1996.

Ambulatory Narrow Excision for Thin Melanoma (≤2 mm): Results of a Prospective Study

Bono A, Bartoli C, Clemente C, et al (Istituto Nazionale Tumori, Milan; Univ of Milan, Italy)

Eur J Cancer 33:1330–1332, 1997 14–2

Objective.—Conservative treatment of clinical stage I thin cutaneous melanoma in selected candidates involves a narrow excision. Results of a prospective study of narrow surgical excision of melanomas and the relation to tumor thickness were evaluated.

Methods.—Between May 1987 and December 1991, 168 patients (63 men), average age 50 years, with clinical stage I invasive melanoma with thickness of 2 mm or less had narrow excision (1-cm margin) with the use of local anesthesia. Patients were followed up for an average of 62 months. Relapse-free survival was estimated using the Kaplan-Meier method.

Results.—Forty (24%) patients had a melanoma thickness between 1 and 2 mm. The probability of relapse-free survival at 5 years was 91%. Eleven patients had relapse and 3 had other neoplasms. The crude incidence of regional metastases was 5.6% and the crude incidence of distant metastases was 1.5%. There were no local recurrences.

Conclusion.—Narrow excision of melanomas is justified for melanomas with thickness of 2 mm or less.

▶ This article indicates that a 1-cm margin for a melanoma up to 2 mm in depth is not associated with an increase in isolated local recurrence. The importance of this article is that it lends more credence to performing an outpatient ambulatory surgical procedure using local anesthesia as effective therapy in patients with relatively thin melanomas of less than 2 mm. It had been routine to consider a 1-cm margin in patients with melanomas of 1 mm or less, but to apply this margin extent to treat depths of 2 mm widens the feasibility to a larger patient population. This study actually confirms a previous report by Veronesi and colleagues[1] that failed to reveal any significant differences in recurrence free or overall survival[1] with comparison of 1-cm margins to 3-cm margins in patients with melanomas up to 2 mm. Clearly, the oncologic considerations are paramount in planning the extent of wide excision; however, the width of margins has significance for the ability to treat patients in an outpatient surgery setting with primary closure obviating the need for local tissue flaps or skin graft.

B.L. Eisenberg, M.D.

Reference

1. Veronesi U, Cascinelli N, Adamus J, et al: Thin stage I primary cutaneous malignant melanoma; Comparison of excision with margins of 1 or 3 cm. *N Engl J Med* 318:1159–1162, 1988.

Computed Tomography in Evaluation of Patients With Stage III Melanoma

Kuvshinoff BW, Kurtz C, Coit DG (Mem Sloan-Kettering Cancer Ctr, New York)

Ann Surg Oncol 4:252–258, 1997 14–3

Objective.—Computed tomography is generally not useful for detecting metastatic disease. Because the value of routine CT for stage III melanoma has not been established, the diagnostic yield in a large homogeneous group of patients with clincial stage III melanoma and the influence of these findings on patient management were assessed.

Methods.—Between 1988 and 1994, 347 patients (140 female) aged 14–93 years, with clinical stage III melanoma received at least 1 CT scan of the chest, abdomen, or pelvis. Results of CT were compared with histologic results.

Results.—Of 788 CT scans, 33 (4.2%) showed metastatic melanoma, and 66 (8.4%) were false positive scans. No head CT scans revealed metastases. Seven (20%) of 35 chest scans revealed metastatic disease in patients with cervical lymph node metastases, however, only 6 (5%) of 120 showed metastatic disease in the thorax vs. patients with axillary adenopathy, and 1 (2%) revealed metastatic pulmonary disease in patients with inguinal adenopathy. Three (8%) of 37 abdominal scans showed metastatic disease from neck primaries, 5 (4%) revealed metastatic disease from patients with axillary disease, and only 4 (4%) of 93 showed metastatic disease in the abdomen in patients with inguinal adenopathy. None of the pelvic scans revealed metastatic disease in patients with presentation of neck or axilla adenopathy, and only 7 (7%) of 94 showed metastatic disease in the clinical setting of groin adenopathy.

Conclusion.—The overall 5% diagnostic yield of CT scans for detection of metastatic disease in patients with stage III melanoma does not justify its routine use.

► The workup and evaluation of patients with newly diagnosed stage III melanoma often includes an extensive array of radiologic screening tests for detection of clinically occult metastatic disease. This retrospective review from Memorial Sloan Kettering Cancer Center addresses the necessity of routine CT scans of the brain, chest, abdomen, and pelvis in detecting occult metastatic disease for this particular patient population. In this day of cost-conscious medical care, it is important to evaluate the efficacy and benefit from routine multiple staging procedures. The conclusion from this review is that CT imaging should be used only in selective instances when there is an absence of any specific symptoms that may indicate systemic involvement. This is in contradistinction to most clinical practices where patients who are seen with node positive melanoma are generally subjected to an array of radiologic tests to prove or disprove the presence of further occult disease. This may be required in a clinical trial evaluating the necessity for adjuvant treatment in the presence of stage III disease. However, with the exception of a chest radiograph, I have found that it is often unrewarding to order a battery of diagnostic tests in the absence of symptoms, because they infrequently show positive results. One can make a compelling argument that routine brain, chest, abdomen, and pelvis CT scans are not indicated in the workup of any asymptomatic patient with stage III melanoma, except in the instance of palpable inguinal femoral nodes where a pelvic CT scan is important in evaluation of the deep pelvis and retroperitoneum for surgical planning.

B.L. Eisenberg, M.D.

Basal Cell Carcinoma of the Face: Surgery or Radiotherapy? Results of a Randomized Study

Avril M-F, Auperin A, Margulis A, et al (Institut Gustave Roussy, Villejuif, France; Centre Hospitalier Louis Pasteur, Colmar, France; Institut Européen d'Oncologie, Milan, Italie, et al)

Br J Cancer 76:100–106, 1997 14–4

Introduction.—Basal cell carcinoma (BCC) of the face is the most common cutaneous cancer in Caucasians. Cure rates with surgery and radiotherapy are high. These treatments have never undergone prospective evaluation. Surgery and radiotherapy were compared in a prospective trial that began in 1982 and included 347 patients with primary BCC of the face measuring less than 4 cm.

Methods.—Patients were randomized to surgical treatment or radiotherapy. Patients were followed at 3, 6, and 12 months after completion of

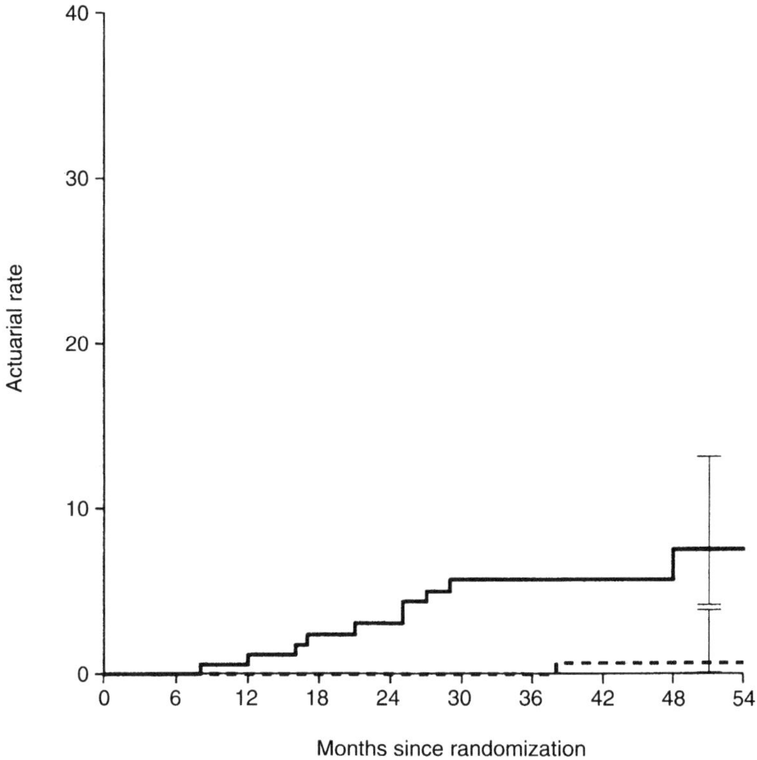

FIGURE 1.—Kaplan-Meier plot of recurrent or persistent basal cell carcinoma in patients treated with surgery or radiotherapy. *Bars* indicate 95% confidence intervals. *Broken line* indicates surgery (n = 174, 1 event); *solid line* indicates radiotherapy (n = 173, 11 events). (Courtesy of Avril M-F, Auperin A, Margulis A, et al: Basal cell carcinoma of the face: Surgery or radiotherapy? Results of a randomized study. *Br J Cancer* 76:100–106, 1997.)

treatment, then yearly until the fourth year. The primary end point was the cure rate after 4 years of follow-up. The secondary end point was cosmetic results, as determined by the patient, the dermatologist, and 3 persons not involved in the trial.

Results.—Of 174 patients in the surgery group, 71% underwent local anesthesia and 91% had frozen section examination. Of 173 patients in the radiotherapy group, 55%, 33%, and 12% underwent interstitial brachytherapy, contactherapy, and conventional radiotherapy, respectively. The 4-year actuarial failure rate for the surgery group was 0.7%, compared with 7.5% (a significant difference) for the radiotherapy group (Fig 1). Four of five judges decided that cosmetic results were significantly better for the surgery group than for the radiotherapy group. Treatment was considered good by 87% of patients who were treated by surgery and 69% of patients who were treated by radiation (a significant difference).

Conclusion.—Surgery was superior to radiotherapy for survival and cosmetic results. Surgery is the recommended course of treatment for patients with BCC of the face of less than 4 cm. Radiotherapy should be reserved for patients for whom surgery is contraindicated.

▶ This is an interesting study that for a variety of reasons I do not think would be investigated in this country. French patients who had BCC on the face were randomized to receive either surgery or radiotherapy. Both in terms of local control and of cosmesis, these patients were better treated by surgical excision. I do not have any trouble with that. On the other hand, one of the important issues is the comparability of these patients and the locations of their tumors. I think there are problems with certain locations—around the ear, for example—where radiation might be preferable to surgery. These sites are relatively uncommon, however. In the near future when photodynamic therapy can be given on a weekly or biweekly basis, perhaps that will be superior to either or both of these 2 forms of treatment. Only time will tell.

E. Glatstein, M.D.

15 Sarcomas

Association of Local Recurrence With Subsequent Survival in Extremity Soft Tissue Sarcoma

Lewis JJ, Leung D, Heslin M, et al (Mem Sloan-Kettering Cancer Ctr, New York)

J Clin Oncol 15:646–652, 1997 15–1

Background.—The appropriate means for treating primary extremity soft-tissue sarcoma is widely debated. A large cohort of patients with this condition was examined. The hypothesis used was that local recurrence was not an adequate prognostic factor because local and systemic failure are influenced by similar biological factors. Thus, the correlation between local recurrence, disease specific survival, and metastasis was investigated.

Method.—Using the Cox Proportional Hazards model, researchers compared the end points—disease specific survival, distant metastasis, and local recurrence—for patients who were treated for soft-tissue sarcoma. All 911 were patients at Memorial Sloan-Kettering Cancer Center from July 1982 to July 1995.

Results.—Thirty-three percent of patients (297 patients) had recurrences. Thirteen percent were local (116 patients); 18% were metastatic (167 patients); and 2% had metastasis with synchronous local recurrence, (13 patients). In 38 of the patients with local recurrence, metastasis developed. Thirty four of these died as a result of metastasis. The patients with local recurrence who had deep (P = 0.02; risk = 2.9) or high-grade (P = 0.005; risk = 3.5) tumors were most likely to have metastasis develop. The patients most likely to die had large (greater than 5 cm; P = 0.01; risk = 3.2) or high grade (P = 0.007; risk = 3.7) initial tumors.

Conclusion.—Not only is local recurrence a prognostic factor for metastasis and tumor mortality, but aggressive local treatment may not impact survival. Conversely, local recurrence cannot be considered a purely causal predictor for metastasis and death.

► Patients with soft-tissue sarcomas present the clinician with 2 separate problems, namely, local recurrence and systemic recurrence. Progress in decreasing local recurrence to the 10% to 20% range with multimodality therapy (wide surgical resection and radiation therapy) has promoted limb-sparing surgery without having a detrimental effect on disease-related mortality. The question, however, remains as to the overall effect of local recurrence on tumor-specific survival.

This paper from Memorial Sloan-Kettering Cancer Center addresses this question with a conclusion that all of us have long suspected; that is, although local recurrence is not directly causally related to survival, there are similar disease-related factors that are significant for each of these end points. These factors include tumor grade and tumor size. Those two factors taken as independent risk factors are related to both local control and disease-free survival. It is interesting to note that of the patients with high-grade tumors who experience local recurrence, approximately 50% will then have metastatic disease within 2 years. This presents a cogent argument for placing these patients in intensive doxorubicin-based adjuvant chemotherapy trials.

B.L. Eisenberg, M.D.

The Impact of Residual Disease on Local Recurrence in Patients Treated by Initial Unplanned Resection for Soft Tissue Sarcoma of the Extremity

Davis AM, Kandel RA, Wunder JS, et al (Univ of Toronto)

J Surg Oncol 66:81–87, 1997 15–2

Introduction.—The use of clinical examination and CT and MRI modalities make it possible to control local disease in 95% of patients with extremity soft-tissue sarcomas (STSs). It is difficult to accurately assess the extent of disease when the patient has undergone complete excision of the macroscopic lesion before appropriate evaluation ("unplanned excision"). If all patients were treated with re-excision of the tumor bed after an unplanned excision, about 35% would have residual sarcomas. Two hundred thirty-nine patients with primary, extremity STSs were evaluated to determine whether unplanned excisions would have an impact on local relapse, even if the tumor bed was re-excised.

Methods.—Of 239 patients, 47 had low-grade tumors and 192 had high-grade tumors. Seventy-eight percent of patients underwent surgery and irradiation. The mean tumor diameter was 7.5 cm. Twenty patients had local recurrence, and 64 had systemic relapse.

Results.—At a mean follow-up of 33 months, 40 (16.7%) patients had died of their disease, 23 (9.6%) were alive with systemic disease, and 165 (69.0%) were disease free. In univariate analysis, margin-positive surgery and prior surgery were significant predictors of local relapse. Multivariate analysis showed that both the margin of resection and the status of the local tumor site at definitive surgery were significant predictors of local relapse.

Conclusion.—Two significant risk factors for local relapse in patients with extremity STSs were resection with microscopic evidence of a tumor at the resection margin and a history of unplanned resections before referral in which the residual sarcoma was detected in the resection of the tumor bed.

► Soft-tissue sarcomas represent a rare and biologically diverse group of malignancies. In some instances, a soft-tissue mass can be misdiagnosed, and the subsequent excisional biopsy does not take the full malignant potential of these cancers into proper perspective, which results in the initial surgery becoming an unplanned resection. This will be manifested by improperly placed surgical scars, particularly in extremity lesions, and a compromised surgical field. The uncommon occurrence of these cancers often leads to an unexpected diagnosis by the initial surgeon. This article supports the fact that inappropriate or unplanned surgical excision of a soft-tissue sarcoma can be a definite risk factor in local recurrence, even if the subsequent definitive surgical procedure provides radically resected wide margins. It is therefore critical that any suspected soft-tissue sarcoma be managed appropriately from the onset with proper biopsy techniques to avoid tumor dissemination and implantation and to avoid improperly placed or oriented biopsy incisions. The patient's ultimate outcome may depend on it.

B.L. Eisenberg, M.D.

CT and MR Imaging in the Local Staging of Primary Malignant Musculoskeletal Neoplasms: Report of the Radiology Diagnostic Oncology Group

Panicek DM, Gatsonis C, Rosenthal DI, et al (Mem Sloan-Kettering Cancer Ctr, New York; Harvard Med School, Boston; Massachusetts Gen Hosp, Boston; et al)

Radiology 202:237–246, 1997 15–3

Background.—Individualized treatment planning for primary malignant bone and soft-tissue tumors requires precise delineation of the local extent of neoplasm in bone, muscle, joints, blood vessels, and nerves. Many clinicians feel that MRI is superior to CT for this purpose. The relative accuracies of these 2 imaging modalities in the local staging of primary malignant bone and soft-tissue tumors were determined.

Methods.—Three hundred sixty-three patients aged 6–89 years were enrolled at 4 centers. Both CT and MRI were performed in the 4 weeks before operation.

Findings.—Data on 316 patients were able to be analyzed. One hundred eighty-three had primary bone tumors, and 133 had primary soft-tissue tumors. The 2 imaging modalities did not differ in their ability to demonstrate tumor involvement of muscle, bone, joints, or neurovascular structures. Combined interpretation of CT and MR images did not increase accuracy significantly. Interreader variability was comparable for CT and MRI (Tables 2 and 3).

Conclusions.—Computed tomography and MRI provide comparable information pertinent to preoperative local staging of primary malignant

TABLE 2.—Primary Bone Tumors: Agreement Between Assessments of Length of Intramedullary Tumor

Comparison	Agreement (%)		Absolute Value of Difference (cm)		Difference (cm)		Mean Difference (cm) ± Standard Deviation
	Tumor ≤2 cm	Tumor ≤5 cm	Median	Range	Median	Range	
CT versus pathology	67 (94 of 141)	89 (125 of 141)	1.5	0–11.0	0.5	−6.0–11.0	1.1 ± 3.1*
MR imaging versus pathology	69 (88 of 127)	88 (112 of 127)	1.5	0–12.9	0.2	−12.9–11.0	0.9 ± 3.3*
CT versus MR imaging	72 (91 of 126)	89 (112 of 126)	1.3	0–10.9	0.0	−10.7–10.9	0.2 ± 3.3†

Note: Tumor length was greater at CT than at pathologic analysis in 58% (82 of 141) of patients and greater at pathologic analysis than at CT in 32% (45 of 141) of patients. Tumor length was greater at MR imaging than at pathologic analysis in 53% (67 of 127) of patients and greater at pathologic analysis than at MR imaging in 35% (44 of 127) of patients. Tumor length was greater at CT than at MR imaging in 49% (62 of 120) of patients and greater at MR imaging than at CT in 40% (51 of 126) of patients.

*$P < 0.001$ (Wilcoxon signed rank test).

†$P = 0.42$ (Wilcoxon signed rank test).

(Courtesy of Panicek DM, Gatsonis C, Rosenthal DI, et al: CT and MR imaging in the local staging of primary malignant musculoskeletal neoplasms: Report of the Radiology Diagnostic Oncology Group. *Radiology* 202:237–246. Copyright 1997, Radiological Society of North America.)

TABLE 3.—Primary Bone Tumors: Descriptive Statistics for Bone, Joint, Muscle, Vessel, and Nerve Involvement and for Skip Lesions

	CT					MR Imaging				
Tumor Location	Sensitivity (%)*	Specificity (%)†	Accuracy (%)	PPV (%)	NPV (%)	Sensitivity (%)*	Specificity (%)†	Accuracy (%)	PPV (%)	NPV (%)
Humerus										
Periosteum	89 (19)	25 (4)	78	85	33	100 (19)	40 (5)	88	86	100
Cortex	89 (19)	25 (4)	78	85	33	94 (18)	33 (6)	79	81	67
Medullary cavity	95 (19)	75 (4)	91	95	75	94 (18)	50 (6)	83	85	75
Pelvis										
Periosteum	100 (24)	98 (45)	99	96	100	88 (25)	89 (19)	89	92	85
Cortex	100 (26)	100 (43)	100	100	100	89 (27)	100 (17)	93	100	85
Medullary cavity	96 (24)	100 (45)	99	100	98	96 (25)	100 (19)	98	100	95
Femur										
Periosteum	96 (57)	64 (39)	83	80	93	98 (52)	50 (36)	78	74	95
Cortex	97 (66)	70 (30)	89	88	91	100 (62)	56 (25)	87	85	100
Medullary cavity	96 (68)	75 (28)	90	90	88	94 (62)	68 (25)	86	88	81
Tibia										
Periosteum	100 (24)	73 (26)	86	77	100	100 (23)	77 (22)	89	82	100
Cortex	100 (28)	86 (22)	94	90	100	96 (26)	89 (19)	93	93	94
Medullary cavity	96 (28)	96 (23)	96	96	96	92 (25)	90 (21)	91	92	90
Fibula										
Periosteum	88 (8)	95 (19)	93	88	95	100 (7)	79 (14)	86	70	100
Cortex	100 (8)	89 (19)	93	80	100	100 (7)	86 (14)	90	78	100
Medullary cavity	100 (9)	100 (18)	100	100	100	88 (8)	100 (13)	95	100	93
Skip lesions	0 (7)‡	97 (151)‡	93	0	95	14 (7)‡	96 (139)‡	92	14	96
Intraarticular extension	67 (24)‡	81 (135)‡	79	39	93	70 (23)‡	80 (124)‡	78	39	93
Muscles										
Arm or shoulder	93 (14)	50 (16)	70	62	89	83 (12)	47 (17)	62	53	80
Pelvis or hip	95 (19)	84 (76)	86	60	98	100 (19)	67 (36)	78	61	100
Thigh or knee	67 (24)	66 (93)	66	33	88	63 (24)	58 (83)	59	30	84
Calf	75 (16)	75 (52)	75	48	91	71 (14)	81 (42)	79	56	89
Vessels	33 (6)‡	95 (164)‡	92	18	97	33 (6)‡	93 (151)‡	91	17	97
Nerves	33 (3)‡	95 (158)‡	94	11	99	50 (2)‡	93 (148)‡	92	08	99

*Numbers in parentheses are true-positives + false-negatives. Differs from † in some instances because of excluded patients.
†Numbers in parentheses are true-negatives + false-positives. Differs from * in some instances because of excluded patients.
‡$P > 0.05$ (McNemar test).
Abbreviations: NPV, negative predictive value; *PPV*, positive predictive value.
(Courtesy of Panicek DM, Gatsonis C, Rosenthal DI, et al: CT and MR imaging in the local staging of primary malignant musculoskeletal neoplasms: Report of the Radiology Diagnostic Oncology Group. *Radiology* 202:237–246. Copyright 1997, Radiological Society of North America.)

musculoskeletal neoplasms in the anatomical sites studied. Combining the reading of the 2 studies provided no objective benefit.

▶ There has always been some controversy about the comparative superiority or lack thereof between CT and MR imaging of musculoskeletal sarcomas. This investigation, carried out prospectively by the Radiology Diagnostic Oncology Group (RDOG), looks at 367 patients at 4 institutions who had malignant bony or soft tissue neoplasms in the extremities. No statistically significant difference can be detected between CT and MR imaging in regards to determining tumor involvement of structures. The addition of CT to MR, or vice versa, did not significantly improve the accuracy.

Some people thought these studies were relatively complementary, but there appears little evidence to support that view in this study. The RDOG has been in existence for about a decade and has carried out multi-institutional studies that look at the role of imaging modalities in the staging of a variety of neoplasms. Their work has been useful and of high quality. This paper is another in their continuing area of activity.

E. Glatstein, M.D.

Adjuvant Chemotherapy for Localised Resectable Soft-Tissue Sarcoma of Adults: Meta-analysis of Individual Data

Tierney JF, for the Sarcoma Meta-analysis Collaboration (MRC Cancer Trials Office, Cambridge, England)

Lancet 350:1647–1654, 1997 15–4

Background.—Whether adjuvant chemotherapy benefits adults with localized resectable soft-tissue sarcoma remains unclear. A meta-analysis of data from previous randomized studies was presented to further explore this issue.

Methods and Findings.—Data on 1,568 patients included in 14 studies of doxorubicin-based adjuvant chemotherapy were analyzed. The hazard ratios were 0.73 for local recurrence-free intervals (RFIs), 0.70 for distant RFIs, and 0.75 for overall recurrence-free survival. These ratios corresponded to absolute benefits of 6%, 10%, and 10%, respectively, at 10 years. The hazard ratio for overall survival (0.89), was nonsignificant but represents an absolute benefit of 4% at 10 years. Prespecified changes in the groups analyzed did not affect these findings. The relative effect of adjuvant chemotherapy did not appear to differ for any subgroup of patients for any end point. However, the strongest evidence of an effect on survival was for patients with sarcomas of the extremities.

Conclusion.—This meta-analysis suggests that adjuvant doxorubicin-based chemotherapy significantly improves time to local and distant recurrence and overall recurrence-free survival. A trend toward improved overall survival was also noted.

► Soft-tissue sarcomas are a heterogenous group of tumors. Although advocation of the routine use of adjuvant chemotherapy for large, high-grade sarcomas has become more routine in clinical practice, there are no published data to support the efficacy of this concept. Most prospective, randomized trials have not been large enough or properly enough designed to detect important adjuvant treatment effect against a control group of patients.

This paper from the Cancer Trials Office in Cambridge presents a well-constructed meta-analysis with full individual patient chart review to verify the reported results. The information is based on 1,568 patients representing 14 trials of the adjuvant use of doxorubucin-based chemotherapy against a suitable control group. Significant differences were noted in local and distant RFIs and overall recurrence-free survival at 10 years in favor of the treated groups. These improvements resulted in absolute benefits from chemotherapy of 6% to 10%. This is an important study because it represents a statistical analysis of combined randomized trial data for a relatively rare tumor for which, in the past, meaningful data collection has been hampered by poor accrual numbers.

Although this information may be subject to some criticism based on methodology, it does represent a substantial work in justification of a change in treatment paradigm for soft-tissue sarcomas, namely, that patients with high-grade sarcomas, particularly in extremity locations, do benefit from adjuvant chemotherapy. Questions related to preoperative vs. postoperative treatment, the use of radiation therapy, and a clear-cut division between effects for low-grade vs. high-grade lesions remain to be answered by combined cooperative group efforts to specifically address these issues within well-controlled clinical trials.

B.L. Eisenberg, M.D.

Randomized Prospective Study of the Benefit of Adjuvant Radiation Therapy in the Treatment of Soft Tissue Sarcomas of the Extremity

Yang JC, Chang AE, Baker AR, et al (Natl Cancer Inst, Bethesda, Md)

J Clin Oncol 16:197–203, 1998 15–5

Background.—In this randomized, prospective study, researchers examined the relationship of local recurrence (LR), quality of life, and overall survival to postoperative external-beam radiation therapy (EBRT) and limb-sparing resection in treating extremity sarcomas.

Method.—All patients with extremity tumors were able to undergo limb-sparing surgery. Patients were randomized to be treated with EBRT or with surgery only. Those patients with high-grade sarcomas were treated with adjuvant chemotherapy. Those with low-grade sarcomas were treated with surgery alone, as were patients with aggressive nonmalignant tumors.

Results.—Forty-seven of 91 patients with high-grade tumors received radiotherapy. Forty-four did not. Although a significant decrease (P =

0.0028) was seen in the radiotherapy patients after a median 9.6-year follow-up, the overall survival was the same in both groups. The same was true for patients with low-grade lesions (50 patients). The 26 patients who received radiotherapy had a lower chance for LR (P = 0.16). Again, overall survival remained constant. Quality-of-life investigations concerning radiotherapy showed weaker limbs and range of motions, as well as edema. However, these symptoms did not persist and were, thus, judged not to have a profound effect on daily life.

Conclusion.—After limb-sparing surgery, many patients with extremity soft-tissue sarcomas, especially those with a low-risk for LR, may not need EBRT, even though this treatment is highly effective in curtailing LRs.

► A recent area of controversy in the management of extremity soft-tissue sarcomas is the issue of the necessity of adjuvant radiation therapy for all patients. This study from the National Cancer Institute concerns a long-term trial evaluating a randomized treatment scheme using postoperative adjuvant radiation therapy vs. surgery alone in the management of both high-grade and low-grade soft-tissue extremity sarcomas. The importance of this study lies in the fact that it is a prospective trial with a medium follow-up of nearly 10 years and includes a quality-of-life study for evaluating the long-term toxicity of adjuvant radiation therapy in this clinical setting.

Notably, patients in both high-grade and low-grade groups benefited from adjuvant radiation therapy in terms of LC. However, this did not result in a survival benefit considering that all patients with high-grade lesions had adjuvant chemotherapy. Of interest, the quality-of-life study indicated early differences in limb function favoring the non–radiation therapy group; however, the long-term effects and differences were inconsequential. It is also of interest that no patient in this study with high-grade sarcoma with widely negative margins and the absence of radiation therapy experienced a local recurrence. This suggests that these selective patients may not require radiation therapy.

It is an apparent conclusion of this study that the majority of patients with high-grade sarcomas who have close or microscopically positive margins do benefit from adjuvant radiation therapy, with enhanced long-term local-disease control and without significant detriment to their quality of life. It is my belief that patients with high-grade extremity sarcomas that otherwise have good prognostic features (i.e., widely negative microscopic margins or no residual sarcoma seen after wide re-excision after initial excisional biopsy) do not, in most instances, require adjuvant radiation therapy. It is also reasonable to consider that for those patients with high-grade large (greater than 8 cm) proximal soft-tissue extremity sarcomas, preoperative radiation therapy may prove to be a more effective therapy choice.

B.L. Eisenberg, M.D.

Radiation Therapy for Rhabdomyosarcoma: Local Failure Risk for Clinical Group III Patients on Intergroup Rhabdomyosarcoma Study II

Wharam MD, Hanfelt JJ, Tefft MC, et al (Johns Hopkins Oncology Ctr, Baltimore, Md)

Int J Radiat Oncol Biol Phys 38:797–804, 1997 15–6

Introduction.—The second Intergroup Rhabdomyosarcoma Study (IRS) enrolled 999 eligible patients from 1978 to 1984. The results of this randomized, prospective trial were published in 1993. A subset of 532 patients (group III) with localized gross residual tumor had either biopsy only or subtotal resection and received radiation therapy (RT) according to IRS-II protocol. A group of 362 patients who received at least 1 day of RT were followed to determine local and regional failure after RT and to ascertain patient, tumor, and treatment factors contributing to the risk for local or regional failure.

Methods.—Patients excluded from the original group had tumors arising in the "special pelvic" primary sites and were required to receive primary chemotherapy (123 patients) or were excluded before RT or were omitted because they did not receive RT (47 patients). Univariate and multivariate analyses were conducted to determine patient, tumor, and treatment factors that contributed to the risk of local and regional failure.

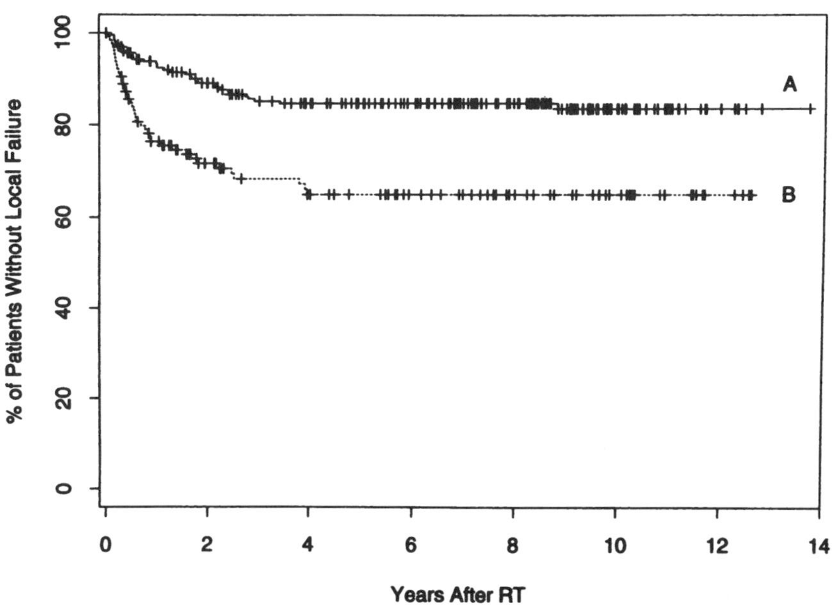

FIGURE 2.—Time to local failure for prognostic groups A and B (log rank test: *P* less than 0.001). Group B was the group with highest risk of local failure. (Reprinted by permission of the publisher from Wharam MD, Hanfelt JJ, Tefft MC, et al: Radiation therapy for rhabdomyosarcoma: Local failure risk for Clinical Group III patients on Intergroup Rhabdomyosarcoma Study II. *Int J Radiat Oncol Biol Phys* 38:797–804, copyright 1997 by Elsevier Science Inc.)

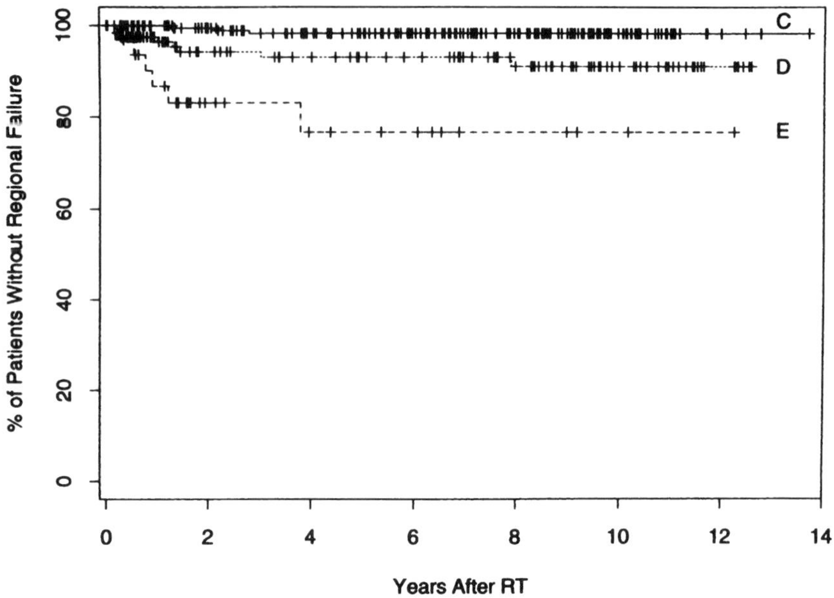

FIGURE 4.—Time to regional failure for risk groups C, D, and E (log rank tests: E was the highest risk group, D the median risk group, and C the lowest-risk group. D vs. C, $P = 0.02$; E vs. D, $P = 0.02$; E vs. D vs. C, P less than 0.001). (Reprinted by permission of the publisher from Wharam MD, Hanfelt JJ, Tefft MC: Radiation therapy for rhabdomyosarcoma: Local failure risk for Clinical Group III patients on Intergroup Rhabdomyosarcoma Study II. *Int J Radiat Oncol Biol Phys* 38:797–804, copyright 1997 by Elsevier Science Inc.)

Results.—The local (only) failure rate was 17% and the local (all) failure rate was 20% for the cohort of 362 patients. The 5-year actuarial risk of local (all) failure was 22% and the risk of regional (nodal) failure was 2%–23%. Increasing tumor size was predictive of a higher risk of local failure. The risk of local failure was lower for primary sites above the clavicle. Patients at highest risk for local failure were those with primary tumors in the chest, pelvic region, extremity, or trunk, or tumors greater than 10 cm in diameter. The local failure rate for this patient subset was 35% (Fig 2), compared with 15% for the remaining patients. Patients at highest risk for regional (nodal) failure had node involvement at diagnosis and a primary tumor originating at a site other than the orbit, parameninges, or trunk (Fig 4). Compliance with RT was almost predictive of local failure but did not achieve significance. Age, race, gender, adenopathy, and histology did not influence local failure risk.

Conclusion.—Local control was possible using RT and chemotherapy for most patients in group III. New treatment strategies can be enhanced with an understanding of the factors that predict an increased risk of local or regional failure.

► This paper from the Intergroup Rhabdomyosarcoma Study demonstrates how effective radiation therapy can be on a wide group basis regarding the problem of pediatric rhabdomyosarcoma. The control figures for this very aggressive tumor are excellent. I think the real problem with this paper (and my only real criticism) is that there is no discussion of the morbidity of treatment. This is obviously age related and also volume and dose related. Nevertheless, the authors must have some data on this point, and because of the difficulty in being able to obtain adequate margins of resections of this particularly invasive tumor, I believe such information would be appropriate.

E. Glatstein, M.D.

Angiographic Response of Locally Advanced Soft-Tissue Sarcoma Following Hyperthermic Isolated Limb Perfusion With Tumor Necrosis Factor

Olieman AFT, van Ginkel RJ, Hoekstra HJ, et al (Univ Hosp Groningen, The Netherlands)

Ann Surg 4:64–69, 1997 15–7

Objective.—Although soft-tissue sarcomas are rare, most are located on the limbs and require amputation or exarticulation for recurrent or locally advanced disease. Because hyperthermic isolated limb perfusion (HILP) with tumor necrosis factor-alpha (TNF-α), melphalan, and interferon-

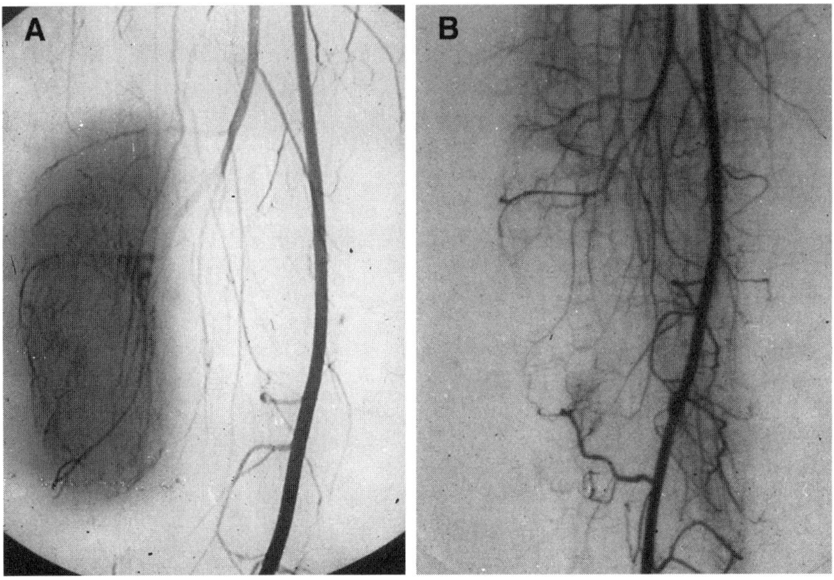

FIGURE 1.—A, angiography of a rhabdomyosarcoma of the right thigh in an 18-year-old woman before tumor necrosis factor–α (TNF-α) perfusion. The tumor shows an abnormal vascular pattern with tumor blush, cork screws, and sclerosis. **B**, angiography in the same patient 7 weeks after TNF-α-perfusion, showing a complete normalization of the previously abnormal vascular pattern. (Courtesy of Olieman AFT, van Ginkel RJ, Hoekstra HJ, et al: Angiographic response of locally advanced soft-tissue sarcoma following hyperthermic isolated limb perfusion with tumor necrosis factor. *Ann Surg Oncol* 4:64–69, 1997.)

gamma (IFN-γ) have been used to salvage the limb and function in such patients, a prospective investigation of the angiographic changes occurring during perfusion and their relation to the histologic response of the resected specimen was conducted.

Methods.—Between July 1991 and January 1995, angiographic studies were performed before and 4 to 14 weeks after a 90-minute arterial perfusion with melphalan, TNF-α, and IFN-γ in 25 patients (11 female), aged 18 to 80, with locally advanced soft-tissue sarcoma. There were no local or systemic reactions. After approximately 8 weeks, the residual tumor mass was excised. Changes in tumor vascularity and tumor stain were recorded. Magnetic resonance imaging was used to determine tumor size.

Results.—All patients had significant tumor neovascularity and stain before treatment. Angiographic results were normal and tumor size was reduced in 18 patients, with 9 having a devitalized tumor and 9 having isolated viable tumor cells or less than 10% viable cells (Fig 1). The remaining 7 patients had persistent tumor vascularity. In the latter group, pathological examination showed a complete response in 1 patient, 10% to 50% viable tumor volume in 4, and no response in 2. The sensitivity and specificity of the procedure were 95% and 100%, respectively. Angiographic and pathologic classification were significantly correlated. Angiographic score and malignancy grade were not.

Conclusion.—After HILP with melphalan, TNF-α, and IFN-γ angiography vascular patterns of soft tissue sarcomas normalize regardless of the pathologic response expected.

► This paper reviews the responsiveness of locally advanced soft-tissue sarcomas of the extremity as assessed by angiography following hyperthermic isolated limb perfusion with tumor necrosis factor. Apparently this technology, which has been around for some time, has really been perfected in terms of getting tumors to shrink. It also employs interferon and melphalan. It seems to be indicated for the sarcomas or melanomas of the extremity, and it really does seem to be associated with impressive shrinkage with a high degree of probability. In this series, 18 of 25 patients developed a normal angiogram following treatment, and all were associated with a complete pathologic response at the time of resection!

As best I can figure, it is a real effort to do this, but it does seem to be worth it in the sense that the majority of patients seem to achieve a very good response. The durability remains in question at this point, but this treatment may have to be moved up in the priority of treatments for extremity problems. I think we will hear more of this in the future as preoperative procedures become more acceptable.

E. Glatstein, M.D.

Prognostic Factors Associated With Long-term Survival for Retroperitoneal Sarcoma: Implications for Management
Heslin MJ, Lewis JJ, Nadler E, et al (Mem Sloan-Kettering Cancer Ctr, New York)
J Clin Oncol 15:2832–2839, 1997 15–8

Objective.—Only 0.1% of cancers in the United States are retroperitoneal soft tissue sarcomas. Little is known about their long-term outcome or patterns of recurrence. Long-term survivors of retroperitoneal soft tissue sarcomas were studied to determine the patterns of recurrence and factors associated with survival.

Methods.—Using a prospective soft tissue sarcoma database, 198 adults treated for retroperitoneal soft tissue sarcoma who had been followed up for at least 5 years were identified. Forty-eight patients were known to be alive 5 years or longer after tumor resection. The long-term outcomes in this group and the relevant prognostic factors were analyzed.

Findings.—Recurrence rate was about 5% per year since the initial operation for retroperitoneal soft tissue sarcoma. Forty percent of patients who were free of disease at 5 or more years after their initial surgery had a recurrence by 10 years postoperatively (Fig 3). The only factor significantly associated with a reduced risk of local recurrence was radiation therapy (Fig 5). Patients aged 50 years or younger and those with high-grade tumors were at significantly increased risk for distant metastasis (Figs 6 and 7). The only factor significantly associated with an increased risk of tumor-related death was incomplete gross resection.

Conclusions.—Patients with retroperitoneal sarcoma who undergo primary complete resection have the best chance of long-term survival. Long-term recurrence is possible; patients who have been disease free for 5 years

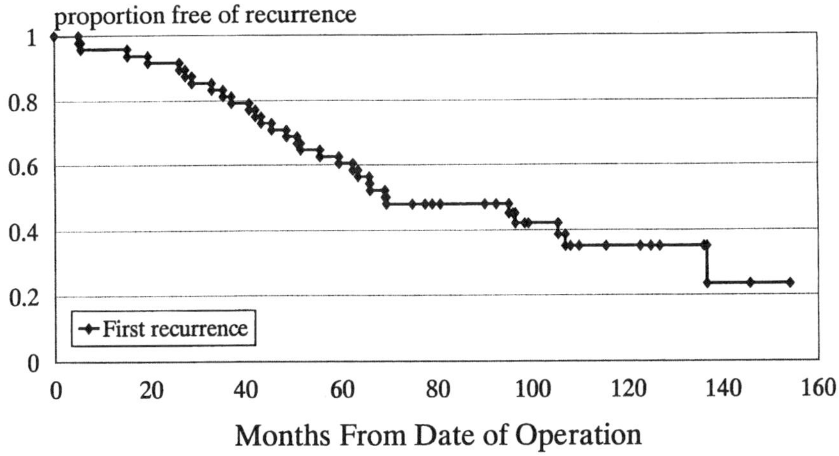

FIGURE 3.—Time to recurrence after operation (n = 48). (Courtesy of Heslin MJ, Lewis JJ, Nadler E, et al: Prognostic factors associated with long-term survival for retroperitoneal sarcoma: Implications for management. *J Clin Oncol* 15:2832–2839, 1997.)

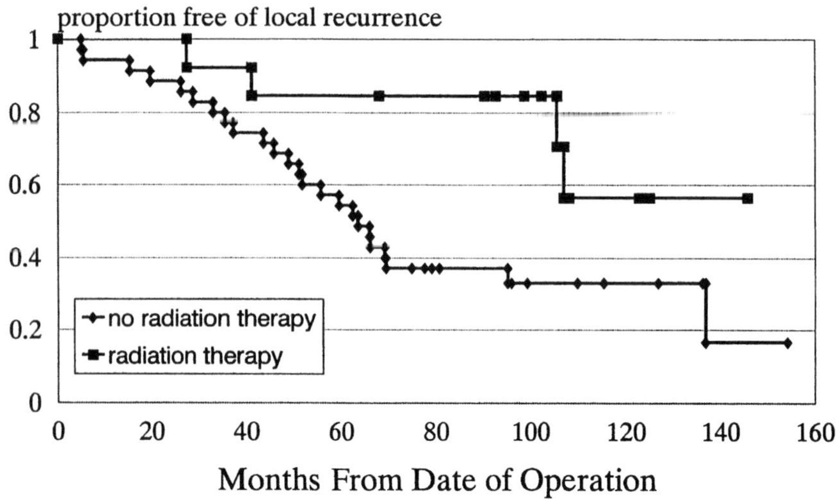

FIGURE 5.—Effect of radiation therapy on the proportion developing a local recurrence. Radiation therapy, n = 13; no radiation therapy, n = 35 ($P = 0.02$, log-rank test). (Courtesy of Heslin MJ, Lewis JJ, Nadler E, et al: Prognostic factors associated with long-term survival for retroperitoneal sarcoma: Implications for management. *J Clin Oncol* 15:2832–2839, 1997.)

cannot be considered cured. Risks are higher for patients who have less-than-complete initial resection, who are younger than 50 years, and who have high-grade tumors; these patients should be considered for experimental adjuvant therapy.

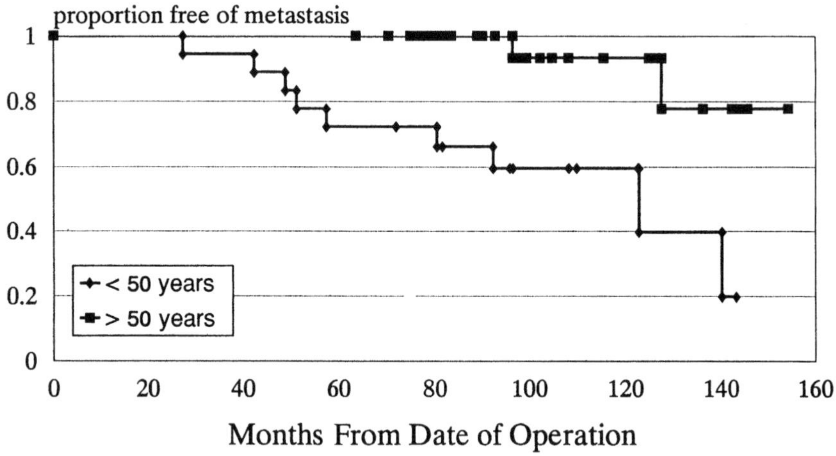

FIGURE 6.—Effect of age on the proportion developing a distant metastasis. Age < 50 years, n =18; age ≥ 50 years, n = 30 ($P < 0.006$, log-rank test). (Courtesy of Heslin MJ, Lewis JJ, Nadler E, et al: Prognostic factors associated with long-term survival for retroperitoneal sarcoma: Implications for management. *J Clin Oncol* 15:2832–2839, 1997.)

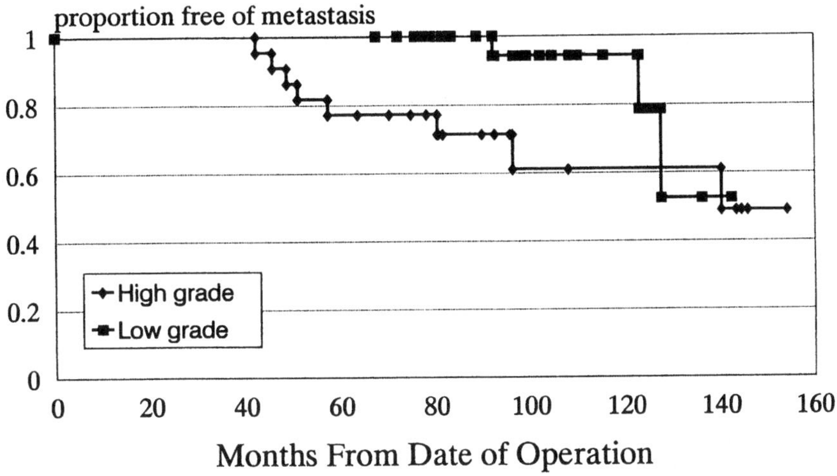

FIGURE 7.—Effect of grade on the proportion developing a distant metastasis. Low grade, n =26; high grade, n = 20 ($P < 0.009$, Wilcoxon test). (Courtesy of Heslin MJ, Lewis JJ, Nadler E, et al: Prognostic factors associated with long-term survival for retroperitoneal sarcoma: Implications for management. *J Clin Oncol* 15:2832–2839, 1997.)

▶ This is an excellent retrospective analysis of retroperitoneal sarcomas from Memorial Sloan-Kettering. The authors have reasonable numbers of patients, and they also accompany their analysis with an excellent flow diagram of what happened to all the patients. I think this retrospective paper is important because it gives a very good quantitative assessment of what really happened at each step along the way. The subsequent data thus become more interpretable. Obviously, the adequacy of the surgery and the surgical grade are still critical factors, although it is interesting to see that at 10 years the importance of the grade is less obvious. Radiation therapy appeared to decrease the rate of local recurrence in a statistically significant way, even though it was administered to a minority of patients, and presumably to the worst group of patients.

These patients continue to have problems, and they continue to be seen with relatively advanced lesions because of the comparatively blind complex of symptoms expressed in their natural history. This paper figures to be a standard reference for at least the next decade, in the management of these difficult and challenging patients. The other point to emphasize is the continuous and unequivocal need for long-term follow-up of these patients. There are many patients who relapse between 5 and 10 years out. Although long-term follow-up is available for more than 13 years, there are only a handful of patients that are available for follow-up beyond 10 years, so that the data in the third 5-year cohort are still evolving.

E. Glatstein, M.D.

Liposarcoma: Outcome and Prognostic Factors Following Conservation Surgery and Radiation Therapy

Zagars GK, Goswitz MS, Pollack A (Univ of Texas, Houston)

Int J Radiat Oncol Biol Phys 36:311–319, 1996 15–9

Introduction.—Only malignant fibrous histiocytoma exceeds the incidence of liposarcoma, one of the more common variants of soft-tissue sarcoma. It is one of the few sarcomas for which outcome is heavily dependent on histologic subtype, yet few clinical reports specifically address this disease. A retrospective review of patients with clinically localized liposarcoma treated with conservation surgery and radiotherapy was conducted because few series report the outcome and prognostic variables for this sarcoma when managed by these therapies.

Methods.—There were 112 patients with liposarcoma treated with conservation surgery and radiotherapy. The outcomes—with local control, metastatic relapse, and survival as end points—were evaluated with univariate and multivariate statistics. Significant prognostic factors were independently delineated.

Results.—Thirty-six patients had preoperative radiation to a mean dose of 50 Gy, and 76 patients had postoperative radiation to a mean dose of 61 Gy. At a median follow-up of 9 years, disease progression at some site had developed in 30% of patients. The actuarial local relapse rate was 13% at 10 years, and local recurrence developed in 13% of patients. In 21% of patients, metastases developed, with an actuarial metastatic rate of 23% at 10 years.. The 5-year survival rate was 79%, the 10-year survival rate was 69%, and the 15-year survival rate was 61%. Tumor histologic subtype was the most important factor influencing outcome A local control rate exceeding 90% at 10 years was seen with well-differentiated and myxoid subtypes Metastases did not develop in any patient with well-differentiated liposarcoma A highly malignant tumor with a high local recurrence rate of 37% was pleomorphic liposarcoma; it had a metastatic rate of 41% at 10 years. The 10-year survival rate was 87% for well-differentiated lesions, 76% for myxoid tumors, and 39% for pleomorphic tumors.

Conclusion.—Results reported for liposarcoma without histologic stratification are likely to be meaningless because it is a highly pleomorphic disease whose outcome is greatly determined by its histologic subtype. Excellent local results are achieved with conservation surgery and radiation, which are also appropriate for pleomorphic liposarcoma. An important goal for this variant of liposarcoma is effective systemic therapy.

▶ This paper from the M.D. Anderson Cancer Center addresses long-term clinical experience and follow-up for patients with liposarcoma. It is clear from this series and others that liposarcoma variants have quite different biological behaviors, and the information necessary for treatment-related decisions must include histologic subtype. This prognosis for well-differentiated and myxoid liposarcoma warrants complete surgical resection and adjuvant radiation therapy, depending on the size and location of the lesion. However, those patients with pleomorphic liposarcoma will often be seen with a rapidly growing proximal extremity mass or retroperitoneal mass and a poor 5-year survival expectancy. It is also interesting to note that the less aggressive variant (myxoid liposarcoma) can present a protracted series of local recurrences, particularly in retroperitoneum, or a dedifferentiation can occur and a more aggressive tumor subtype emerge with subsequent rapid progressive disease.

B.L. Eisenberg, M.D.

16 Bone Marrow Transplantation and Stem Cell Support

Incidence and Risk Factors for Invasive Fungal Infections in Allogeneic BMT Recipients
Jantunen E, Ruutu P, Niskanen L, et al (Helsinki Univ; Kuopio Univ, Finland)
Bone Marrow Transplant 19:801–808, 1997 16–1

Introduction.—Treatment of invasive fungal infections (IFI) after bone marrow transplantation (BMT) is frequently unsuccessful; mortality ranges from 60% to 95%. The role of graft-versus-host-disease (GVHD), particularly the effects of regimens used in GVHD prophylaxis or treatment, have not been examined as risk factors for IFI. The incidence of and risk factors for IFI after allogeneic BMT were retrospectively evaluated in 142 consecutive adult BMT recipients.

Findings.—Eleven unrelated donors and 131 sibling donors were evaluated. Twenty-one patients had either definite or probable IFI. Causative organisms were *Aspergillus* (15 patients), *Candida* (4 patients), *Fusarium* (1 patient), and *Absidia* (1 patient). The median interval between BMT and IFI was 136 days. Fourteen percent of IFIs were detected during the neutropenic period after BMT. In the pretransplant period, hematologic disease and unrelated donor were significant risk factors for IFI. Acute GVHD grade III-IV and extensive chronic GVHD were significant risk factors for IFI. There were 3 (14%) long-term survivors of IFI.

Conclusion.—The cause of IFI was *Aspergillus* in most patients, and the infections occurred late after BMT. The infection was associated with GVHD and its treatment in most patients. The mortality rate was high. There was an association between high risk of IFI and having an unrelated donor, grade III–IV acute GVHS, and extensive chronic GVHD. A more effective prophylaxis for GVHD could reduce the risk of IFI after allogeneic BMT.

▶ Invasive fungal infections remain a complication after allogeneic BMT. As these procedures are carried out more frequently, the characteristics associated with the development of such infection are important to identify. This study is useful because it documents that only a minority of IFIs occur during the neutropenic period. Pretransplant characteristics associated with the development of IFIs include myelodysplastic syndromes, unrelated donor transplantation, and both acute and chronic GVHD. The most common organism in this series was *Aspergillus*, and when such infections occur in this setting, the infection is usually fatal. Improved methods for preventing such potentially fatal infection are needed.

M.S. Tallman, M.D.

European Results of Matched Unrelated Donor Bone Marrow Transplantation for Chronic Myeloid Leukemia: Impact of HLA Class II Matching

Devergie A, for the Chronic Leukemia Working Party of the European Group for Blood and Marrow Transplantation (Hopital Saint Louis, Paris)

Bone Marrow Transplant 20:11–19, 1997 16–2

Objective.—Unrelated donor (UD) bone marrow transplantation is an alternative treatment for patients with chronic myeloid leukemia (CML). In the past, UDs were selected according to serologic identification of HLA-A, HLA-B, and HLA-DR alleles. However, gene sequencing studies have shown that many serologically matched pairs have previously unrecognized mismatches. This retrospective study analyzed the effects of advances in HLA class II typing on the results of UD bone marrow transplantation.

Methods.—The analysis included 366 patients undergoing UD bone marrow transplantation for CML from 1985 through 1994. There were 211 males and 155 females with a median age of 34 years. The transplant was performed in first chronic phase in 238 patients and in advanced phases in 116 at a median of 827 days after diagnosis. For prophylaxis of graft-versus-host disease (GVHD), 202 patients received cyclosporin A plus methotrexate and 129 underwent T-cell depletion (TCD). In recent years, UD selection was performed with DNA-based methods of HLA-class II typing. Further analysis compared 300 patients according to specific HLA-DRB1 donor/receipient compatibility: 210 received marrow from HLA-DRB1–identical donors (group 1), 31 from HLA-DRB1–mismatched donors (group 2), and 59 from donors in whom HLA-DRB1 typing was not performed.

Results.—In the overall experience, the 2-year survival rate was 37% and the leukemia-free survival rate was 31%. Factors associated with a good prognosis on univariate analysis were transplant in first chronic phase, less than the median time from diagnosis to bone marrow transplant, nonuse of TCD for GVHD prophylaxis, acute GVHD of less than grade IIII, and HLA-DRB1 donor/recipient matching.

Transplant-related mortality was related to HLA-DRB1 matching: 49% in group 1, 79% in group 2, and 80% in group 3. On multivariate analysis, the variable with the greatest impact on survival, leukemia-free survival, and transplant-related mortality was HLA-DRB1 matching. The findings were used to define a good-risk group of UD transplant patients: those transplanted in first chronic phase, receiving marrow from an HLA-DRB1–matched donor, and not undergoing TCD. Patients in this group had a 2-year leukemia-free survival rate of 51%, transplant-related mortality rate of 47%, and a relapse rate of 2%.

Conclusion.—In UD bone marrow transplantation, patients receiving marrow from an HLA-DRB1–matched donor and having other favorable prognostic features have long-term outcomes similar to those of patients receiving identical sibling marrow. In contrast, those receiving nonidentical marrow during advanced-phase disease have very high transplant-related mortality rates. Alternative therapies are needed for patients in this category.

▶ Attempts have increased for refining the technique of matched UD transplantation. This report is of significant interest because the outcome of a large cohort of patients treated over a 10-year period is presented. The leukemia-free survival at 2 years was 31%, which is what others have reported. Interestingly enough, on multivariant analysis, HLA-DRB1 matching was the most significant factor influencing survival. The most favorable group identified—HLA-DRB1–matched patients undergoing transplantation in the first chronic phase without TCD as prophylaxis against GVHD—had a leukemia-free survival rate of 51%. Despite this optimistic outcome, the treatment-related mortality rate, even in patients in this favorable group, was 47%. This paper is important because it shows that subsets of patients can be identified for whom UD transplantation may or may not be indicated.

M.S. Tallman, M.D.

Marrow Transplantation for Chronic Myeloid Leukemia: The Influence of Plasma Busulfan Levels on the Outcome of Transplantation

Slattery JT, Clift RA, Buckner CD, et al (Fred Hutchinson Cancer Research Ctr, Seattle; VA Med Ctr, Seattle)

Blood 89:3055–3060, 1997 16–3

Objective.—An evaluation was made of the influence of plasma busulfan (BU) levels on relapse and survival in patients with chronic myelogenous leukemia (CML) treated with BU plus cyclophosphamide before receiving allogenic marrow transplants from HLA-identical related donors.

Methods.—Between 1991 and 1995, 45 patients with CML—39 in the chronic phase (CP) and 6 in the accelerated phase (AP)—were treated for 4 days with BU, 1.0 mg/kg 4 times daily, followed by 2 days with IV cyclophosphamide, 60 mg/kg. Steady-state concentrations of BU were determined in each patient during dosing.

Results.—Mean and median BU levels were 917 ng/mL. Regimen-related toxicity included mucositis in 95% of patients and veno-occlusive disease of the liver in 34%. There was 1 death in the latter group. All 7 patients with relapses (5 in the CP and 2 in the AP group) had steady state BU levels below the median level. Three patients with relapse died. The difference between relapse rates for patients above and below the median steady state BU levels was significant. Nine CP and 2 AP patients have died. Four of these had steady state BU values above the median level, and 7 had values below the median level. There were 8 deaths among patients who had not relapsed. There was no significant difference in survival or nonrelapse mortality between patients with steady state BU levels above the median and those with levels below the median.

Conclusion.—Low BU levels are associated with an increased risk of relapse in patients with CML treated with BU before receiving allogenic marrow transplants.

▶ This paper is important because it is one of the first which systematically explores the importance of plasma levels of chemotherapy achieved with high-dose chemotherapy administration in preparation for allogeneic bone marrow transplantation. The authors observed that low BU plasma levels were associated with the increased risk of relapse. It appears clear that monitoring plasma levels of BU—as well as other agents included in high-dose chemotherapeutic preparative regimens—has important implications with respect to outcome.

M.S. Tallman, M.D.

Influence of Age on the Outcome of 500 Autologous Bone Marrow Transplant Procedures for Hematologic Malignancies

Kusnierz-Glaz CR, Schlegel PG, Wong RM, et al (Stanford Univ, Calif)

J Clin Oncol 15:18–25, 1997 16–4

Background.—Although age plays a major role in the outcome of allogeneic bone marrow transplantation, the effect of age on the outcome of high-dose therapy and autologous bone marrow transplantation is unclear. Results of autologous bone marrow transplantation in patients older than 50 are important because diseases such as acute myelogenous leukemia, non-Hodgkin's lymphoma, and multiple myeloma are more common in older patients.

Methods.—A retrospective analysis was conducted of 500 consecutive patients who had autologous bone marrow transplantation for Hodgkin's disease, non-Hodgkin's lymphoma, multiple myeloma, or acute myelogenous leukemia. Patients were categorized into minimal- or advanced-disease groups. Patients were between 1 year and 65 years old.

Results.—At 5-year follow-up, the event-free survival rate was 44%, the relapse rate was 47%, and regimen-related mortality was 8.6%. The strongest predictor of event-free survival and relapse was disease status at the time of transplantation. In patients with minimal disease, the event-free survival rate was 48% and the relapse rate was 43%. In patients with advanced disease, the event-free survival rate was 30% and the relapse rate was 72%. The rate of event-free survival was 46% in patients younger than 50 years and 34% in patients 50 years or older. Age was predictive of event-free survival. The regimen-related mortality rate was 7.4% in patients younger than 50 years and 12.7% in patients 50 years or older. The factors most predictive of regimen-related mortality were age and period of transplantation.

Discussion.—Although older patients have a lower long-term event-free survival rate after autologous bone marrow transplantation, a high percentage of patients have a disease-free outcome. This treatment should not be limited based only on the age of the patient. The upper age limit for autologous bone marrow transplantation remains to be determined.

▶ Since many patients are excluded from the potential benefit of high-dose chemotherapy with autologous stem cell transplantation because of age, this article is of significant interest. This study has the limitations of being a retrospective analysis and of including patients with various hematologic malignancies. However, the results do show that, although age is associated with an inferior outcome, age itself does not appear to be a reason to exclude patients from this approach. The recent advances in the technique of carrying out high-dose chemotherapy with autologous stem cell transplantation, including the use of peripheral blood stem cells and post-transplant hematopoietic growth factors, have enabled this treatment to be used in patients of older ages.

M.S. Tallman, M.D.

Hematopoietic Recovery After Allogeneic Blood Stem-Cell Transplantation Compared With Bone Marrow Transplantation in Patients With Hematologic Malignancies

Pavletic ZS, Bishop MR, Tarantolo SR, et al (Univ of Nebraska, Omaha)
J Clin Oncol 15:1608–1616, 1997 16–5

Objective.—Hematopoietic recovery, duration of hospitalization, and early outcome were compared for patients receiving allogenic-blood stem cells (BSCs) and conventional allogenic bone marrow transplantation (BMT).

Methods.—Between December 1994 and August 1995, outcomes of 21 patients in a prospective phase II trial who received allogenic BSC transplantation were compared with outcomes of 22 patients treated historically with allogenic BMT. The BSCs were obtained from healthy HLA-matched relatives given recombinant granulocyte colony-stimulating factor (G-CSF), 5 µ/kg/day subcutaneously for 5 days. Cyclosporine (2 mg/kg IV every 12 hours beginning on day −3 and followed by oral cyclosporine, 6.25 mg/kg every 12 hours) was administered as graft-versus-host-disease (GVHD) prophylaxis. Beginning 2 hours after transplantation all patients received G-CSF (10 μ/kg/day subcutaneously) until neutrophil count exceeded 500/μL for 3 days.

Results.—The most common side effects included myalgias/arthralgias, fever, headache, and chills. All toxicities were grade I and transient. The median CD34+ cell dose was 7.73 × 10^6/kg and the median granulomacyte-macrophage colony-forming unit value was 41.6 × 10^4/kg. The median time for neutrophil recovery (greater than 500/μL) after BSC transplantation was 11 days, whereas the median time for neutrophil recovery after BMT was 16.5 days. The median number of days to platelet recovery was 13 after BSC transplantation and 24 after BMT. The median number of days to hemoglobin recovery was 12 after BSC transplantation and 24 after BMT. Median days of hospitalization were 25 after BSC transplantation and 31.5 after BMT. Survival at 100 days was similar for both groups. The incidence of GVHD was similar for both groups.

Conclusion.—Whereas BSC transplantation may result in faster engraftment and a shorter hospital stay, 100-day survival is similar to that for BMT.

▶ Allogeneic peripheral BSC transplantation is being increasingly explored as an alternative to allogeneic BMT. This study is among the first to demonstrate potential benefits from this approach. Patients undergoing allogeneic peripheral BSC transplantation had a faster time to neutrophil recovery and a trend toward a faster platelet and red blood cell recovery. In addition, such patients received less platelet transfusions. Finally, the duration of hospitalization was significantly shorter for patients undergoing allogeneic peripheral BSC transplantation. Although not statistically significantly different, there was a trend toward a higher incidence of acute GVHD (grades II–IV) among patients undergoing peripheral BSC transplantation compared with conventional BTM (57% and 45%, respectively). There appear to be a number of benefits from the use of allogeneic peripheral BSC transplantation, although the ultimate benefits of greater relapse-free survival and overall survival are, as yet, undetermined.

M.S. Tallman, M.D.

Superiority of Tandem Autologous Transplantation Over Standard Therapy for Previously Untreated Multiple Myeloma

Barlogie B, Jagannath S, Vesole DH, et al (Univ of Arkansas, Little Rock; Natl Cancer Inst, Bethesda, Md; Arizona Cancer Ctr, Tucson; et al)

Blood 89:789–793, 1997 16–6

Background.—Standard therapy (ST) for multiple myeloma (MM) remains ineffective. Total therapy (TT) for MM consists of a series of non–cross-resistant induction regimens, followed by a double autotransplant. TT and ST were compared in a group of MM patients.

Methods.—Total therapy consisted of vincristine, doxorubicin, and dexamethasone; followed by high-dose cyclophosphamide and granulocyte-macrophage colony-stimulating factor for peripheral blood stem cell collection and then etoposide, dexamethasone, cytarabine, and cisplatin. After the induction phase, patients underwent autotransplant with high-dose melphalan (MEL 200). If at least a partial remission was present, patients underwent a second autotransplant with MEL 200. Patients without remission underwent MEL 140 plus total body irradiation or high-dose combination chemotherapy. Interferon maintenance was continued until disease relapse. The TT group consisted of 123 MM patients. These patients were compared with 116 patients from the Southwest Oncology Group trials who received ST and were matched for age, $b_2$microglobulin levels, and serum creatinine concentrations. Median follow-up for ST patients was 63 months and for TT patients was 31 months.

Results.—Total therapy induced complete remission in 40% of the 123 patients in the TT group. By 12 months, 7% of the TT patients had died. Median duration of event-free survival was 49 months and of overall survival was more than 62 months. Abnormalities of chromosomes 11q and 13 were associated with poor prognosis, while complete remission within 6 months of induction therapy was associated with good prognosis. Total therapy induced significantly higher remission rates than ST, and induced significantly longer event-free survival and overall survival.

Conclusions.—A group of MM patients who underwent a complex treatment of non–cross-resistant remission induction regimens followed by double autologous transplants were compared to a group of matched MM patients who underwent ST. Despite the complexity of the TT regimen, treatment-related mortality was low, and both short-term and long-term efficacy were high. Compared to ST, TT extended event-free survival and overall survival and had a higher remission rate. For those patients who do not respond to TT, new treatment approaches are needed.

▶ This study is important because it compares the outcome of patients undergoing the tandem autologous transplantation for myeloma to the outcome of patients undergoing what is regarded as standard therapy. Although this was not a prospective randomized trial, the results of the outcome of a relatively large number of patients undergoing transplantation are reported. Compared to standard therapy, tandem autologous transplantation, preceded by standard dose cytoreductive chemotherapy (which included vincristine, adriamycin and dexamethasone, high-dose cyclophosphamide and etoposide, dexamethasone, ara-C, and cisplatin), resulted in improved event-free and overall survival. Nevertheless, the majority of patients continued to relapse and faired poorly, particularly the 15% of patients who presented with abnormalities of chromosomes 11 and/or 13. Therefore, continued evaluation of these strategies is in order.

M.S. Tallman, M.D.

High-Dose Chemotherapy With Autologous Transplantation for Persistent/Relapsed Ovarian Cancer: A Multivariate Analysis of Survival for 100 Consecutively Treated Patients

Stiff PJ, Bayer R, Kerger C, et al (Loyola Univ, Maywood, Ill)

J Clin Oncol 15:1309–1317, 1997 16–7

Purpose.—Studies suggest that high-dose platinum-based chemotherapy, at intensities about 5 times higher than conventional doses, may be of some benefit for patients with advanced ovarian cancer. These patients need stem cell support to protect against marrow damage caused by such intensive therapy. In the authors' experience with transplantation in more than 100 patients with advanced ovarian carcinoma, platinum sensitivity and tumor bulk <1 cm appear to be the most important prognostic factors. The prognostic factors associated with survival after autologous stem cell transplantation for advanced ovarian cancer were analyzed in detail.

Methods.—One hundred patients (median age, 48 years) underwent autologous stem cell transplantation after chemotherapy for advanced ovarian cancer. The chemotherapy regimen was high-dose carboplatin, mitoxantrone, and cyclophosphamide, with or without cyclosporine, in 70 patients; melphalan and mitoxantrone, with or without paclitaxel, in 25; and other drugs in 5. The tumors were of papillary serous type in 70% of patients, grade III in 62%, platinum resistant in 66%, and 1 cm or larger in 61%. The patients had received a median of 2 previous chemotherapy

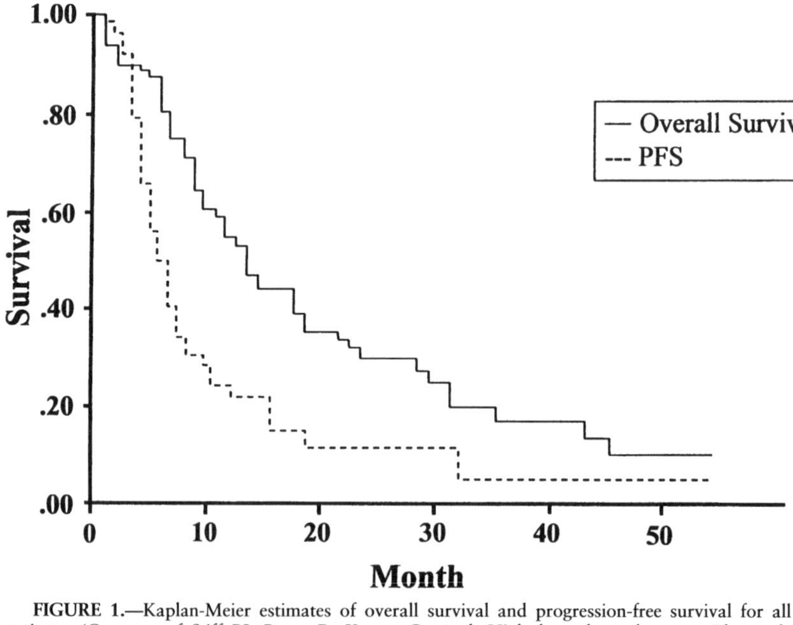

FIGURE 1.—Kaplan-Meier estimates of overall survival and progression-free survival for all 100 patients. (Courtesy of Stiff PJ, Bayer R, Kerger C, et al: High-dose chemotherapy with autologous transplantation for persistent/relapsed ovarian cancer: A multivariate analysis of survival for 100 consecutively treated patients. *J Clin Oncol* 15:1309–1317, 1997.)

regimens. Prognostic factors were evaluated by univariate and multivariate analyses, including age, disease stage, initial bulk, histologic type, grade, response to initial therapy, number of previous chemotherapy regimens, time since diagnosis, transplant regimen, platinum sensitivity, and tumor bulk at transplantation. The main outcome measures were progression-free survival (PFS) and overall survival (OS).

Results.—Median PFS was 7 months, and median OS 13 months (Fig 1). On stepwise Cox proportional hazards modeling, the main predictors of PFS were tumor bulk and cisplatin sensitivity. The best predictors of OS were age, tumor bulk at transplant, and platinum sensitivity. Twenty patients had platinum-sensitive tumors with bulk of 1 cm or less; their median PFS was 19 months; and median OS, 30 months. Overall survival was unaffected by the use of chemotherapy or surgery to minimize the extent of disease present.

Conclusions.—High-dose chemotherapy may be effective in the treatment of recurrent or persistent advanced ovarian cancer. However, it does not appear to be appropriate in patients with platinum-resistant, bulky disease. High-dose chemotherapy and autologous stem cell transplantation may be best suited for patients with minimal disease that is responsive to initial chemotherapy.

► Autologous transplantation appears to be increasingly used in the treatment of patients with persistent or relapsed ovarian cancer. Unfortunately, there is no prospective data to support the contention that it is superior to treatment with active agents in conventional doses. In this highly selected group of 100 patients with ovarian cancer treated with high-dose carboplatin, mitoxantrone, and cyclophosphamide, only two conclusions can be reached. First is that such an approach is unlikely to have any benefit in patients who have either platinum-resistant or bulky disease, and these patients should unequivocally not undergo transplantation. In patients who responded to prior platinum-based chemotherapy and who have small amounts of disease at the time of transplantation, the survival was encouraging. However, there is no evidence that it is superior to that which could be achieved with retreatment with active agents in this same drug-sensitive group of patients. Consequently, outside of a clinical trial situation, there is no accepted role for high-dose chemotherapy with transplantation in patients with persistent or recurrent ovarian cancer.

R.F. Ozols, M.D., Ph.D.

Prognostic Factors for Survival After High-Dose Therapy and Autologous Stem Cell Transplantation for Patients With Relapsing Hodgkin's Disease: Analysis of 280 Patients From the French Registry

Brice P, Bouabdallah R, Moreau P, et al (Hôpital Saint-Louis, Marseille, France; Centre Hospitalier de l'Hotel Dieu, Nantes, France; Hôpital Henri Mondor, Créteil, France; et al)

Bone Marrow Transplant 20:21–26, 1997 16–8

Purpose.—Most patients with Hodgkin's disease (HD) can be cured by chemotherapy and/or radiotherapy. However, the prognosis is poor for patients who have a relapse. One suggested approach to the treatment of relapsed HD is high-dose therapy with autologous stem cell transplantation (ASCT). The results of ASCT for relapsed HD were analyzed using registry data.

Methods.—A total of 280 patients, identified from the French bone marrow transplantation registry, were studied. All had a relapse after initial therapy for HD, including chemotherapy. Males outnumbered females 5 to 1, and the median age was 30 years. Forty-three percent of patients had stage I or II disease, and 57% had stage III or IV disease. Initial treatment consisted of chemotherapy in 32% of patients and chemotherapy plus radiotherapy in 68%. All patients had a relapse after going into complete remission in response to initial therapy. High-dose therapy with ASCT was administered a median of 34 months after diagnosis. In 78% of patients, the initial relapse developed within 18 months after the end of treatment. Salvage chemotherapy was given before high-dose therapy with ASCT, with high-dose therapy starting a median of 5 months after relapse.

Results.—After salvage chemotherapy, 84% of patients were judged to have chemosensitive relapse. Sixty percent of patients received BEAM conditioning therapy, while 26% received CBV/BEAC therapy. Six percent of patients had transplant-related mortality. The patients were followed up a median of 3 years after high-dose therapy. Four-year overall survival was 66%, while progression-free survival at the same time was 60%. Survival was unaffected by conditioning therapy and stem cell source. Patients with a chemosensitive relapse and those treated for an initial rather than later relapse had a better prognosis.

Additional factors related to survival in 214 patients treated for their first relapse were a time to relapse of less than 12 months and extranodal rather than nodal relapse. The combination of these 2 factors in a prognostic model identified 3 different subgroups with differing 4-year survivals. Survival was 93% for patients with neither factor, 59% for those with 1 factor, and 43% for those with both factors.

Conclusions.—The findings suggest that high-dose therapy with ASCT is indicated for all patients with relapsed HD who are not cured by second-line radiotherapy or who have early relapse. The role of high-dose therapy in patients without adverse prognostic factors remains to be determined. For patients in first relapse, conventional treatment can be used in the good-prognosis group, high-dose therapy for those who respond to second-line therapy, and more intensive treatment for those in the bad-prognosis group. Even with ASCT, the outlook is very bad for patients with disseminated or very early relapse who do not respond to second-line chemotherapy.

▶ Although it is generally accepted that patients with HD who relapse after initial therapy should strongly be considered for high-dose chemotherapy with ASCT, all the prognostic factors that impact on the outcome of such an approach have not been clearly identified. This report is useful because it evaluates a large cohort of patients who underwent high-dose chemotherapy with ASCT for relapsed HD. All patients received salvage cytoreductive chemotherapy before the high-dose treatment. With this approach, 84% of patients had chemotherapy-sensitive disease. Interestingly, the transplant-related mortality was quite low (6%), and the progression-free survival at 4 years was 60%. The following factors may be used to guide the therapeutic strategy; (1) whether the disease is chemosensitive at the time of relapse; (2) whether the patient is in first relapse or not; (3) whether the interval from complete remission to relapse is less than 12 months; and (4) whether there is extranodal disease. Three prognostic groups can be identified with quite different outcomes. This study suggests that patients with a good prognosis may do well with chemotherapy at relapse, those with 1 abnormal prognostic factor may do well with high-dose therapy, and those patients with 2 abnormal prognostic factors may require additional novel approaches.

M.S. Tallman, M.D.

17 Basic Radiation Therapy and Radiation Biology

Radiation Biology in Brachytherapy
Brenner DJ (Columbia Univ, New York)
J Surg Oncol 65:66–70, 1997 17–1

Background.—There is renewed interest in the use of brachytherapy for cancer treatment. Key technical advances have included afterloading, which greatly reduces the radiation dose to individuals other than the patient. The biological rationale for brachytherapy was reviewed, focusing on low-dose rate (LDR) brachytherapy.

Advantages of Brachytherapy.—The main advantages of LDR brachytherapy are the ability to position the radioactive source close to or within the tumor, short treatment times, and low-dose rate. Source positioning within or close to the tumor permits a high dose of radiation to be delivered to the target tissues while avoiding radiation damage to adjacent tissues. This good dose distribution spares not only early responding normal tissues, but also the late responding tissues that are often the dose-limiting effect of external beam radiotherapy. It also permits a much shorter treatment time than possible with external radiotherapy.

The lower dose rate of brachytherapy reduces radiobiological damage. The lower the dose rate, the better the balance between tumor control and late sequelae. Recent years have seen a trend toward high-dose rate (HDR) brachytherapy, in which higher activity sources are implanted but for a shorter time. The intent is generally to permit outpatient treatment, with the understanding that part of the therapeutic advantage will be compromised. In some unusual situations, such as intracavitary implants for cervical cancer, HDR brachytherapy might even offer better results than LDR brachytherapy.

Advances in Brachytherapy.—Remote afterloading is the main advance leading to the recent resurgence of brachytherapy. Other innovations have been proposed to strike an even more favorable balance between tumor control and late sequelae. One of these is pulsed brachytherapy (PDR), which simulates a continuous LDR treatment with a series of brief HDR irradiations, exploiting the potential of remote afterloader technology. This offers numerous advantages, including keeping the patient free from radiation most of the time, cutting down on the inventory of sources, and easy correction for radioactive source decay without changing the overall treatment time. If it proves possible to use PDR only during "office hours," it may become a major treatment approach in the United States. Through temporal optimization, PDR may offer a therapeutic advantage over continuous LDR brachytherapy by giving a higher dose in the early and late pulses and a lower dose in the intervening pulses. This technique results in differential sparing of late vs. early responding tissues, including the target tumor. This approach would exploit the flexibility of computer-controlled PDR to replace continuous LDR brachytherapy with a series of pulses.

Discussion.—Spurred by the development of remote afterloaders, the use of brachytherapy is on the rise in the United States. Where practical, it has become the treatment of choice for many sites. Brachytherapy offers important advantages over external beam radiotherapy, and has the potential for significant improvement over currently achieved clinical outcomes.

► It seems to me we are seeing quite a resurgence in brachytherapy as part of radiation treatment these days, and this article reviews the biological rationale for its use. The reasons for this resurgence are complex, but they include remote afterloading techniques that protect the physician, the development of the computer for quick and accurate calculations, and the arrival of newer isotopes. This review gives an excellent rationale for the use of brachytherapy, and also briefly covers pulsed or high-dose rate brachytherapy. For those who are interested, this is an excellent review that is well worth reading.

E. Glatstein, M.D.

Dynamics of Pear-Shaped Dimensions and Volume of Intracavitary Brachytherapy in Cancer of the Cervix: A Desirable Pear Shape in the Era of Three-Dimensional Treatment Planning

Kim RY, Caranto JF, Pareek PN, et al (Univ of Alabama, Birmingham)

Int J Radiat Oncol Biol Phys 37:1193–1199, 1997 17–2

Background.—Intracavitary brachytherapy is still the mainstay of treatment for cervical cancer. The traditional principle of this form of therapy, based on specific source-loading rules, is to achieve a constant dose rate at point A with a uniform pear-shape isodose distribution centered on the cervix. Computerized dosimetry is now used to reduce radiation exposure of the rectum and bladder; however, this can change the pear-shaped isodose distribution to a less desirable configuration, even with no change in the dose to point A. The dynamics of pear-shaped dimensions and volumes in intracavitary brachytherapy for cervical cancer were examined,

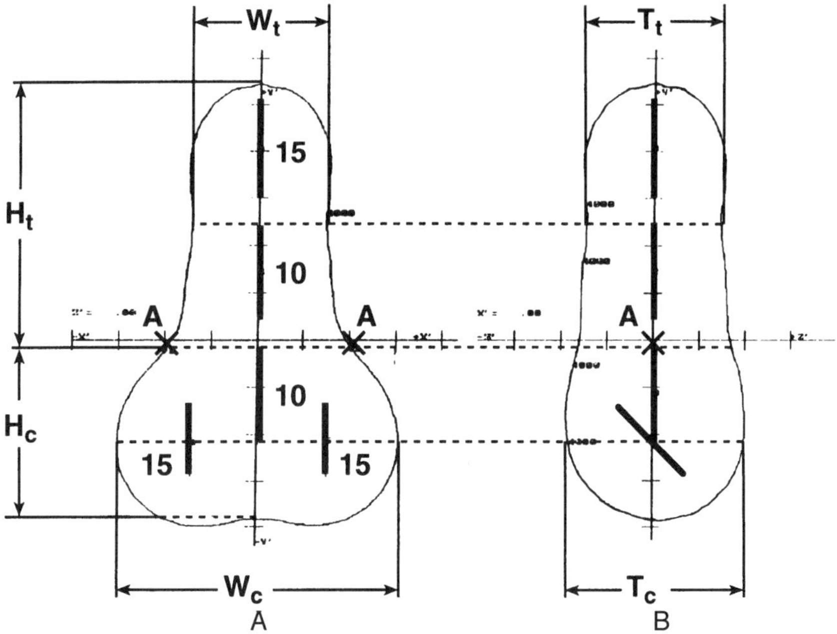

FIGURE 1.—Measurements of pear-shaped dimensions on frontal (**A**) and sagittal plane (**B**). Width (W_t), height (H_t), and thickness (T_t) at the tandem portion, and width (W_c), height (H_c), and thickness (T_c) at the colpostat portion of pear shape are shown. (Courtesy of Kim RY, Caranto JF, Pareek PN, et al: Dynamics of pear-shaped dimensions and volume of intracavitary brachytherapy in cancer of the cervix: A desirable pear shape in the era of three-dimensional treatment planning. *Int J Radiat Oncol Biol Phys* 37:1193–1199. Copyright 1997, Elsevier Science Inc. Reprinted by permission.)

including the definition of a desirable pear shape from the context of 3-dimensional treatment planning.

Methods.—A new technique for evaluating the dimensions and configuration of the pear shape was used. Changes in this shape were assessed by artificially dividing it into tandem and colpostat portions—defined as those parts above and below, respectively, a reference line between both the right and left of point A on the frontal and sagittal plane (Fig 1). The model defined width, height, and thickness at the tandem portion on the frontal plane (W_t, H_t, and T_t, respectively) and at the colpostat portion on the sagittal plane (W_c, H_c, and T_c, respectively). The pear-shaped isodose line and dose-volume histogram were generated using 12 variations of applicator geometry and source loading so as to assess the dynamics of the pear-shape configuration.

Results.—Reducing the source strengths in the colpostat portion for optimization reduced W_c, H_c, and T_c, even though there was no change in the dose to point A. At the same time, even though the overall pear-shaped volume was unchanged, W_c, H_c, and T_c increased. Increasing the separation of the colpostats without changing the source strength led to an increase in W_c and reductions in H_c and T_c. W_t, H_t, and T_t were unchanged

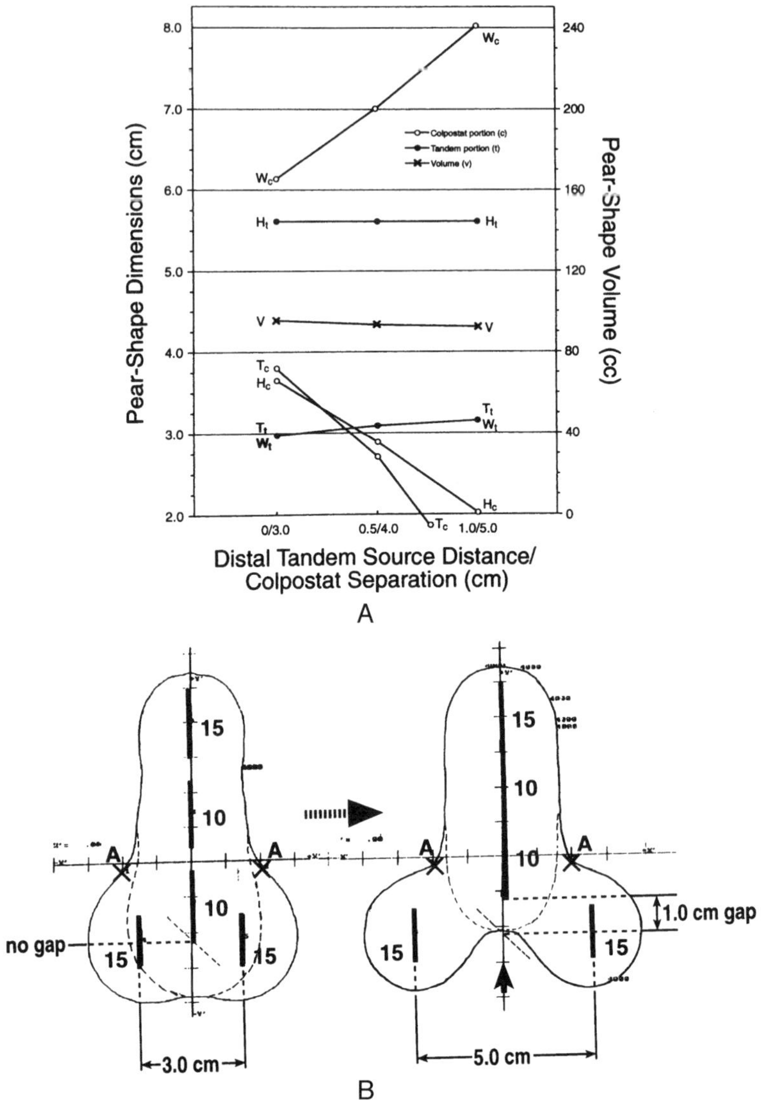

FIGURE 3.—**A**, effects of source separation between the colpostats and the distal tandem in addition to the colpostat separation on pear-shaped dimensions and volume. Note that H_c and T_c are reduced rapidly. **B**, increasing sources separation between colpostats and distal tandem to creating a cold spot between colpostats quickly (*arrow*) (*solid line,* frontal plane; *dotted line*, sagittal plane). (Courtesy of Kim RY, Caranto JF, Pareek PN, et al: Dynamics of pear-shaped dimensions and volume of intracavitary brachytherapy in cancer of the cervix: A desirable pear shape in the era of three-dimensional treatment planning. *Int J Radiat Oncol Biol Phys* 37:1193–1199. Copyright 1997, Elsevier Science Inc. Reprinted by permission.)

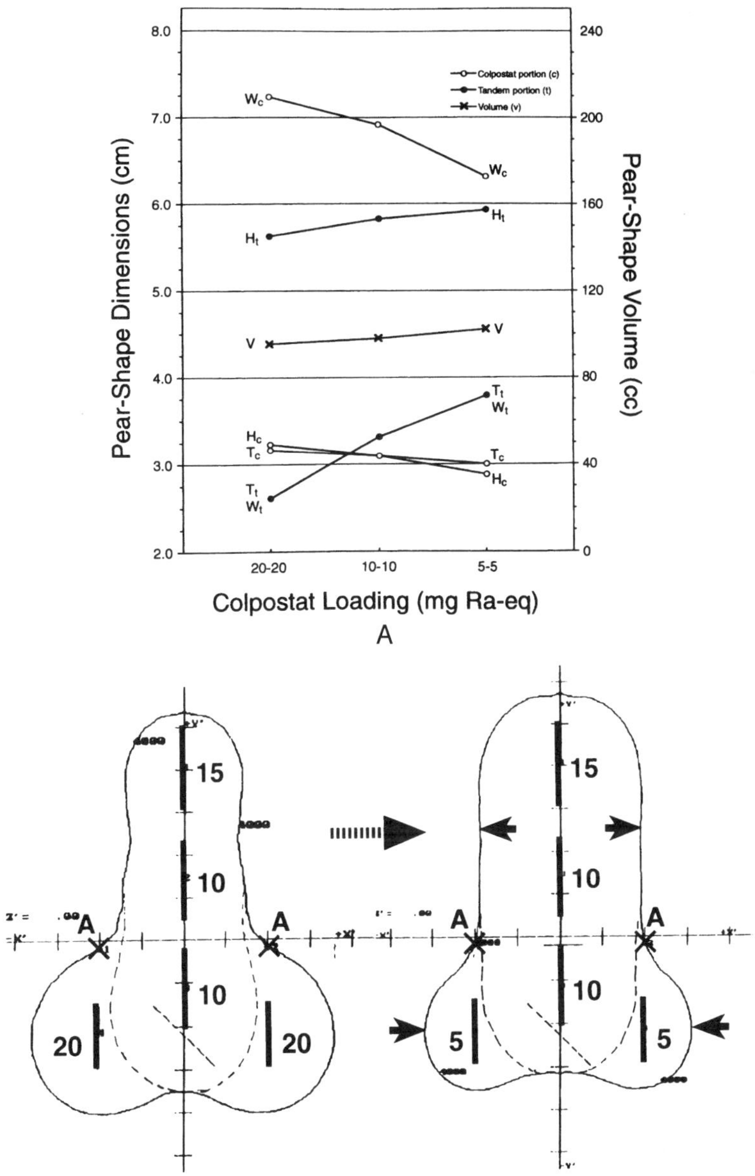

FIGURE 4.—**A,** effects of colpostats loading on pear-shaped dimensions and volume. Note that W_c, H_c, and T_c are smaller and W_t, H_t, T_t are larger in dimensions without affecting the pear-shaped volume. **B,** reducing colpostats loading affecting the configuration at both sides of the pear shape: decreasing the dimensions at the colpostat portion (*arrow*) and increasing the dimensions at the tandem portion (*arrow*) (*solid line*, frontal plane; *dotted line*, sagittal plane). (Courtesy of Kim RY, Caranto JF, Pareek PN, et al: Dynamics of pear-shaped dimensions and volume of intracavitary brachytherapy in cancer of the cervix: A desirable pear shape in the era of three-dimensional treatment planning. *Int J Radiat Oncol Biol Phys* 37:1193–1199. Copyright 1997, Elsevier Science Inc. Reprinted by permission.)

under these conditions, as was the overall pear-shape volume. Separating the colopostats and distal tandem source amplified these changes (Fig 3). Proportional increases in both colpostat separation and source strength yielded proportional increases in W_c, H_c, and T_c and in volume (Fig 4).

Conclusions.—In intracavitary brachytherapy for cervical cancer, the radiation dose to point A must be accompanied by a desirable pear shape surrounding the tumor. Knowledge of the dynamics of the pear shape under the conditions of 3-dimensional treatment planning promises to improve the ability to individualize radiation dosimetry to the tumor size and location. Understanding the relationship between the pear shape and the tumor coverage it provides can enhance the reliability of dose specification for cervical cancer.

► This interesting paper is worth reading, even though I think that the authors have really missed a point here. The purpose of defining point A in treating cervix cancer is simply that the brachytherapy treatment evolved in an era when there was no imaging available to indicate where the cancer was. As a consequence, the idea of the inverted pear distribution of radiation dosimetry for cervix cancer developed, and point A was arbitrarily defined and usually taught to imply that it is where the uterine artery and ureter cross. Given the complex treatment plans that are available to be generated today, in conjunction with modern imaging techniques, the need to define point A has been effectively eliminated. In fact, it is really a vestige of another era. With the imaging techniques that are now available; the whole idea of radiation therapy is to define the target volume in 3 dimensions, and put an appropriate isodose curve around that volume in all 3 dimensions. That is really what radiation therapy is about, and with our imaging techniques, we do not need to define point A anymore.

E. Glatstein, M.D.

The Effect of Combined External Beam Radiotherapy and Brachytherapy on Local Control and Wound Complications in Patients With High-grade Soft Tissue Sarcomas of the Extremity With Positive Microscopic Margin

Alekhteyar KM, Leung DH, Brennan MF, et al (Mem Sloan-Kettering Cancer Ctr, New York)

Int J Radiat Oncol Biol Phys 36:321–324, 1996 17–3

Background.—In a previous study, authors from the Memorial Sloan-Kettering Cancer Center showed that adjuvant brachytherapy (BRT) gives local control advantages when used for entirely resected high-grade soft-tissue sarcoma (STS). Recently, patients with positive margins of resection have been treated with a combination of BRT boost and wide field external beam radiotherapy (EBRT). The effect on local control of BRT boost used with EBRT for patients who fall into this subset was investigated. The study also investigated the effect of these procedures on wound complication rates.

Method.—Researchers studied 105 patients who had extremity-based recurrent high-grade STS (primary or local) and were treated from 1987 through 1992. Eighty-seven patients were treated with only BRT and wide local excision (dose: 45 Gy). Eighteen patients were treated with a combination of BRT and EBRT (dose:15–20 Gy BRT and 45–50 Gy EBRT). Ten of 18 BRT+EBRT patients had positive margins of resection. In the BRT-only group, 17 of 87 had a positive margin of resection. Researchers followed up with patients at a median of 22 months after treatment. Three categories were established for wound complications. The first was "major," or needing more operative intervention. The second was "moderate," or having purulent discharge, a 2-cm or greater wound separation, and hematoma greater than 25 mL. Anything less than moderate was considered "minor."

Results.—The actuarial local control rate for 2 years was predicted to be 86% and this control rate did not differ between the BRT+EBRT group (90%) and the BRT-only group (82%) ($P = 0.32$). In the patients with positive resection margins, the local control rate did differ markedly, almost significantly. ($P = 0.08$) (BRT+EBRT, 90%; BRT, 59%). This difference was not observed in patients with negative margins. The overall wound complication rate and the combined wound complication rate for major and moderate subsets showed no significant differences (26 vs. 16% for BRT; 38 vs. 27% for BRT+EBRT; $P = 0.31$ and 0.39, respectively).

Conclusion.—This study suggests that the optimal treatment for STS with positive resection margins is BRT boost + BRT. Wound complication rates do not differ between the 2 techniques.

► Functional limb-sparing surgical efforts have become part of the standard therapy for extremity STS within the last decade. Previous publications from the Memorial Sloan-Kettering Cancer Center[1] have established the usefulness of BRT in conjunction with limb-sparing surgery to enhance local control. This recent paper from the Memorial Sloan-Kettering Cancer Center expands the previous work combining BRT and surgery to include BRT as a tumor-bed boost dose, surgery, and postoperative EBRT for those specific patients with high-grade STS with positive resection margins.

In this study, there was a 90% local control rate with BRT + EBRT vs. BRT alone (59%) in patients with positive resection margins. The number of patients was not large enough to draw a statistically significant effect from the combined treatment, however. It is likely that with a large, high-grade, extremity STS in which margins are either microscopically positive or close, a combined approach of a BRT tumor boost and a planned course of EBRT should result in optimal local control.

We routinely use this treatment paradigm in patients with this profile. We agree with the findings of the Memorial Sloan-Kettering Cancer Center group that even with the addition of EBRT, the wound complication rate does not exceed that seen with a major STS resection alone.

B.L. Eisenberg, M.D.

Reference

1. Harrison LB, Franzese F, Gaynor J, et al: Long-term results of a prospective randomized trial of adjuvant brachytherapy in the management of completely resected soft tissue sarcomas of the extremity and superficial trunk. *Int J Radiat Oncol Biol Phys* 27:259–265, 1993.

Dose Escalation for Non–Small Cell Lung Cancer Using Conformal Radiation Therapy

Robertson JM, Ten Haken RK, Hazuka MB, et al (Univ of Michigan, Ann Arbor)

Int J Radiat Oncol Biol Phys 37:1079–1085, 1997 17–4

Objective.—For patients with non–small cell lung cancer (NSCLC), radiation therapy (RT) can achieve clinical local control rates of 50% to 70%. Reports suggest that increasing the radiation dose could improve local control. Three-dimensional radiation therapy treatment planning (3D RTP) offers a way to improve targeting and understanding of the dose-volume relationship within the normal lung. This technique was used to design an RT dose-escalation trial for NSCLC, in which the dose was determined by the effective volume of normal lung irradiated and the estimated risk of complications.

Methods.—Reported normal tissue parameters were used to graph the isonormal tissue complication probability (NTCP) levels associated with a radiation dose and effective volume (V_{eff}). In the resulting dose-escalation schema, patients were assigned to 1 of 5 treatment "bins," depending on the V_{eff} of the optimal treatment plan. The treatment bins, with starting doses ranging from 63 to 84 Gy, were escalated separately, as in phase I dose-escalation studies. The dose-limiting complication was grade 3 or higher radiation pneumonitis. In each bin, at least 3 patients were followed up for at least 6 months. Using 3D RTP, radiation was administered only to the radiographically abnormal areas. The dosage was 2.1 Gy/day, corrected for lung inhomogeneity. No prophylactic treatment was given for clinically uninvolved lymph nodes.

Results.—Preliminary data on 48 patients with NSCLC were reported. Eighteen had stage I/II disease, 28 had stage III disease, and 2 had mediastinal recurrence after surgery. Thirty patients with more than 6 months' follow-up were evaluable; none had radiation pneumonitis.

At least 1 dose escalation was carried out in each treatment bin, with current doses of 69.3, 69.3, 75.6, 84.0, and 92.4 Gy. There were 15 patients with 30% or greater NTCP, none of whom had clinical radiation pneumonitis. The actual risk of this complication was therefore less than 20%, with a β error rate of 5%. No patient had failure in the untreated mediastinum as the sole site of first failure, even though high-risk, clinically negative lymph nodes were untreated. Ten patients received 84 Gy or more of radiation; 3 had biopsy-proven residual or locally recurrent disease.

Conclusions.—Three-dimensional radiation treatment planning permits successful dose escalation for patients with NSCLC undergoing RT. Including the effective volume of irradiated tissue in the treatment plan has permitted some patients to receive a total radiation dose more than 50% higher than traditional doses. The risk of radiation pneumonitis does not seem prohibitive, and leaving out elective lymph node radiation has had no apparent negative impact. The final results of this trial will define the maximum tolerable dose of RT as the sole form of treatment of NSCLC, and identify the appropriate radiation dose for phase II trials.

► This is certainly a fascinating paper to read. It looks at 3-dimensional treatment planning and escalating the dose from 69 to over 90 Gy. The authors say they have not seen any clinical radiation pneumonitis in these groups. Radiation pneumonitis was not seen among the 15 patients who were evaluated. The particular technology here included 3-dimensional treatment planning along with multileaf collimators. It is certainly not clear to me that escalation of dose could possibly be done without all the elaborate technology, at least with patients tolerating the treatment well. Our decision to limit ourselves to a traditional "tolerance" level is, to a major degree, arbitrary.

All this does not necessarily mean that with conventional treament we have to stand pat. It surely is impressive to see the dose increase reported here. On the other hand, the concept of tolerance requires many patients to be followed for a very long time before any meaningful conclusion can be made about the efficacy and safety of higher doses.

E. Glatstein, M.D.

Hypofractionated Radiotherapy for Invasive Bladder Cancer

Scholten AN, Leer J-WH, Collins CD, et al (Univ of Leiden, The Netherlands; St Thomas' Hosp, London)

Radiother Oncol 43:163–169, 1997 17–5

Introduction.—The optimal radical treatment for patients with invasive transitional cell cancer of the bladder is controversial. The advantages of hypofractionation are a decreased number of treatment sessions, thus less traveling for the patient, and better use of limited resources. The results of hypofractionated radiotherapy with curative intent in the treatment of 123 patients with T2–T3 transitional cell carcinoma of the bladder were compared with those of conventional radiotherapy described in the literature.

Methods.—Local control rate, crude and cancer-specific survival, and morbidity were evaluated. The biological effectiveness of hypofractionated radiotherapy in this patient series was compared with that of the literature, using the biologically equivalent dose for antitumor efficacy and the biologically equivalent dose for late normal tissue effects.

Results.—Local failure was observed in 69 (59%) patients. The actuarial local cure rate was 31% and 29%, for 5 and 10 years, respectively

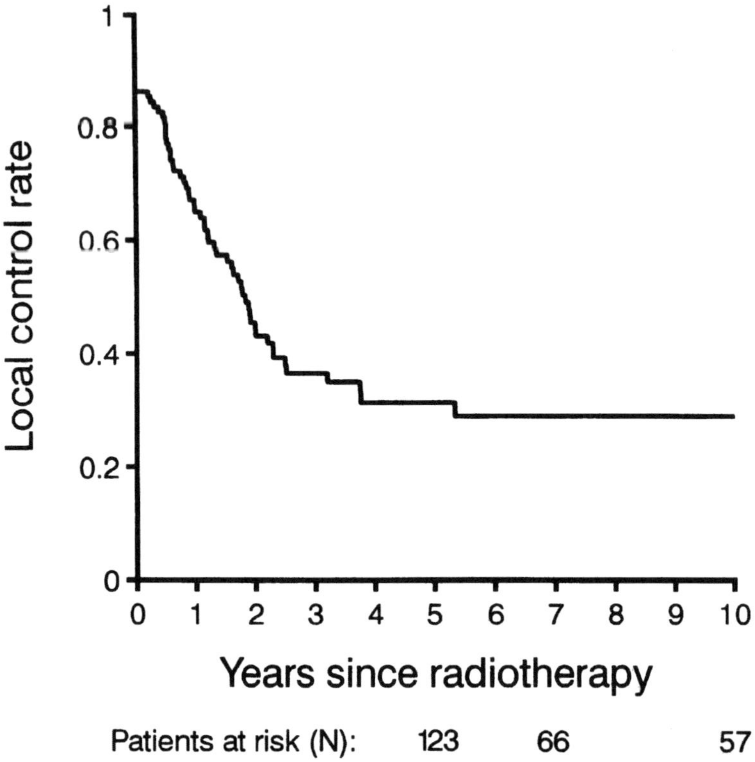

FIGURE 1.—Local control rate after hypofractionated radiotherapy, and the number of patients at risk before and 2 and 5 years after irradiation, in 123 patients with T2–T3 transitional cell carcinoma of the urinary bladder. (Courtesy of Scholten AN, Leer J-WH, Collins CD: Hypofractionated radiotherapy for invasive bladder cancer. *Radiother Oncol* 43:163–169, 1997. Copyright 1997. Reprinted with kind permission of Elsevier Science-NL, Sara Burgerhartstraat 25, 1055 KV Amsterdam, The Netherlands.)

(Fig 1). The actuarial cancer-specific 5-year survival rate was 48%. The 10-year rate was 39% (Fig 2). The cause of death of 100 patients was distributed as follows: 32 local bladder cancer, 34 metastatic disease (most also had local bladder disease), 25 intercurrent disease, and 9 unknown causes (Table 2). Eighty-seven percent of patients experienced acute, but not severe, side effects during or immediately after treatment. Late side effects occurring 3 or more months after irradiation completion were 33% at 5 years. Nine percent of patients experienced severe late side effects.

Conclusion.—Local control, survival, and early side effects were comparable in this patient series to those observed in the literature. Hypofractionated radiotherapy was associated with more late radiation side effects than conventional radiotherapy schedules.

▶ This British series for invasive bladder cancer uses hypofractionation radiation therapy to minimize the commitment. It basically puts all patients in a palliative category, which I have some trouble with because there is a

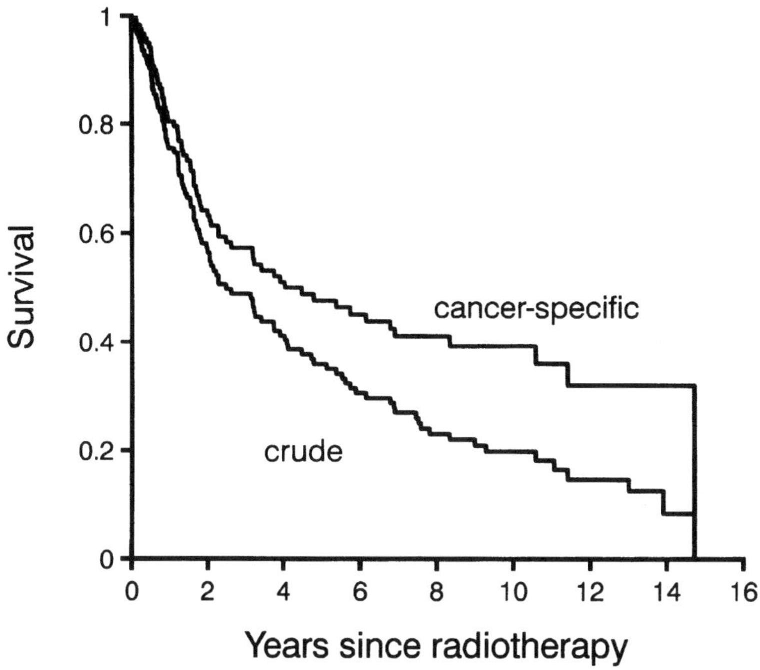

FIGURE 2.—Crude and cancer-specific survival after hypofractionated radiotherapy in 123 patients with T2–T3 transitional cell carcinoma of the urinary bladder. (Courtesy of Scholten AN, Leer J-WH, Collins CD: Hypofractionated radiotherapy for invasive bladder cancer. *Radiother Oncol* 43:163–169, 1997. Copyright 1997. Reprinted with kind permission of Elsevier Science-NL, Sara Burgerhartstraat 25, 1055 KV Amsterdam, The Netherlands.)

TABLE 2.—Cause of Death

		Patients (*N*)
Local bladder cancer		32
Metastatic disease		34
Intercurrent disease		25
Heart failure	8	
Bronchopneumonia	5	
Renal failure	5	
Ca. stomach	2	
Ca. kidney/pelvis	2	
Ca. lung	1	
Pulmonary embolus	1	
Burst aneurysm	1	
Not known		9
Loss to follow-up/still alive		23
Total		123

(Courtesy of Scholten AN, Leer J-WH, Collins CD: Hypofractionated radiotherapy for invasive bladder cancer. *Radiother Oncol* 43:163–169, 1997. Copyright 1997. Reprinted with kind permission of Elsevier Science-NL, Sara Burgerhartstraat 25, 1055 KV Amsterdam, The Netherlands.)

finite success rate with optimally fractionated treatment, albeit modest. The authors show their actuarial local control rate at 10 years to be about 30%. They acknowledge that the reduction in the number of fractions may result in a higher incidence of later morbidity. On the other hand, the real reason for including this paper is to remind other physicians that this treatment has some usefulness and can effectively control a certain proportion of patients for a long term.

E. Glatstein, M.D.

Advances in Prevention of Radiation Damage to Visceral and Solid Organs in Patients Requiring Radiation Therapy of the Trunk

Ritter EF, Lee CG, Tyler D, et al (Duke Univ, Durham, NC)

J Surg Oncol 64:109–114, 1997 17–6

Introduction.—In the adjuvant treatment of many malignancies, radiation therapy has assumed an increasingly prominent role. However, radiation damage can often occur to the gastrointestinal tract, bladder, kidneys, liver, spleen, and lungs. Mechanical strategies to avoid radiation exposure to sensitive organs have been proposed, such as omental slings, polyglycolic acid mesh slings, tissue expanders, or gel implants. The use of saline-filled, silicone-shelled breast implants has been incorporated as a method of organ displacement before radiation therapy. Two illustrative cases were reported.

Methods.—To displace visceral and solid organs away from the radiation field, saline breast implants were placed in polyglycolic acid mesh sheets in 2 patients. One patient had the implant placed in the retroperitoneum after resection of a primary retroperitoneal sarcoma. The other patient had the implant placed in the pelvis after resection of a radiation-induced soft tissue sarcoma of the suprapubic area. A surgical team placed the implants in collaboration with a radiation oncologist. The implants were inflated and manipulated to displace radiation-sensitive tissues not felt to be at risk for tumor

Results.—Uninvolved organs were successfully displaced away from the radiation fields by this technique, which minimizes the radiation dose to such organs and tissues. By decreasing exposure of radiation-sensitive tissues, such as the small bowel, while delivering a high dose of radiation to the tumor or tumor bed, placement of tissue implants can potentially increase the therapeutic index of such treatment. Using the external beam approach resulted in an improved therapeutic index with the saline-filled implant in place (Fig 3).

Conclusions.—To prevent radiation damage to visceral and solid organs adjacent to trunk tumor sites, this safe and efficacious method involves placement of a silicone-shelled, saline-filled breast prosthesis in a polyglycolic acid mesh pocket.

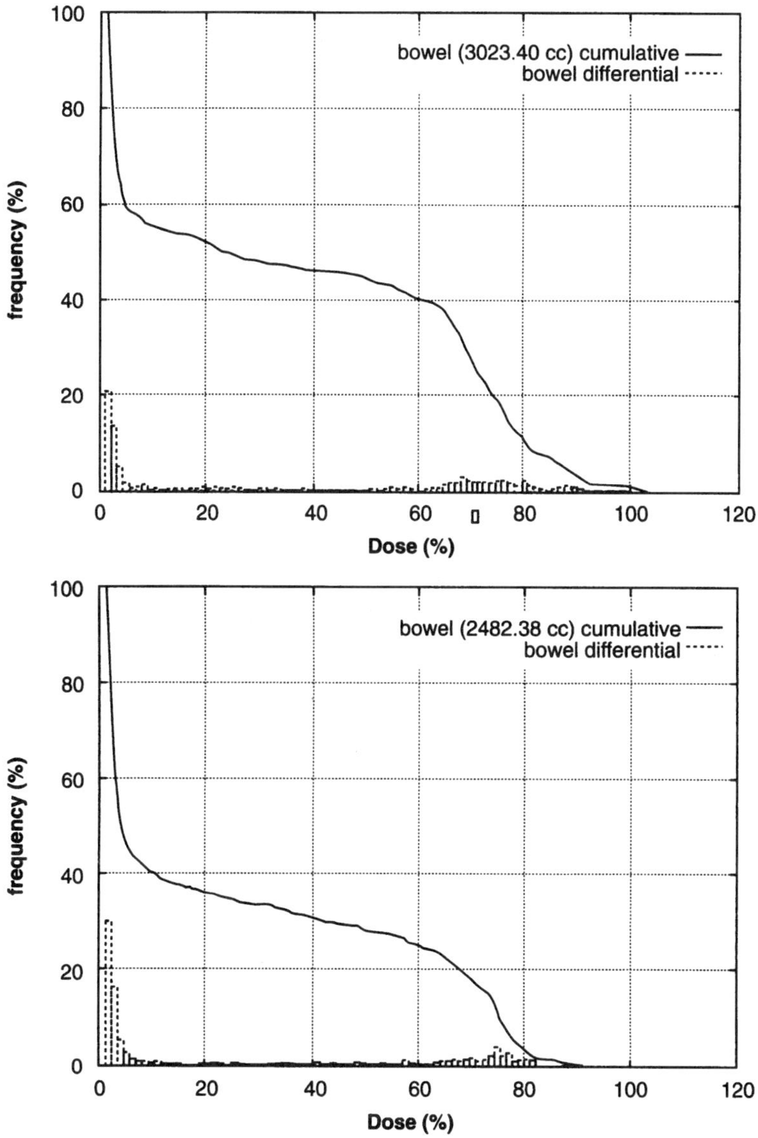

FIGURE 3.—**Top**, dose volume histogram (DVH) showing cumulative (*solid*) and differential (*dash*) bowel doses (cGy) without saline-filled implant in place (patient 1). **Bottom**, DVH, which shows markedly decreased cumulative (*solid*) and differential (*dash*) bowel doses (cGy) with saline-filled implant in place (patient 1). (Courtesy of Ritter EF, Lee CG, Tyler D, et al: Advances in prevention of radiation damage to visceral and solid organs in patients requiring radiation therapy of the trunk. *J Surg Oncol* 64:109–114, 1997. Reprinted by permission of Wiley-Liss, Inc., a subsidiary of John Wiley & Sons, Inc.)

► This paper deals with issues of trying to prevent radiation injury when using high-dose radiation therapy to the torso. It is basically about case reports, rather than real analysis of a procedure used by the authors. They used a saline breast implant placed in a polyglycolic acid mesh sheet which was used to displace viscera away from the radiation field in the torso. This has been going on for some time, and I just wish someone could give us a real overview of this experience, rather than giving us case reports. Questions really have to do with long-term follow-up in terms of how effective this kind of intervention is in preventing stochastic problems. Unfortunately, this paper does not answer those questions.

E. Glatstein, M.D.

Radiotherapy in Addition to Radical Surgery in Rectal Cancer: Evidence for a Dose–Response Effect Favoring Preoperative Treatment

Glimelius B, Isacsson U, Jung B, et al (Univ of Uppsala, Sweden)

Int J Radiat Oncol Biol Phys 37:281–287, 1997 17–7

Introduction.—More than 7,000 patients have been included in randomized trials evaluating treatment approaches for rectal cancer. Results have been variable. The relationship between preoperative and postoperative radiation doses and the reduction in local recurrence rates was assessed in prospective randomized trials that included a surgery-only group.

Methods.—All randomized trials before 1988 that compared preoperative and postoperative radiotherapy with surgery alone or with each other

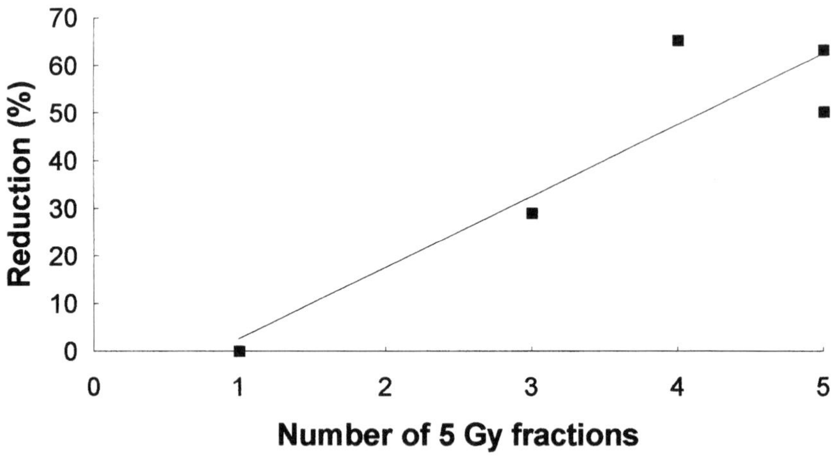

FIGURE 2.—Relationship between number of fractions and reduction in local recurrence rates in trials giving the radiation with 5 Gy fractions preoperatively. A weighted least-squares fit was made to a linear regression line. (Reprinted by permission of the publisher from Glimelius B, Isacsson U, Jung B, et al: Radiotherapy in addition to radical surgery in rectal cancer: Evidence for a dose–response effect favoring preoperative treatment. *Int J Radiat Oncol Biol Phys* 37:281–287, copyright 1997 by Elsevier Science Inc.)

were assessed. Local failure rates for 5,626 randomized patients were examined. The linear quadratic formula was applied to compensate for differences in radiotherapy schedules.

Results.—A definite dose–response relationship could be established for preoperative radiotherapy. The range of doses for postoperative radiotherapy was narrow, and a dose–response relationship was not determined. At similar doses, preoperative radiotherapy seemed more efficient in decreasing the local failure rate than postoperative radiotherapy. The 1 trial that compared preoperative and postoperative radiotherapy was in agreement with these findings. The average local recurrence rates were 28% for the surgery group alone, 16% for the preoperative radiotherapy group, and 20% for the postoperative radiotherapy group. There was no reduction in recurrence rates in trials with only 1 fraction, an intermediate reduction with 3 fractions, and a clear reduction with 4 and 5 fractions (Fig 2). It may be that a dose that is 15–20 Gy higher may be needed postoperatively than preoperatively to achieve similar efficacy.

Conclusion.—Preoperative radiotherapy may be more dose effective than postoperative radiotherapy in treating rectal cancer. The relative decrease in local failure rates with similar doses in linear quadratic times was about twice as large as with postoperative radiotherapy.

▶ This paper from a group in Sweden addresses the controversial subject of preoperative vs. postoperative radiation for patients with rectal cancer. All prospective, randomized trials initiated before 1988 comparing preoperative and postoperative radiotherapy with either surgery alone or to each other were included in this analysis. The authors conclude that preoperative radiotherapy is more efficacious, in terms of both the dose-response relationship and evidence of the beneficial effect on local control rates, than postoperative radiation or surgery alone. The preoperative radiation dose in these studies varied but was approximately 25.5–38 Gy in multiple split fractions or hyperfractionation schemes. In addition, multiple fields were used to decrease both short- and long-term toxicity. As noted in Figure 2, there is a linear relationship between the preoperative radiotherapy dose and the reduction of local recurrence rates. Although trials using preoperative radiotherapy alone have only suggested a survival benefit, it is likely that the addition of chemotherapy will provide enhanced survival rates. Certainly, preoperative radiotherapy promotes better patient compliance and obviates the problem of a prolonged delay in initiation of postoperative treatment, as has been seen in trials using postoperative radiotherapeutic regimens.

B.L. Eisenberg, M.D.

18 Pharmacology

Microfilament Depletion and Circumvention of Multiple Drug Resistance by Sphinxolides

Zhang X, Minale L, Zampella A, et al (Fox Chase Cancer Ctr, Philadelphia; Università di Napoli "Federico II", Italy)

Cancer Res 57:3751–3758, 1997 18–1

Objective.—Some natural cytotoxins that induce changes in microfilament organization of eukaryotic cells may be useful as anticancer drugs. Sphinxolides from the sponge *Neosiphonia superstes* are cytotoxic toward tumor cells. The ability of these compounds to kill drug-resistant cells and their effects on microfilament structure were examined.

Methods.—The cytotoxicity of varying concentrations of sphinxolides and tolytoxin were evaluated in MCF-7 human breast carcinoma cells; MCF-7/ADR (a P-glycoprotein-overexpressing subline); HL-60 human promyelocytic leukemia cells; HL-60R cells, which overexpress multidrug resistance-associated protein; A-10 rat aortic smooth muscle cells; and SK-OV-3 human ovarian carcinoma cells (Fig 1). Analysis of cell cycle, actin isolation and polymerization, and apoptosis, immunofluorescence, adenosine triphosphatase activity of actomyosin, and cleavage complex formation assays were performed.

Results.—Tolytoxin was slightly more cytotoxic and cytochalasins significantly less cytotoxic than the 4 sphinxolide compounds, which had similar inhibition potencies. Both tolytoxin and sphinxolide C affected decreased cell production in the G_2M-phase in a dose-dependent manner, and both induced apoptosis. The antiproliferative effects of sphinxolide C, tolytoxin, and cytochalasin were reversed when the drugs were removed. Addition of sphinxolides and tolytoxin resulted in irreversible disorganization of microfilaments, but the sphinxolides left the microtubules intact. Sphinxolides (1 μmol sphinxolide B) inhibited polymerization of 20 μmol actin by 75%, and 5 μmol inhibited polymerization completely. Sphinxolides inhibited adenosine triphosphatase activity in a dose-dependent manner and also inhibited topoisomerase.

Conclusion.—Sphinxolides inhibit actin polymerization by reversibly disorganizing microfilaments. They are associated with cell cycle arrest in the G_2 phase and induction of apoptosis. Overexpression of multidrug resistance-associated protein does not result in resistance to sphinxolides. This new class of drugs may be useful in treating drug-resistant tumors.

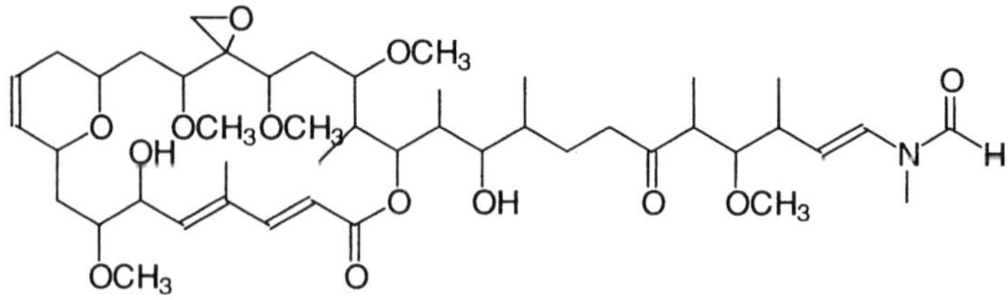

Tolytoxin

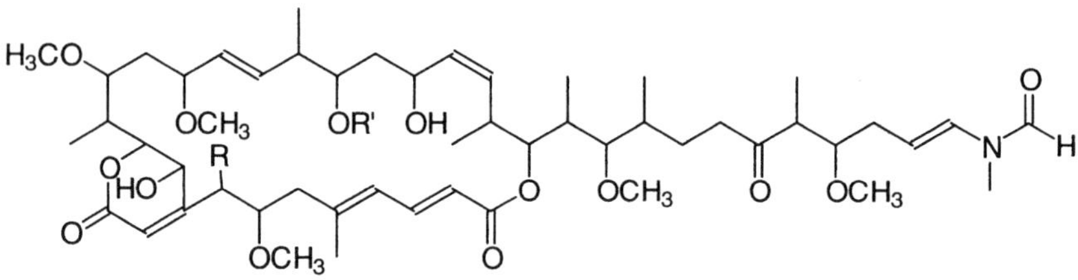

Sphinxolide:	R = OCH_3	R' = H
Sphinxolide B:	R = H	R' = H
Sphinxolide C:	R = OCH_3	R' = CH_3
Sphinxolide D:	R = H	R' = CH_3

FIGURE 1.—Structures of tolytoxin and sphinxolides. (Courtesy of Zhang X, Minale L, Zampella A, et al: Microfilament depletion and circumvention of multiple drug resistance by sphinxolides. *Cancer Res* 57:3751–3758, 1997.)

▶ Drug resistance remains a major obstacle to successful chemotherapy. Tumors that express P-glycoprotein or the multidrug resistance-associated protein are resistant to natural products on the basis of increased drug efflux. Sphinxolides are novel compounds whose cytotoxicity is caused by cell arrest in G_2-M and induction of apoptosis. In contrast to other natural products, sphinxolides' cytotoxicity is independent of P-glycoprotein or multidrug resistance-associated protein expression. Consequently, these agents may be particularly useful in drug-resistant tumors.

R.F. Ozols, M.D., Ph.D.

Topotecan Increases Topoisomerase IIα Levels and Sensitivity to Treatment With Etoposide in Schedule-dependent Process

Whitacre CM, Zborowska E, Gordon NH, et al (Case Western Reserve Univ, Cleveland, Ohio)

Cancer Res 57:1425–1428, 1997 18–2

Background.—Topoisomerases (Topos), enzymes that control the conversion of one DNA topologic isomer to another, are divided into 2 classes: Topo I, which breaks 1 strand of double-stranded DNA, permitting the remaining intact strand to pass through the break, resulting in DNA relaxation, and Topo II, which catalyzes transient double-strand breaks and passage of double-stranded DNA in an ATP-dependent reaction. Thus, topo inhibitors should be effective in combination chemotherapy regimens. The sequential use of Topo I and II inhibitors may be the best combination, as Topo I inhibition may result in a compensatory increase in Topo II levels, rendering tumors more sensitive to a subsequent dose of Topo II inhibitors. However, the activity of this sequence and the molecular basis for its effect has not yet been demonstrated in vivo.

Methods.—The effect of Topo I inhibitors in the modulation of Topo II levels and sensitivity to Topo II–directed drugs were investigated in a murine model. Athymic mice bearing SW480 human colon cancer xenografts were treated with simultaneous, subsequent, or distant doses of topotecan and etoposide.

Findings.—Simultaneous administration of topotecan and etoposide produced an antagonistic response. By contrast, Topo I inhibition by topotecan resulted in a compensatory increase in Topo IIα levels associated with increasing sensitivity of tumors to subsequent treatment with the Topo II inhibitor etoposide. Five days after the last dose of topotecan, Topo IIα levels declined, resulting in restoration of the original response of the xenografts to etoposide.

Conclusion.—These data provide the biochemical basis for optimizing combination chemotherapy with Topo I- and II-active agents. The role of schedule dependency is critical for achieving the best result.

▶ Both topotecan, a topoisomerase I inhibitor, and oral etoposide, a topoisomerase II inhibitor, are active in the treatment of recurrent ovarian cancer. For these drugs to make an impact upon the overall survival of patients with ovarian cancer, it is likely that they will have to be incorporated as part of upfront combination regimens. However, other drugs have recently been identified as active in recurrent ovarian cancer, including encapsulated doxorubicin and vinorelbine. Studies such as this which examine the biochemical synergy between different combinations of agents will be useful in identifying specific combinations that will be further evaluated in phase I and phase II clinical trials.

R.F. Ozols, M.D., Ph.D.

Phase I and Pharmacologic Study of Oral Topotecan Administered Twice Daily for 21 Days to Adult Patients With Solid Tumors

Creemers GJ, Gerrits CJH, Eckardt JR, et al (Rotterdam Cancer Inst, The Netherlands; Univ Hosp, Rotterdam, The Netherlands; Univ of Texas, San Antonio; et al)
J Clin Oncol 15:1087–1093, 1997 18–3

Background.—Topotecan is a specific inhibitor of topoisomerase I, a nuclear enzyme that resolves topologic problems of the supercoiled DNA. Bioavailability of an oral formulation of about 30% with limited variability has been reported. A phase I and pharmacokinetic study of this oral topotecan formulation was conducted to characterize the maximum-tolerated dose, toxicities, and antitumor effects in patients with refractory malignancies.

Methods.—Thirty-one patients were enrolled in the study. Treatment consisted of oral topotecan given twice daily for 21 days. Cycles were repeated every 28 days. The dose was escalated from 0.15 to 0.6 mg/m^2 twice daily in subsequent cohorts. Pharmacokinetic studies were done on days 1 and 8 of the first course. A total of 59 courses were delivered to the 30 evaluable patients.

Findings.—Dose-limiting toxicity occurred at 0.6 mg/m^2 twice daily. It consisted of diarrhea, which began subacutely at a median onset on day 15 and resolved after a median of 8 days. Other toxicities—leukocytopenia, thrombocytopenia, nausea, and vomiting—were mild. The maximum tolerated dose was 0.5 mg/m^2 twice a day. There were no responses. A marked variation of the area under the plasma concentration-time curve was observed at time point "t" (AUC[t]) of topotecan and ring-opened product hydroxyacid. There was a significant association between the percentage of reduction in white blood cell count vs. the AUC(t) of topotecan, modeled by a sigmoidal maximal effect concentration function.

Conclusion.—In this phase I study, the dose-limiting toxicity of chronic oral topotecan given for 21 days was diarrhea. For phase II studies, the recommended dose is 0.5 mg/m^2 2 times a day.

► Dose-limiting toxicity of IV topotecan is myelosuppression. This phase I study of oral topotecan came up with diarrhea as the dose-limiting toxicity. Topoisomerase inhibitors, such as topotecan, are highly S-phase–specific, and in preclinical models, cytotoxicity is a function of exposure time to the drug above a critical concentration. It is possible that 21 days is not necessary and that a shorter exposure time, such as 5–10 days, or oral administration might produce the necessary drug levels for observing antitumor activity but, at the same time, decrease the gastrointestinal toxicity (e.g., diarrhea).

R.F. Ozols, M.D., Ph.D.

Overexpression of a Rabbit Liver Carboxylesterase Sensitizes Human Tumor Cells to CPT-11

Danks MK, Morton CL, Pawlik CA, et al (St Jude Children's Research Hosp, Memphis, Tenn)

Cancer Res 58:20–22, 1998 18–4

Background.—CPT-11 (7-ethyl-10-[4-(1-piperidino)-1-piperidino]carbonyloxycamptothecin) is a chemotherapy drug whose active metabolite, SN-38, inhibits topoisomerase I, causes DNA damage, and induces apoptosis. Conversion of CPT-11 to SN-38 takes place through carboxylesterases (CEs). Animal studies suggest that relatively small increases in tolerance of or tumor sensitivity to CPT-11 could be of therapeutic benefit. Whether expression of a CE capable of converting CPT-11 to SN-38 in tumor cells can make tumors more sensitive to CPT-11 was determined.

Methods and Findings.—In in vitro studies, partially purified rabbit liver CE converted CPT-11 to SN-38 in concentration-dependent fashion. Reaction products of CPT-11 incubated with active CE produced significant inhibition of pediatric rhabdomyosarcoma cells, confirming the biological activity of the metabolite. In cancer cells that were stably transfected with the CE cDNA to CPT-11, cell sensitivity to the prodrug was elevated more than eightfold.

Conclusions.—CPT-11 is converted to its active metabolite by a CE, and mammalian cells transfected with a cDNA encoding a CE have increased sensitivity to the chemotherapy agent CPT-11. The findings suggest a potentially valuable prodrug/enzyme combination approach, analogous to the ganciclovir/herpes simplex virus thymidine kinase and 5–fluorouracil/cytosine deaminase combinations currently being studied. The authors are attempting to clone the human homologue of the cDNA used in this study, and are conducting preclinical studies of CPT-11 sensitivity in mice bearing CE-expressing xenografts.

▶ CPT-11 is a topoisomerase-1 inhibitor with activity in colorectal cancers, even those that exhibit a resistance to 5–fluorouracil. The clinical utility of the agent has been somewhat limited by its toxicity, particularly diarrhea. CPT-11 requires metabolic activation to produce the cytotoxic metabolite, SN-38. This reaction is facilitated by carboxylesterases. Because CPT-11 also has an apparent steep dose-response relationship in experimental tumors, it is possible that increased expression of specific carboxylesterases in tumors may sensitize them to CPT-11 and allow for administration of doses that are not associated with diarrhea.

R.F. Ozols, M.D., Ph.D.

Phase I and Pharmacologic Study of Docetaxel and Cisplatin in Patients With Advanced Solid Tumors

Pronk LC, Schellens JHM, Planting AST, et al (Univ Hosp, Rotterdam, The Netherlands; Rhône-Poulenc Rorer, Antony, France)

J Clin Oncol 15:1071–1079, 1997 18–5

Background.—The new antimicrotubule agent docetaxel has shown activity against various types of tumors in humans and animals. Noncumulative neutropenia is the major dose-limiting toxic effect. Docetaxel is a good candidate for combination with cisplatin; both drugs are active against a wide range of solid tumors, with only minimal overlap between their toxicity profiles. A phase I trial of docetaxel and cisplatin in combination against various solid tumors was conducted.

Methods.—The study included 64 patients with documented solid tumors for whom no first- or second-line treatment was available. The patients had received no treatment with taxanes or cisplatin derivatives, and no more than 1 regimen of combination chemotherapy or 2 regimens of single-agent chemotherapy. Patients were treated with 1 of 2 regimens: schedule A, 1-hour infusion of docetaxel plus 3-hour infusion of cisplatin; or schedule B, cisplatin followed by docetaxel. The dose of docetaxel ranged from 55 to 100 mg/m^2, and the dose of cisplatin from 50 to 100 mg/m^2. The maximum tolerated doses were determined. Toxicity evaluated focused on sequence-dependent side effects.

Results.—Leukocytopenia and granulocytopenia occurred in 90% of patients, reaching grade 3 or 4 severity in 87%. These complications were transient and depended on the docetaxel dose. Ten percent of courses were complicated by infection, and 4.5% by neutropenia. Nonhematologic toxic effects were mild to moderate, including alopecia, nausea, vomiting, diarrhea, mucositis, neurotoxicity, fluid retention, and skin and nail effects. The pharmacokinetics of the 2 schedules were similar. One patient had a complete response, and 9 had partial responses. Docetaxel 100 mg/m^2 plus cisplatin 75 mg/m^2, and docetaxel 85 mg/m^2 plus cisplatin 100 mg/m^2 were considered tolerable dose levels. These doses represented a high median relative dose intensity, with 81% to 88% of cycles given at full intended dosage.

Conclusions.—Preliminary results of combination therapy with docetaxel and cisplatin in patients with solid tumors suggest that, for convenience sake, docetaxel should be given before cisplatin. The schedule A regimen used in this study is recommended for further evaluation. Proper patient selection, based on performance score, will be essential for these studies.

► The dose-limiting toxicity of docetaxel has been significant fluid retention and myelosuppression. The fluid retention is ameliorated by steroids and diuretics. The myelosuppression has been thought to be a significant limiting factor in evaluating docetaxel combinations with other myelosuppressive agents. This study demonstrates, however, that docetaxel can be administered at therapeutic doses (85–100 mg/m²) together with cisplatin at standard doses (75–100 mg/m²) with acceptable toxicity. A similar combination is currently being tested by the Eastern Cooperative Oncology Group in patients with metastatic non-small-cell lung cancer. In this trial, patients are randomized to either docetaxel plus cisplatin, cisplatin plus paclitaxel, carboplatin with paclitaxel, or gemcitabine plus cisplatin. Such prospective randomized comparisons are essential to determine the comparative efficacy and toxicity of platinum compounds together with new classes of antineoplastic agents, including the taxanes and the topoisomerase inhibitors.

R.F. Ozols, M.D., Ph.D.

Growth Inhibitory Effects of Sodium Phenylacetate (NSC 3039) on Ovarian Carcinoma Cells *in Vitro*

Ferrandina G, Melichar B, Loercher A, et al (Univ of Texas MD Anderson Cancer Ctr, Houston; Catholic Univ, Rome)

Cancer Res 57:4309–4315, 1997 18–6

Introduction.—The third most common gynecologic malignancy is ovarian cancer. Tumors recur in most patients, even those who have surgically confirmed complete responses to primary chemotherapy. For the treatment of chemotherapy-refractory tumors, new and less toxic therapeutic agents are being sought. A new class of growth-inhibitory compounds may be sodium phenylacetate, present in micromolar concentrations in human plasma. The antiproliferative activity of sodium phenylacetate against ovarian carcinoma cell lines was determined.

Methods.—A large panel of ovarian cell lines and freshly obtained tumor cells from patients with ovarian cancer were used to investigate the effects of sodium phenylacetate. Cell cycle-specific events were determined, as well as modulation of p21/ras and apoptosis-related genes, along with modulation of MHC expression and tumor growth factor β1 and β2. The growth-inhibitory effects of the combination of sodium phenylacetate and cisplatin in vitro were also evaluated.

Results.—A dose-dependent inhibition of all ovarian carcinoma cell lines was induced by sodium phenylacetate, although there was variance of the sensitivity of individual lines to sodium phenylacetate. A response to sodium phenylacetate was seen with cisplatin-sensitive and cisplatin-resistant cell lines. There was a detection of growth activity against cells that were freshly isolated from previously treated patients who had a malignant ascites. A maximum effect was seen at 72 hours with the growth inhibitory effects produced by sodium phenylacetate. There was no association with cytotoxic action. The effects produced by sodium phenylacetate on growth inhibition were reversible. A reduction in the percentage of cells in the S-phase was seen after 48 and 72 hours of exposure to sodium phenylacetate. There was also recruitment of cells in the G0-G1 phase. The proportion of cells in apoptosis did not increase significantly with treatment with sodium phenylacetate after different exposure times. There was a significant reduction in the percentage of cells positive for bcl-2 and the percentage of cyclin-D1– and p21/ras-positive cells with sodium phenylacetate. There was an increase in the percentage of bax/p21-positive cells. In HLA class I and transforming growth factor β1 antigens, there were minimal if any alterations with sodium phenylacetate. After exposure to sodium phenylacetate, the percentage of transforming growth factor β2 decreased.

Conclusions.—An additive inhibitory effect was seen in the combination of sodium phenylacetate and cisplatin. The growth of ovarian carcinoma cell lines and the cells from malignant ascites of chemotherapy-treated patients with ovarian carcinoma were inhibited with sodium phenylacetate. In patients with ovarian carcinoma, there could be possible new therapeutic potential with the growth-inhibitory properties of sodium phenylacetate.

► Sodium phenylacetate (NaPa) has already undergone clinical trials in patients with prostate cancer and gliomas. Antitumor activity was observed in these trials even though the mechanism of this effect remains an area of active investigation. Sodium phenylacetate, a product of phenyalanine metabolism, is present in micromolar concentrations in human plasma. Why such a ubiquitous compound should have an effect on cell growth and differentiation of malignant cells remains a mystery. This study demonstrates that NaPa inhibits growth of human ovarian cancer cells and may provide a stimulus for further clinical evaluation of this compound, either for treatment or possibly as a chemopreventive agent.

R.F. Ozols, M.D., Ph.D.

Dose-Effect Study of Carboplatin in Ovarian Cancer: A Danish Ovarian Cancer Group Study

Jakobsen A, Bertelsen K, Andersen JE, et al (Odense Univ, Denmark; Aarhus Univ, Denmark; Herning Hosp, Denmark; et al)

J Clin Oncol 15:193–198, 1997 18–7

Objective.—Most epithelial ovarian cancers are sensitive to chemotherapy at the beginning of treatment, but resistance can develop later. Though the mechanisms of resistance vary, it seems likely that resistance can be overcome by increased exposure to cytotoxic drugs. For some drugs, such as anthracyclines and carboplatin, the area under the concentration-vs.-time curve (AUC) appears to be a better measure of exposure and effect than milligrams per square meter. This measure was used in a study of carboplatin dose intensity in ovarian cancer.

Methods.—The randomized trial included 222 women with stages II to IV epithelial ovarian cancer. All underwent laparotomy. All received 6 courses of cyclophosphamide 500 mg/m^2, given every 4 weeks. They also received carboplatin at an AUC of 4 or 8 (AUC4 or AUC8), with AUC

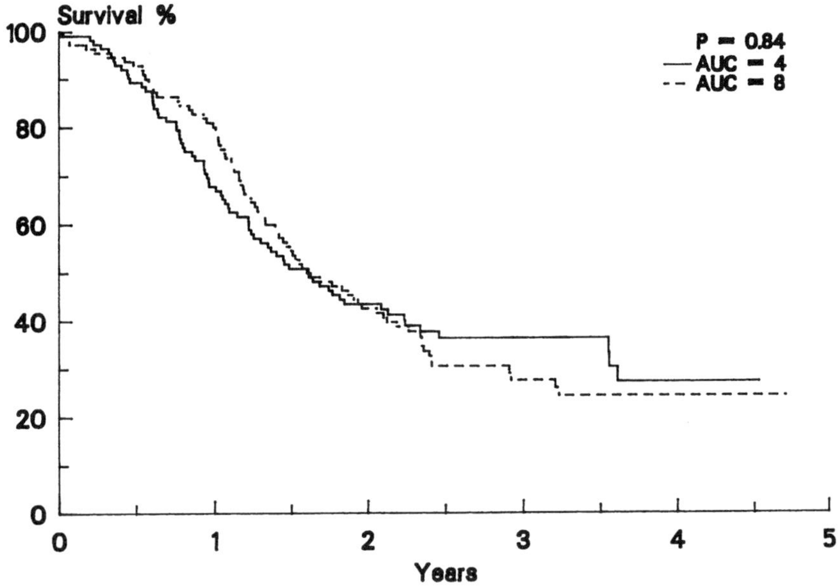

FIGURE 1.—Crude survival according to treatment arm. (Courtesy of Jakobsen A, Bertelsen K, Andersen JE, et al: Dose-effect study of carboplatin in ovarian cancer: A Danish Ovarian Cancer Group study. *J Clin Oncol* 15:193–198, 1997.)

calculations made according to Calvert's formula. In addition, 123 patients underwent measurement of the carboplatin AUC using a single-sample method, and the results were compared with the calculated AUC. The 2 groups were compared for their rates of complete pathologic remission and crude survival.

Results.—Second-look surgery was performed in about half of each group. Complete pathologic remission was achieved in 32% of the AUC4 group and 30% of the AUC8 group. The survival curves were similar in the 2 groups: 4-year survival was 27% in the AUC4 arm and 24% in the AUC8 arm (Fig 1). There was little difference in the dose intensity of cyclophosphamide. However, the dose intensity of carboplatin was 1.86 times greater in the AUC8 group than in the AUC4 group. For most patients, there was good agreement between the calculated and measured AUC values. Patients in the AUC8 group had greater bone marrow toxic effects.

Conclusions.—In patients with epithelial ovarian cancer, doubling the dose intensity of carboplatin while holding the dose of cyclophosphamide stable does not offer any significant improvement in pathologic remission rate or survival. The AUC of carboplatin can be estimated with reasonable accuracy using Calvert's formula. The higher dose intensity of carboplatin is associated with greater bone marrow toxicity. Growth factor or stem cell support would be needed to achieve any further increase in carboplatin dosage.

► The importance of dose intensity in ovarian cancer has been debated for a long time. This study demonstrates that there is no clinical benefit in patients with advanced ovarian cancer when they were treated with carboplatin dosed to an AUC of 8 compared with those who received an AUC of 4. All patients in this study received cyclophosphamide as well, and were treated for 6 cycles. This large randomized trial, together with a previous study from the Gynecologic Oncology Group as well as several other trials, clearly demonstrates that doubling the dose of platinum compounds past an effective range is not associated with any significant improvement in clinical outcome. Consequently, in ovarian cancer the recommended dose for cisplatin is 75 mg/m^2 and for carboplatin AUC dosing between 5.0 and 7.5. The most widely used regimen in the United States consists of the combination of paclitaxel at 175 mg/m^2 together with carboplatin dosed to an AUC of 7.5. While previous randomized trials have failed to demonstrate a significant advantage for more than 6 cycles of chemotherapy with a platinum-based regimen, it is unclear what the optimal number of cycles of paclitaxel-based chemotherapy should be in previously untreated patients with advanced disease. It is possible that the number of cycles and the duration of treatment may be more important than the actual dose of chemotherapy administered with each cycle.

R.F. Ozols, M.D., Ph.D.

Phase I and Pharmacologic Study of the Combination Paclitaxel and Carboplatin as First-line Chemotherapy in Stage III and IV Ovarian Cancer

Huizing MT, van Warmerdam LJC, Rosing H, et al (Antoni van Leeuwenhoek Hosp/Netherlands Cancer Inst, Amsterdam; Academic Med Ctr; Slotevaart Hosp, Amsterdam; et al)

J Clin Oncol 15:1953–1964, 1997 18–8

Background.—Because of its reduced toxicity, carboplatin has recently been used instead of its parent, cisplatin, in chemotherapy for patients with ovarian cancer. Previous studies have shown that a combination of paclitaxel and cisplatin improved survival and prolonged the disease-free interval. But would these advantages remain for a combination of paclitaxel with carboplatin? The maximum tolerated dose, antitumor efficacy, and any drug-drug interactions for paclitaxel and carboplatin were examined in a phase I trial.

Methods.—Thirty-five patients less than 70 years old with stage II or IV ovarian cancer who had not been exposed to chemotherapy were enrolled. Paclitaxel (starting dose 125 mg/m^2) was given as a 3-hour infusion immediately followed by carboplatin (starting dose 300 mg/m^2) for 30 minutes. Each course of treatment lasted 4 weeks, with a planned series of 6 courses. Doses were increased until dose-limiting toxicity occurred. The tumor response was evaluated at the end of every second course. Those with normal serum CA 125 levels and complete resolution of measurable disease for at least 4 weeks were considered to have complete remission. A partial remission was defined as at least a 50% decrease in the sum of the products of the diameters of measurable lesions for at least 4 weeks. Blood samples for determining the pharmacokinetics of both drugs were drawn at regular intervals.

Findings.—Doses of paclitaxel and carboplatin ranged from 125 to 225 mg/m^2 and from 300 to 600 mg/m^2, respectively, over a total of 11 dose levels. Data from 214 courses of therapy were available for analysis. Neutropenia and thrombocytopenia developed and were more pronounced during later cycles at higher doses; this effect was cumulative. Neutropenic fever, thrombocytopenia requiring platelet transfusion, and neuropathy were causes of dose-limiting toxicity. A complete or partial response was seen in 26 of 33 assessable patients (78%). No drug-drug interactions between paclitaxel and carboplatin were observed.

Conclusions.—The maximum tolerated dose was paclitaxel, 200 mg/m^2 and carboplatin, 550 mg/m^2 every 4 weeks. At these doses, no dose reductions or treatment delays were needed because of neutropenia or anemia. Furthermore, the 2 drugs exhibited no drug-drug interactions. Future studies will examine the role of a 3-week dosing schedule.

▶ This study confirms the safety and efficacy of combining paclitaxel and carboplatin as initial chemotherapy for patients with advanced ovarian cancer. Previous studies by Bookman et al.[1] have demonstrated a similar result. However, these investigators had used carboplatin area under the curve (AUC) dosing instead of dosing carboplatin on body surface area. Several prospective randomized trials are currently in progress now comparing the combination of paclitaxel and carboplatin vs. paclitaxel and cisplatin as first-line chemotherapy for patients with advanced ovarian cancer. The prospective randomized trials all utilize AUC dosing for carboplatin. A widely accepted regimen for the treatment of ovarian cancer consists of paclitaxel at a dose of 175 mg/m^2 in a 3-hour infusion followed by carboplatin dosed to an AUC of 7.5, and this is a regimen that is being tested in a large Gynecologic Oncology Group trial in the United States.

R.F. Ozols, M.D., Ph.D.

Reference

1. Bookman MA, McGuire WP III, Kilpatrick D, et al: Carboplatin and paclitaxel in ovarian carcinoma: A phase I study of the Gynecologic Oncology Group. *J Clin Oncol* 14:1895–1902, 1996.

p53 Status Does Not Affect Sensitivity of Human Ovarian Cancer Cell Lines to Paclitaxel

Debernardis D, Siré EG, De Feudis P, et al (Istituto di Ricerche Farmacologiche "Mario Negri," Milan, Italy; Istituto Nazionale per la Ricerca sul Cancro, Genova, Italy)

Cancer Res 57:870–874, 1997 18–9

Background.—In some cell types, the blockade of mitosis by paclitaxel results in apoptosis. Another cause of apoptosis is an increased level of p53. And research has shown that cells with a disrupted wild-type p53 have increased sensitivity to paclitaxel compared to cells having wild-type p53. So is p53-induced apoptosis involved in the actions of paclitaxel? Paclitaxel-induced cytotoxicty in ovarian cell lines with differing p53 status was examined.

Methods.—Nine human ovarian cancer cell lines were selected as having wild-type p53 (n = 4) or having no or mutated p53 (n = 5). Also, a p53 null-cell line was transfected with a temperature-sensitive murine p53 or with a human wild-type p53 controlled by a tetracycline-dependent promotor (SKT4). Both cells treated with paclitaxel (after 6 or 24 hours of dosing) and those not treated underwent RNA extraction, fractionation, and blotting. Paclitaxel concentrations that inhibited growth by 50% (IC_{50}) were calculated after 72 hours of recovery in drug-free medium. Levels of the genes *p21/WAF1*, and *GADD45* mRNA, and *bax* were also measured, as these substances are directly activated by p53 (i.e., downstream genes). Apoptosis was evaluated as the amount of ^{14}C-labeled DNA present in the lysis fraction compared with total intracellular ^{14}C-labeled DNA.

Findings.—In all the cell lines except A2780 (which expressed wild-type p53), paclitaxel had comparable IC_{50} values. Furthermore, introducing a temperature-sensitive or tetracycline-dependent mutant p53 did not change the IC_{50} value. After 6 or 24 hours of paclitaxel, p53 levels increased in the cells expressing wild-type p53, whereas cells expressing no or mutant p53 had reduced or undetectable p53 levels. *WAF1* and *GADD45* mRNA expression was increased in most of the cell lines with wild-type p53, and *bax* expression was higher in 1 of these 4 cell lines. Conversely, no or only slight increases in these substances were seen in cells without p53. At concentrations close to the IC_{50}, paclitaxel caused no cell death.

Conclusions.—The presence or absence of p53 had no effect on paclitaxel sensitivity. This lack of effect held true even in the cells that showed increased expression of p53 downstream genes. Furthermore, paclitaxel caused no apoptosis. Thus, the p53 level is not a marker of paclitaxel-induced cytotoxicity in ovarian cancer.

▶ The mechanism by which paclitaxel exerts its antineoplastic effect is not completely established. It has been shown to cause polymerization of microtubules, which interferes with mitosis. In addition, there is some evidence that paclitaxel may exert an antiangiogenic effect. These novel mechanisms of action may account for the observation reported in this article that p53 status does not affect the sensitivity of human ovarian cell lines to paclitaxel. In most other tumor systems, it has been demonstrated that p53, by virtue of its effect on inducing apoptosis after exposure to DNA-damaging drugs, is a major determinant of chemosensitivity. In the absence of wild-type p53 or in the presence of p53 mutations, the apoptotic pathway may not be activated after exposure to cytotoxic agents and, consequently, tumor cells can continue to proliferate if their damage can be repaired.

R.F. Ozols, M.D., Ph.D.

Phase I and Pharmacologic Study of Paclitaxel Administered Weekly in Patients With Relapsed Ovarian Cancer

Fennelly D, Aghajanian C, Shapiro F, et al (Memorial Sloan-Kettering Cancer Ctr, New York)

J Clin Oncol 15:187–192, 1997 18–10

Introduction.—Paclitaxel has shown antitumor activity against both heavily and minimally pretreated advanced ovarian cancer. However, the optimal dose and schedule remain to be established. Fractionated, brief infusions of paclitaxel may be more effective than 24-hour infusion, recent in vitro studies suggest. A new schedule of weekly paclitaxel treatment using 1-hour infusions was evaluated in a phase I trial.

Methods.—The study included 18 patients, (mean age, 54 years) with recurrent ovarian cancer after paclitaxel and cisplatin therapy. The patients had received a median of 3 previous regimens of chemotherapy, and had been free of paclitaxel for a mean of 10 months. All patients were put on a weekly, 1-hour infusion paclitaxel regimen in which the dose was escalated from 40 to 50 to 60 to 80 to 100 mg/m^2. Standard premedication was used in all patients.

Results.—The evaluation included 194 weekly cycles of paclitaxel, for a mean of 10 per patient. None of the patients had mucositis or grade III neuropathy; 1 had alopecia. The mean low point of neutrophil count was 4.0×10^9/L. At the 100 mg/m^2 dose, 90.75% of the planned dose intensity was actually delivered, more than double the standard dose intensity.

Four of 13 assessable patients had partial responses, a rate of 30%. This included 2 patients who had had disease progression with the standard 3-week paclitaxel schedule. There was a significant correlation between increasing paclitaxel dose and the measured area under the curve. The maximal, 100 mg/m^2 dose caused dose-limiting toxic effects, causing a delay in treatment in 2 of 3 patients. Thus, the maximum tolerated dose on a weekly paclitaxel regimen in heavily pretreated patients was 80 mg/m^2.

Conclusions.—This phase I trial shows that a weekly, 1-hour infusion schedule of paclitaxel is well tolerated. This new regimen does not cause cumulative myelosuppression, and may permit a more intensive dosage of paclitaxel. The results in a heavily pretreated group of patients are encouraging. Weekly paclitaxel may be a useful part of future combination chemotherapy regimens.

▶ Paclitaxel is an active agent in a wide variety of malignancies, including ovarian cancer, lung cancer, and breast cancer. Many questions, however, still remain regarding how best to use this agent, including what the optimal dose and schedule are. In this study, paclitaxel was administered weekly in patients who had received prior therapy with paclitaxel on a more traditional schedule, every 3 to 4 weeks. Partial responses were observed in 30% of the patients. It was of particular interest that paclitaxel administered as a 1-hour weekly infusion was very well tolerated without any evidence of cumulative myelosuppression. Furthermore, there were responses observed in patients with progression of disease on standard 3-week paclitaxel schedules when they were switched to a weekly schedule. These studies suggest that this form of therapy deserves further evaluation not only for ovarian cancer but for any other solid tumors in which paclitaxel has marked clinical activity.

R.F. Ozols, M.D., Ph.D.

19 Novel Therapy

Modulation of Cancer Chemotherapy by Green Tea
Sadzuka Y, Sugiyama T, Hirota S (Univ of Shizuoka, Japan)
Clin Cancer Res 4:153–156, 1998 19–1

Background.—Biochemical modulation in cancer chemotherapy has been studied extensively. The effects of green tea and its components on the antitumor activity of doxorubicin were investigated in the current study.

Methods and Findings.—The combination of green tea and doxorubicin on Ehrlich ascites tumor-bearing mice was assessed, along with the effects of the green tea components theanine and caffeine, which are known to enhance the activity of antitumor agents. The combination increased the doxorubicin concentration in the tumor. By contrast, there was no increase in doxorubicin concentration in normal tissue after the green tea combination was given. The tea-induced enhancement of doxorubicin's antitumor activity was also noted in M5076 ovarian sarcoma, which has low sensitivity to doxorubicin.

Conclusions.—Drinking green tea appears to enhance the efficacy of chemotherapy. This effect may help improve the quality of life of patients with cancer.

► Green tea is an important part of oriental culture with psychological and physiologic attributes. Laboratory studies have identified that green tea contains an ingredient that is also effective for the chemoprevention of cancer. This current study demonstrates that green tea may also be a biochemical modulator of anti-cancer activity of the commonly used drug, doxorubicin. Can it be that we actually have an agent that can increase the quality of life of a cancer patient while at the same time increasing the effectiveness of chemotherapy? Almost sounds too good to be true.

R.F. Ozols, M.D., Ph.D.

Clinicians' Attitudes to Clinical Trials of Cancer Therapy

Fallowfield L, Ratcliffe D, Souhami R (Univ College London)

Eur J Cancer 33:2221–2229, 1997 19–2

Introduction.—Accrual of patients in clinical trials of cancer therapy is low despite many patients' eligibility to participate. The primary reason for poor recruitment of patients has been cited as doctor-related variables. There has been no systematic study of the different attitudes and trial behaviors of clinicians who work with cancer patients in Britain. A survey of oncologists was conducted to determine their attitude toward cancer trials, and these attitudes were compared to those of US oncologists who were previously surveyed.

Methods.—Five hundred fifty-three clinical radiation, medical, and surgical oncologists were mailed a 45-item questionnaire about their attitudes toward trial participation. There was a 65% response rate of 357 clinicians. The questionnaire included such items as the importance of increasing survival vs. the importance of improving the quality of patients' lives; how the clinician reacts if the patient refuses to participate in a trial; level of pressure from the hospital to participate in a trial; reasons for patient referral; and time devoted to publications, lectures, and research compared to time devoted to clinical work.

TABLE 2.—Stepwise Discriminant Function. Items Which Loaded Above 0.3 Are Listed. Function 1. Medical vs. Clinical + Surgical Oncologists

	Medical	Clinical	Surgical
q29 I spend the following amount of my time in research-related activities:			
(a) less than one-third	30%	88%	85%
(b) one-third or more	70%	12%	15%
q13 The time I devote to publications, lectures and research commitments, compared to clinical work is relatively:			
(a) low	37.5%	88%	77%
(b) high	62.5%	12%	23%
q38 In the past 3 years, I have authored-coauthored:			
(a) 0 publications			
(b) 1–5 publications	16%	66%	58.5%
(c) 6–9 publications	84%	34%	41.5%
(d) 10 or more publications			
q8 Currently, I am the principal investigator on one or more research grants:			
(a) no	20%	66%	69%
(b) yes	80%	34%	31%
q12 I participate more actively in professional organisations that are based on:			
(a) my clinical speciality	46%	82%	88%
(b) my research activities	54%	18%	12%
q28 It is more important for me to be well-known among:			
(a) local colleagues	55%	81%	74%
(b) national/international colleagues	45%	19%	26%

(Courtesy of Fallowfield L, Ratcliffe D, Souhami R: Clinicians' attitudes to clinical trials of cancer therapy. *Eur J Cancer* 33:2221–2229, 1997. Copyright 1997 kind permission from Elsevier Science Ltd., The Boulevard, Langford Lane, Kidlington OXS IGB, UK.)

TABLE 3.—Function 2. Surgeons Significantly Different to Clinical and Medical Oncologists on the Following Items

	Surgical	Clinical	Medical
q9 In my hospital setting, doctors are given more reward for:			
(a) clinical skills with patients	84%	62%	63%
(b) contributing to scientific knowledge	16%	38%	37%
q10 When a patient on a protocol relapses or progresses and the protocol dictates additional treatment that the patient does not want, I:			
(a) encourage the patient to stay on the trial	34%	15%	5%
(b) remove the patient from the trial	66%	85%	95%
q30 A major reason for my participation in randomised clinical trials is that it benefits my institution:			
(a) agree	29%	48%	46%
(b) disagree	71%	52%	54%
q45 When there is controversy in the literature as to which treatment is best:			
(a) I enter the patient in a clinical trial if one exists	76%	90%	91%
(b) I personally select a treatment for the patient	24%	10%	9%

(Fallowfield L, Ratcliffe D, Souhami R: Clinicians' attitudes to clinical trials of cancer therapy. *Eur J Cancer* 33:2221–2229, 1997. Copyright 1997 with kind permission from Elsevier Science Ltd., The Boulevard, Langford Lane, Kidlington OX5 1GB, UK.)

Results.—Trial participation was seen in 353 respondents (99%), but 269 of the clinicians (75%) entered fewer than 50% of eligible patients. The clinicians were participating in a median of 3 trials. Within oncology, differences were seen among professional groups. More emphasis on research than on clinical activities was placed by medical oncologists who also were more likely to value being known by national and international colleagues, and who felt greater pressure to participate in trials than did radiation oncologists or surgeons (Table 2). Surgeons were more likely to keep patients on study following relapse, and were more likely to rely on clinical experience rather than to enter patients into a trial (Table 3).

Conclusion.—Communication difficulties, conflicts between the roles of clinician and scientist, were cited as constraints, imposed by the healthcare system, which impeded trial participation. When trials are designed, these factors should be considered. There were broad similarities between British and US data. Encouraged recruitment and a greater commitment to keep patients on trials may be seen in the more protocol-driven culture of the United States.

▶ Clinical trials play an important role in the treatment armentarium of oncologists. Unfortunately, it is estimated that less than 5% of all eligible patients with cancer are entered upon clinical trials in this country. The obstacles are many and varied. This is a very interesting article which helps to define these obstacles and characterizes the differences between surgical and medical oncologists in this country and in Great Britain. Data from this article may help us to overcome some of the obstacles for the betterment of patient care.

P.J. Loehrer, Sr., M.D.

A Phase I Study of TNP-470 Administered to Patients With Advanced Squamous Cell Cancer of the Cervix

Kudelka AP, Levy T, Verschraegen CF, et al (Univ of Texas, Houston; Baylor College of Medicine, Houston; Mahidol Univ, Bangkok, Thailand; et al)

Clin Cancer Res 3:1501–1505, 1997 19–3

Objective.—TNP-470 is a less toxic synthetic analogue of the angiogenesis inhibitor fumagillin. In a phase I study, the effect of TNP-470 was tested in patients with advanced and recurring squamous cell cancer of the cervix.

Methods.—Twenty-one women aged 27–55 years, with recurrent or metastatic cervical cancer, were given TNP-470 in an IV infusion of 9.3 mg/m^2 over 60 minutes every other day for 28 days followed by a 14-day rest period. The dose was escalated at 50% increments until biological activity was observed and then at 25% increments. Patients whose disease stabilized or responded received at least 2 treatment cycles. Treatment was discontinued for intolerable toxicity, disease progression, or at the patient's request. Toxicity was evaluated.

Results.—Three patients did not complete the study, 1 because of disease progression, and 2 because of intolerable toxicity. The 18 assessable patients had a median Zubrod performance status of 1 (range 0–2). Grade 3 neurologic toxicity was reached at a dose of 71.2 mg/m^2. At this level, patients had weakness, vertigo, nystagmus, diplopia, dysmetria, and truncal ataxia. Two patients experienced cognitive impairment. Three patients tolerated a dose of 60 mg/m^2 well. Gastrointestinal toxicity included grade 1 and 2 nausea, grade 1 diarrhea, and grade 1 and 2 stomatitis. One patient had grade 3 nausea. Other side effects included skin rash, itching, and grade 1 and 2 fever. There was no myelosuppression, retinal hemorrhage, weight loss, or significant alopecia. Three patients had stabilized disease, and 1 had a complete response.

Conclusion.—An IV infusion of TNP-470 at 60 mg/m^2 over 60 minutes every other day was well tolerated. A dose of 60 mg/m^2 3 times a week will be used for phase II studies. Neurologic toxicity was dose-limiting, dose-related, and apparently reversible. There was 1 complete response, and disease stabilized in 3 patients.

▶ Inhibition of angiogenesis is an important new strategy in the management of a variety of malignancies. In many solid tumors, multimodality therapy is highly effective in achieving a complete remission. Unfortunately, a majority of patients with solid tumors who achieve a complete remission ultimately have a recurrence. Recurrent disease for solid tumors is usually not associated with a significant cure rate. The development of an active angiogenesis inhibitor can potentially lead to a new paradigm of treatment in which patients would be treated with standard modalities of treatment to decrease their tumor burdens followed by perhaps life-long maintenance therapy with an inhibitor of angiogenesis, which would prevent tumor regrowth to a symptomatic situation. Consequently, oncologists perhaps should be treating metastatic cancer more as a chronic disease that can be controlled instead of as a disease in which the only hope for long-term survival rests in complete tumor eradication. TNP-470 is among the first angiogenesis inhibitors to undergo clinical trial. This phase I study demonstrated that neurotoxicity was dose-limiting, which may be a problem if the chronic model of treatment is found to be useful. However, a phase II study with this agent is currently in progress for patients with squamous cell cancer of the cervix and a better definition of this toxicity will soon be available.

R.F. Ozols, M.D., Ph.D.

Phase I Study of Continuous-infusion L-*S,R*-Buthionine Sulfoximine With Intravenous Melphalan

Bailey HH, Ripple G, Tutsch KD, et al (Univ of Wisconsin, Madison)
J Natl Cancer Inst 89:1789–1796, 1997 19–4

Objective.—Increased intracellular glutathione is associated with resistance to irradiation and chemotherapy. L-*S,R*-buthionine sulfoximine (BSO), an inhibitor of glutathione biosynthesis, has been shown to reduce drug resistance in tumor cells that overexpress glutathione. The effect on the clinical effectiveness of melphalan (L-PAM) of continuous infusion of BSO was examined in a phase I study.

Methods.—A 30-minute infusion of BSO at 3.0 g/m^2 followed by a continuous infusion lasting 24–72 hours was administered to 4 patients with advanced cancer at 0.75 g/m^2 for 24 hours, to 4 patients at 0.75 g/m^2 for 48 hours, to 10 patients at 0.75 g/m^2 for 72 hours, and to 3 patients at 1.5 g/m^2 for 48 hours during week 1. Patients received BSO plus melphalan (15 mg/m^2 during weeks 2 and 3, and then BSO plus melphalan every 4 weeks. Glutathione levels in peripheral mononuclear cells, serum BSO levels, and glutathione levels in tumor biopsy specimens were determined.

Results.—Buthionine sulfoximine infusion resulted in minimal toxicity. Buthionine sulfoximine plus L-PAM resulted in myelosuppression in most patients that was severe in some patients and frequent nausea and vomiting. Peripheral blood lymphocyte glutathione levels were 30% to 40% of control levels. Tumor glutathione levels showed consistent and marked depletion to less than 10% of baseline values.

Conclusion.—Continuous infusion of BSO results in marked depletion of tumor glutathione levels and minimal toxicity.

► Tumor cell resistance is multifactorial. Individual mechanisms have been identified in well-defined in vitro systems after exposure to specific antineoplastic agents. Glutathione (GSH) is a ubiquitous tripeptide that has been shown to be markedly elevated in tumor cells with resistance to alkylating agents and platinum compounds. Glutathione may protect tumor cells by several mechanisms. It has been shown in the past to protect tumor cells by detoxifying chemotherapeutic agents, such as melphalan, via conjugation reactions catalyzed by GSH S-transferase. In addition, GSH may quench drug DNA adducts and also decrease intracellular drug accumulation through the GS-X pump or the multidrug resistance-related protein. Buthionine sulfoximine increases the cytotoxicity of chemotherapeutic agents in vitro and in vivo by inhibiting GSH biosynthesis. On the basis of the study reported here, as well as previous phase I trials, BSO is being studied together with IV melphalan in phase II trials in patients with resistant ovarian cancer. Pharmacologic studies already have demonstrated that GSH levels can be reduced in tumor cells by BSO. Whether or not this leads to significant potentiation clinically of alkylating agents remains to be determined in the ongoing phase II trials.

R.F. Ozols, M.D., Ph.D.

Phase I Clinical and Pharmacokinetic Study of Oral Carboxyamidotriazole, a Signal Transduction Inhibitor

Berlin J, Tutsch KD, Hutson P, et al (Univ of Wisconsin, Madison)

J Clin Oncol 15:781–789, 1997 19–5

Background.—Carboxyamidotriazole (CAI) is a signal transduction inhibitor being evaluated as a treatment for neoplastic diseases. It inhibits calcium influx and possibly angiogenesis, with cytostatic rather than cytotoxic effects. The dosing, pharmacokinetic, and toxicity parameters of an oral gelcap form of CAI were examined in a phase I trial.

Methods.—Carboxyamidotriazole (50 mg/m^2) was given to 29 patients with histologically proven malignancy for 28-day courses. Chemotherapy or radiation or combined treatments had been stopped for at least 4 weeks, and calcium-channel blockers, glucocorticoids, and nonsteroidal anti-inflammatory drugs had been stopped for at least 2 weeks (to avoid interactions with CAI). A standard phase I trial design was followed, and doses were increased until the disease progressed or dose-limiting toxicity occurred. Blood samples were drawn for characterizing the drug plasma pharmacokinetics, and high-performance liquid chromatography was used to assess CAI and its metabolites.

Findings.—The 29 patients completed 84 full 28-day cycles of CAI therapy. Ultimately, 3 doses of CAI were used (50, 75, and 100 mg/m^2), but all 3 patients taking the highest dose had cerebellar neurotoxicity that resolved after the discontinuation of CAI. At all doses, most (23 of 29) reported mild nausea or vomiting or both and almost two thirds reported mild to moderate fatigue; in 6 and 5 patients, respectively, the symptoms resolved when the CAI was switched to nighttime dosing. Plasma concentrations peaked at 2.4 ± 1.5 hours after administration and weekly measurements varied an average of 12.4% ± 5.3%. Trough steady-state concentrations were reached by days 8–15 and remained relatively constant. Progressive disease occurred in 22 patients, 5 refused to continue therapy, and 1 each had neurocortical toxicity or bradycardia unrelated to therapy.

Conclusions.—Carboxyamidotriazole in a gelcap formulation was generally well tolerated, with a maximum tolerated dose of 75 mg/m². Gastrointestinal side effects and fatigue were common but resolved in some patients with nighttime dosing. The pharmacokinetics of CAI were linear and steady-state levels remained relatively constant.

► Carboxyamidotriazole (CAI) was shown in preclinical studies to inhibit tumor proliferation, invasion, and metastases. The agent's ability to modulate calcium-mediated signal transduction leads to inhibition of angiogenesis. It also produces expression of matrix metalloproteinase-2, thereby inhibiting the metastatic cascade. These interesting bichemical effects of CAI have led to phase I trials. Ultimately, such agents will have to be combined with cytotoxic drugs to produce a new paradigm of treatment. Cytotoxic agents perhaps will be used to induce remissions and then agents such as CAI will be used as secondary preventive agents to prevent regrowth and metastases of any residual disease.

R.F. Ozols, M.D., Ph.D.

Phase I Trial and Pharmacologic Trial of Sequences of Paclitaxel and Topotecan in Previously Treated Ovarian Epithelial Malignancies: A Gynecologic Oncology Group Study

O'Reilly S, Fleming GF, Baker SD, et al (Johns Hopkins Oncology Ctr, Baltimore, Md; Univ of Chicago; Fox Chase Cancer Ctr, Philadelphia; et al)

J Clin Oncol 15:177–186, 1997 19–6

Background.—Topotecan given alone or combined with other active agents may be beneficial in patients with ovarian carcinoma, either as a salvage treatment or possibly in earlier stages. In this phase I study, paclitaxel was combined with topotecan with and without granulocyte colony-stimulating factor (G-CSF) in women with recurrent or refractory ovarian cancer.

Methods.—Twenty-two patients were treated. Topotecan was given as a 30-minute infusion daily for 5 days, and paclitaxel as a 24-hour infusion either before topotecan on day 1 or after topotecan on day 5. Every patient received both schedules on an alternating basis every 3 weeks. A total of 109 courses of treatment were administered.

Findings.—Dose-limiting myelosuppression consistently occurred at the first topotecan/paclitaxel dose level of 0.75/135 mg/m², without G-CSF support. Adding G-CSF resulted in decreased rates of complicated neutropenia. However, the incidences of dose-limiting neutropenia and thrombocytopenia were unacceptably high after doses of topotecan or paclitaxel were raised. Hematologic toxicities were similar for the 2 sequences of drug administration. Drug sequencing did not affect the pharmacologic behavior of either agent. Forty percent of the patients with measurable, evaluable disease had major antitumor responses, including 45% and 9%

of patients with potentially cisplatin-sensitive and resistant tumors, respectively.

Conclusion.—Topotecan, 0.75 mg/m^2, on a daily times 5 schedule, combined with paclitaxel, 135 mg/m^2, given as a 24-hour infusion with C-CSF support is recommended for this patient population. Further research on this regimen in women with refractory or recurrent ovarian cancer is needed before the regimen can be recommended for previously treated patients in this setting.

► Paclitaxel and topotecan have both been shown to be active agents in the treatment of patients with ovarian cancer. They have markedly different mechanisms of action and, consequently, are a logical combination for evaluation in the initial chemotherapeutic regimens of untreated patients with advanced disease. This study demonstrates the difficulties, at times, in combining chemotherapies. These drugs have overlapping toxicities and, consequently, major dose reductions are required to produce a combination with acceptable toxicity, even with G-CSF support. In the future, clinical trials may require using regimens of these agents that are less myelosuppressive, such as a 3-hour infusion of paclitaxel instead of a 24-hour infusion. Alternatively, sequential treatment of either single agents or doublets may be necessary to produce acceptable toxicity.

R.F. Ozols, M.D., Ph.D.

Recombinant Methionyl Human Stem Cell Factor and Filgrastim for Peripheral Blood Progenitor Cell Mobilization and Transplantation in Non-Hodgkin's Lymphoma Patients: Results of a Phase I/II Trial

Moskowitz CH, Stiff P, Gordon MS, et al (Mem Sloan Kettering Cancer Ctr, New York; Loyola Univ, Maywood, Ill; Indiana Univ, Indianapolis; et al)

Blood 89:3136–3147, 1997 19–7

Introduction.—In patients undergoing peripheral blood progenitor cell (PBPC) transplantation, cells are more efficiently collected and engraftment occurs more rapidly if the PBPCs are mobilized. This may be achieved by a number of different methods; however, it remains to be determined which approach is most effective. The combination of recombinant-methionyl human stem cell factor (r-metHuSCF) and filgrastim was evaluated for safety and efficacy in PBPC mobilization.

Methods.—The randomized trial included 38 patients with intermediate-grade or immunoblastic high-grade non-Hodgkin's lymphoma. They were assigned to receive the combination of r-metHuSCF (5, 10, 15, or 20 µg/kg/day) and filgrastim (10 µg/kg/day) or filgrastim alone for PBPC mobilization before autologous transplantation. The quality and quantity of PBPCs collected were analyzed, together with their ability to promote engraftment after myeloablative therapy.

Results.—Given with a multiagent premedication protocol, the subcutaneous r-metHuSCF injections were well tolerated. The most frequent associated problems were local injection site reactions. The 2 approaches gave similar results in terms of total mononuclear cell count, CD34+ cell content, granulocyte-macrophage colony-forming cells (GM-CFCs), and burst-forming units–erythroid (BFU-Es) per kilogram in the apheresis product. However, significant differences appeared when previous chemotherapy was taken into account. A group of patients receiving extensive prior therapy was identified, i.e., those receiving 2 or more cycles of the stem cell toxic agents procarbazine, nitrogen mustard, melphalan, or nitrosoureas, or more than 7.5 g of cytosine arabinoside. Eighteen such patients received r-metHuSCF plus filgrastim and 5 received filgrastim alone. Patients in the combination group had more CD34+ cells (1.76 vs. 0.28 $\times$ 10^6/kg; more GM-CFCs (20.5 vs. 5.0 $\times$ 10^4/kg; and more BFU-Es (36.9 vs. 8.9 $\times$ 10^4/kg. Times to reach an untransfused platelet count of 20 $\times$ 10^9/L were 12.5 and 23.0 days, respectively. The differences were not statistically significant but were thought to be clinically relevant.

Conclusion.—In hematopoietic progenitor cell mobilization, the combination of r-metHuSCF and filgrastim is safe and effective. For patients with a history of extensive previous therapy, the combination approach appears to be superior to filgrastim alone. A growing number of patients at risk for poor PBPC mobilization will be seen as treatment dose intensities increase. The authors plan further prospective studies of r-metHuSCF plus filgrastim in extensively pretreated patients with non-Hodgkin's lymphoma, Hodgkin's disease, or multiple myeloma.

► Evaluation of new cytokines is important for patients undergoing high-dose chemotherapy with autologous stem cell transplantation. This prospective, randomized trial is one of the first to evaluate r-metHuSCF for mobilization. Among patients with extensive prior exposure to cytotoxic agents, those receiving a combination of r-metHuSCF and filgrastim had an increased number of CD34+ cells compared with patients receiving filgrastim alone. In addition, these patients had a decreased time to platelet independence. These observations become more important as more patients who have been previously exposed to potentially stem cell–damaging cytotoxic chemotherapy undergo this intensive approach.

M.S. Tallman, M.D.

Radioimmunoguided Surgery for Colorectal Cancer

Manayan RC, Hart MJ, Friend WG (Swedish Hosp Med Ctr, Seattle)

Am J Surg 173:386–389, 1997 19–8

Introduction.—Radioimmunoguided surgery (RIGS) provides surgeons with intraoperative localization of occult malignancy. Preliminary trials with the monoclonal antibody (mAb) B72.3 have shown 82% localization of antibody in patients with recurrent colorectal cancer. Even more promising results have been observed with mAb CC49. The safety and efficacy of the ^{125}I-radiolabeled anti-TAG mAb CC49 as a component of RIGS was assessed in a phase III multiinstitutional trial.

Methods.—Twenty-eight patients with either primary or recurrent colorectal cancer underwent injection of mAb CC49 labeled with ^{125}I. A hand-held gamma-detecting probe was used during the procedure to detect radiolabeled antibody. During surgery, patients underwent both traditional and RIGS explorations.

Results.—Radiolabeled antibody was detected by RIGS in 73% of patients (14 of 19) with primary colorectal cancer and 100% of patients (7 of 7) with recurrent disease. Using RIGS findings, 26% of patients (5 of 19) with primary cancer were upstaged from stage I/II to III/IV.

Conclusions.—Data from this phase III trial indicate that ^{125}I CC49 with RIGS is safe and gives immediate, useful information not currently available using traditional methods. This approach can be used to determine disease stage so that therapeutic management can be optimized.

▶ This paper from the group in Seattle presents a clinical evaluation of the potential usefulness of RIGS surgery utilizing the CC49 monoclonal antibody. As has been noted in other patient series using the RIGS technology, approximately 25% of patients had their disease upstaged unexpectedly because of positive intraoperative findings of detectable radiolabeled antibody. This technology and its enhancement and clinical evaluation has the potential of providing the surgeon with more accurate intraoperative staging of disease and affecting decision making relative to radical resection. This may be evident in a surgical decision not to perform a hepatic metastasectomy because of a RIGS-positive portal lymph node, or it may enhance nodal clearing and subsequent completeness of surgical resection in a primary colorectal surgical procedure. Additionally, RIGS appears to be very sensitive in detecting micrometastatic disease in nodal areas within the upper abdomen (celiac axis, porta hepatis, upper periaortic area). This is an anatomical area where surgical exploration is problematic by traditional evaluation. As the technology of RIGS improves and as tagged monoclonal antibodies become more specific with more efficient clearing through the systemic circulation, this procedure has the potential to enhance the surgical evaluation and staging of gastrointestinal cancers.

B.L. Eisenberg, M.D.

Photodynamic Therapy as Adjuvant Therapy in Surgically Treated Pleural Malignancies

Baas P, Murrer L, Zoetmulder FAN, et al (Netherlands Cancer Inst, Amsterdam; Dr Daniel Den Hoed Cancer Centre, Rotterdam, The Netherlands; Inselspital, Berne, Switzerland)

Br J Cancer 76:819–826, 1997 19–9

Purpose.—Malignant mesothelioma and other pleural malignancies are usually regarded as incurable at diagnosis. Although radical resection may achieve apparently complete removal of tumor cells, cells are still seen on microscopic examination. Adjuvant radiation therapy has failed to improve survival. The use of intraoperative adjuvant photodynamic therapy (PDT) for patients with pleural malignancies was reported.

Methods.—The study included 5 patients, 4 with malignant mesothelioma and 1 with a localized, low-grade carcinoid. After the tumor had been resected as much as possible, intraoperative adjuvant PDT was performed using meta-tetrahydroxyphenylchlorin as the photosensitizer and 652 nm light supplied by a high-power diode laser. In situ isotropic light detectors were used to monitor light delivered to the thoracic cavity, with adjustment to achieve the maximal distribution of light.

Results.—In the 30 days after surgery, there were no deaths. There was 1 major complication (diaphragmatic rupture with hematopericardium). Adjuvant PDT increased operative time by no more than 1 hour. The hemithoracic surface was illuminated with 10 J cm^{-2} light, including incident and scattered light. Thorascopic biopsy specimens obtained the day after surgery showed necrosis and other damage of marker lesions with remaining malignancy. In contrast, normal tissue showed only polymorphonuclear cell infiltration and striated muscle edema. At 9 to 11 months' follow-up, 4 patients were alive with no sign of tumor recurrence. In the other patient, tumor dissemination developed around the thoracoscopy scar, and the patient died of abdominal tumor spread.

Conclusion.—Promising results are reported with adjuvant intraoperative PDT in patients with malignant pleural tumors. The study shows the feasibility of delivering light over large surfaces during surgery in a relatively short time. With in situ dosimetry, optimal light distribution is ensured and total light dose can be monitored from different points within the thoracic cavity. The authors are planning dose escalation and phase II trials of adjuvant PDT for pleural malignancies.

▶ I like this paper very much because it shows how a new kind of treatment can be used for specific problems when the current results of treatment remain poor. These investigators from Holland have treated 5 patients with pleural-based malignancies with intraoperative PDT used as an adjuvant after maximal surgical ablation. We know that surgery alone for these problems gives poor results, and we also know that postoperative radiation adds little, if anything. The role of chemotherapy is still somewhat obscure. Thus, what phototherapy can contribute is not clear, but the authors describe a detailed approach to applying PDT to the pleural surface, and I believe that this is the kind of approach that needs to be taken.

Exactly what it can do remains unclear, but the point I would emphasize is that these patients do not really have good alternatives. This is important investigational work because it attempts to use phototherapy in a way that, up to now, has not been done. Up to now, the phototherapy has been used almost entirely for skin problems and for mucous membranes that can be invaded endoscopically. I think that serosal-based tumors can be approached by phototherapy, and they may turn out to be the most important use for this kind of treatment. Reading this paper is worthy of your time.

E. Glatstein, M.D.

20 Complications of Therapy

Osteoporosis After Orchiectomy for Prostate Cancer

Daniell HW (Univ of California, Redding)

J Urol 157:439–444, 1997 20–1

Introduction.—Up to 20% of men with spinal osteoporosis have hypogonadism. Osteoporosis after castration for prostate cancer is not usually recognized in the literature. The possibility of increased osteoporosis and osteoporotic fractures after therapeutic orchiectomy was assessed in men with nonstage A prostate cancer diagnosed between 1983 and 1990.

Methods.—Hospital records of 235 men were analyzed for therapeutic orchiectomy, other osteoporotic risk fractures, and hospital treatment for vertebral and femoral fractures. The 17 castrated men still alive in 1995 were interviewed and results of femoral neck bone mineral density were compared with those of 23 controls of similar age.

Results.—Castrated men more frequently had advanced disease, tumors with a high Gleason grade, osteoporotic fractures, a history of heavy smoking, testicular atrophy, and slender habitus. The increased incidence of fractures in men with orchiectomy was independent of smoking habits, obesity, age, and degree of testicular atrophy. Ten of 235 men had osteoporotic fractures: 8 of 59 men treated with orchiectomy and 2 of 176 not treated with orchiectomy Fractures among men treated by orchiectomy were significantly higher than among those who were not (13.6% vs. 1.1%). Osteoporotic fractures occurred more frequently than pathologic fractures or traumatic fractures. The average bone mineral density was 0.91 gm/cm^2 in 9 controls without prostate cancer, 0.84 gm/cm^2 in 14 men with prostate cancer before orchiectomy, 0.79 gm/cm^2 in 9 men 8–60 months after orchiectomy, and 0.66 gm/cm^2 in 8 men at 60–115 months after orchiectomy. Of 16 men alive longer than 60 months after orchiectomy 6 had osteoporotic fractures, 5 of 6 had bone mineral density of less than 0.70 gm/cm^2, and 5 of 7 had bone mineral density of less than 75% of normal for their age.

Conclusion.—Men who undergo orchiectomy for prostate cancer frequently experience severe osteoporosis, particularly those whose bone mineral content was depleted before castration. Determination of bone mineral density is recommended before onset of androgen ablation and at periodic intervals thereafter.

► In women, osteoporosis is a well-documented and well-recognized complication after menopause. This trial provides provocative evidence that osteoporosis associated with hypogonadism is not gender specific. In men who have undergone orchiectomy, the incidence of osteoporotic fractures was greater than that of pathologic fractures. Use of hormonal therapy in early stages of prostate cancer may prolong survival but also may select for an increased risk of osteoporosis. Recognition of this should be considered for preventive measures and treatment of nonmalignant osseous disorders.

P.J. Loehrer, Sr., M.D.

Fusarium, a Significant Emerging Pathogen in Patients With Hematologic Malignancy: Ten Years' Experience at a Cancer Center and Implications for Management

Boutati EI, Anaissie EJ (Univ of Texas, Houston)

Blood 90:999–1008, 1997 20–2

Objective.—*Fusarium* is emerging worldwide as an increasingly common cause of fatal fungal infection that frequently mimics aspergillosis. A retrospective study of 43 patients with hematologic cancer and invasive *Fusarium* infection and a literature review of the pathogenesis, prevention, and treatment of *Fusarium* infection were presented.

Methods.—Between January 1986 and December 1995, 43 patients (19 females), aged 14 to 78 years, with hematologic cancer and invasive (n = 3) or disseminated (n = 40) *Fusarium* infection were treated at M.D. Anderson Cancer Center in Houston. Another 54 patients with fusarial infection and hematologic cancer were found by searching MEDLINE and CANCERLIT databases between 1976 and 1995.

Results.—Thirty of the 43 M.D. Anderson patients had acute leukemia. All were immunocompromised. Most had persistent fever. Eleven had sinusitis, 6 had skin lesions, 6 had pneumonia, 3 had myalgia, and 1 had hemoptysis and altered mental status. Infection was present in the bloodstream of 18 patients and in the nails of 5. There were 39 patients with skin lesions, and 18 of those had positive blood cultures. Three of 12 patients who underwent bone marrow transplantation had infection before engraftment. All 43 patients received antifungal therapy; 13 responded and 30 died. Responders tended to be in remission and have sufficient circulating neutrophils and no graft-versus-host disease. Of the 54 patients whose cases were reported in the literature, most had acute leukemia and neutropenia and were immunocompromised. The ports of entry in most patients were the skin or respiratory tract. Infection was documented in the bloodstream in 56% and in skin lesions in 72%. There were 26 patients who responded to therapy. All responders had resolving myelosuppression.

Conclusion.—Patients with hematologic cancer are at increased risk of fatal fusarial infection. Modes of infection included skin and respiratory pathways. Most patients do not respond to standard antifungal therapy; new agents need to be developed. Immunocompromised patients have a very poor prognosis.

▶ This very well-written paper describes a common opportunistic pathogen which is increasing in incidence. *Fusarium* has been reported in a few dozen patients to date and is a highly lethal disease. Although infections may mimic aspergillosis, there are notable differences. Patients with these infections are often seen with persistent fever, which is refractory to antibacterial antifungal therapy, and they may have sinusitis, painful skin lesions, and/or pneumonia. Pulmonary involvement is seen in the vast majority of patients, manifested as either nonspecific infiltrates or nodular lesions. In addition, over 90% of the patients are seen with skin lesions. These infections are highly resistant to the typical antifungal agents.

Boutati et al. suggest that lipid-soluble amphotericin B, granulocyte colony-stimulating factor plus granulocyte transfusions, as well as surgical debridement to affected areas, may provide the best opportunity for successful treatment. This is an entity that should be considered in all patients who are immunocompromised and have a fever not responding to initial antibiotic treatment.

P.J. Loehrer, Sr., M.D.

Nocardiosis After Bone Marrow Transplantation: A Retrospective Study

van Burik J-A, Hackman RC, Nadeem SQ, et al (Univ of Washington, Seattle; Univ of South Florida, Tampa; Mem Sloan-Kettering Cancer Ctr, New York)

Clin Infect Dis 24:1154–1160, 1997 20–3

Background.—Nocardiosis is a rare infection that can occur opportunistically after bone marrow transplantation. The medical records of marrow recipients with positive cultures or diagnoses of nocardiosis were reviewed to determine the incidence after marrow transplantation.

Study Design.—Records of patients with nocardiosis were obtained from the Fred Hutchinson Cancer Research Center in Seattle, the H. Lee Moffitt Cancer Center in Tampa, and the Memorial Sloan-Kettering Cancer Center in New York. Three cases derived from the literature were also reviewed.

Findings.—The patients were predominantly male and older than 18 years. The median time to diagnosis after transplantation was 210 days. *Nocardia asteroides* complex was detected in 96% of isolates. There were 25 invasive infections in this series and all occurred in allogeneic marrow recipients. Ten of these patients were receiving sulfamethoxazole prophylaxis. Treatment included sulfonamides plus synergistic agents. Survival from the infection was 84%. The overall 6-year survival was 34%. The incidence of nocardiosis among allogeneic bone marrow recipients was 0.3% over 25 years.

Conclusions.—This review of a large series of patients receiving bone marrow transplantation patients over a 25-year period indicated that nocardiosis is a relatively rare infection. It can occur long after the transplantation, even when patients are receiving trimethoprin-sulfamethoxazole prophylaxis. Therapy consists of sulfonamide plus synergistic agents. The outcome is favorable, but long-term survival is slightly decreased in marrow recipients with nocardiosis.

► Patients undergoing bone marrow transplantation are susceptible to infections, particularly opportunistic infections. Although infrequent, nocardial infections do occur but have been rarely analyzed in this setting in a systematic way. Therefore, this retrospective report of 25 patients who had invasive nocardial infections is important. The majority of patients (84%) survived the infection and although the treatment often includes sulfonamides, 40% of patients who had nocardiosis were already receiving double-strength oral trimethoprim-sulfamethoxazole as prophylaxis for *Pneumocystis carinii* pneumonia. Fortunately, the overall incidence of nocardiosis among patients undergoing allogeneic bone marrow transplantation averages only 0.3% over 25 years.

M.S. Tallman, M.D.

The Incidence of Breast Cancer Following Mantle Field Radiation Therapy as a Function of Dose and Technique

Tinger A, Wasserman TH, Klein EE, et al (Mallinckrodt Inst of Radiology, St Louis; Washington Univ, St Louis; Univ of Washington, Seattle, et al)

Int J Radiat Oncol Biol Phys 37:865–870, 1997 20–4

Introduction.—The most frequently reported second malignancy in patients treated for Hodgkin's disease (HD) is acute nonlymphocytic leukemia. Recent reports indicate that there may be an increased incidence of breast cancer in women who received mantle field radiation therapy for treatment of HD. The radiation records for 152 women treated with mantle field irradiation for HD between 1966 and 1985 were reviewed for data on the development of breast cancer and treatment-related factors.

Methods.—Patients were grouped into early or current treatment eras (1966 to 1974 and 1975 to 1985, respectively). Each was evaluated for HD status and development of a second malignancy. Patients who developed breast cancer were evaluated for stage, pathology, age at diagnosis, interval since treatment of HD, mediastinal dose, axillary dose, maximum dose from the anterior field (anterior d_{max} dose), the anterior-posterior:posterior-anterior ratio, length of follow-up, and history of splenectomy.

Results.—Of 32 second malignancies, 10 were breast cancer. Eight breast cancers were located in the upper outer quadrant. There was a significant correlation between breast cancer and axillary dose. Patients

TABLE 6.—Observed vs. Expected Development of Breast Cancer

Treatment era	Number at risk	Mean time at risk (years)	Observed	Expected	O/E ratio	Significant at the 0.05 level
1966–1974	69	19	8	1.7	4.7	Yes
1974–1985	83	13	2	0.93	2.2	No
Anterior d_{max} dose	Number at risk	Mean time at risk (years)	Observed	Expected	O/E ratio	Significant at the 0.05 level
>40 Gy	54	19	8	1.3	6.2	Yes
≤40 Gy	98	14	2	0.76	2.6	No

Abbreviation: O/E, observed/expected.

(Reprinted by permission of the publisher from Tinger A, Wasserman TH, Klein EE, et al: The incidence of breast cancer following mantle field radiation therapy as a function of dose and technique. *Int J Radiat Oncol Biol Phys* 37:865–870. Copyright 1997 by Elsevier Science Inc.)

in the early treatment era group were at increased risk for development of breast cancer because of high anterior d_{max} and breast doses from weighting the fields anteriorly on a low–energy linear accelerator (Table 6). Current radiation therapy doses were not correlated with increased risk of breast cancer (median follow-up, 13 years).

Conclusion.—The risk of breast cancer in patients with HD treated with mantle field radiation is lower when lower radiation doses are used. Current radiation doses are not associated with a significantly higher incidence of breast cancer.

▶ A number of recent reports have looked at the frequency of breast cancer after mantle radiotherapy for Hodgkin's disease, and this is another such report, from the Mallinckrodt Institute of Radiology in St. Louis. The key to this research is exactly what kinds of blocks are used. Stanford developed the use of a wing block to define the lower extent of the axillary field and flare out laterally, thereby protecting breast tissue. This is a good technique and one that should have a major impact on the frequency of induced breast cancer in young women. The real message of this article is that we need data to compare to using modern techniques.

E. Glatstein, M.D.

Increased Risk of Breast Cancer in Splenectomized Patients Undergoing Radiation Therapy for Hodgkin's Disease

Chung CT, Bogart JA, Adams JF, et al (State Univ of New York, Syracuse)
Int J Radiat Oncol Biol Phys 37:405–409, 1997 20–5

Background.—As outcomes improve for people with Hodgkin's disease, there are more late complications, including secondary cancers. Previous studies have suggested that women receiving radiotherapy for the treatment of Hodgkin's disease are at increased risk of breast cancer. The risk of subsequent breast cancer for Hodgkin's disease patients treated with splenectomy was evaluated.

TABLE 1.—Age Distribution With or Without Splenectomy

Age (yr.) at Dx.	Splenectomy	No splenectomy
< 10	3	0
10–19	18	9
20–29	31	24
30–39	11	13
40–49	7	3
50–59	4	3
>60	0	10
Total	74	62

(Reprinted by permission of the publisher from Chung CT, Bogart JA, Adams JF, et al: Increased risk of breast cancer in splenectomized patients undergoing radiation therapy for Hodgkin's disease. *Int J Radiat Oncol Biol Phys* 37:865–870. Copyright 1997 by Elsevier Science Inc.)

Methods.—136 women and girls were treated for histologically confirmed Hodgkin's disease over a 23-year period. Treatment included mantle or mediastinal irradiation for all patients; 74 underwent splenectomy and 62 did not (Table 1). Splenectomy was evaluated by multiple linear

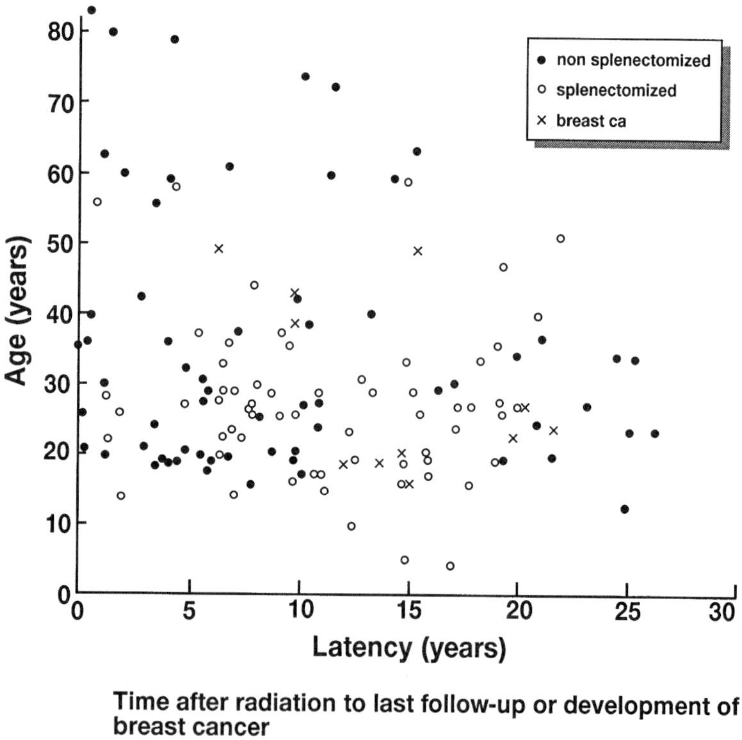

FIGURE 1.—Age at treatment, splenectomy, latency, and breast cancer status. (Reprinted by permission of the publisher from Chung CT, Bogart JA, Adams JF, et al: Increased risk of breast cancer in splenectomized patients undergoing radiation therapy for Hodgkin's disease. *Int J Radiat Oncol Biol Phys* 37:865–870. Copyright 1997 by Elsevier Science Inc.)

regression analysis for its effect on subsequent breast cancer risk, along with patient age, stage, dose and extent of radiation field, time since radiation therapy, and chemotherapy. The splenectomized patients were followed up for a mean of 13 years and the nonsplenectomized patients for nearly 17 years.

Results.—Fifteen percent of patients in the splenectomy group had breast cancer, compared with 0% of those who did not undergo splenectomy. Of the 11 cases of breast cancer, 9 were invasive and 2 were ductal carcinoma in situ. The only factor independently related to breast cancer was splenectomy. The combination of age, latency, and splenectomy also was associated with an increased risk of breast cancer (Fig 1). Survival was better for nonsplenectomized patients, probably reflecting their more advanced disease, which obviated the need for staging laparotomy.

Conclusion.—Hodgkin's disease patients who undergo splenectomy are at increased risk of subsequent breast cancer. A multicenter study is needed to define this relationship more clearly. Breast cancer risk should be a consideration when staging laparotomy is recommended in women with Hodgkin's disease. All female survivors of Hodgkin's disease should be followed up closely, and all should have mammograms.

▶ This paper suggests that the risk of breast cancer in patients who undergo radiotherapy for the treatment of Hodgkin's disease is markedly increased in those who have had a splenectomy. This is a complicated subject because the main risk of such an event is a function of the patient's age at the time of initial treatment. Table 1 clearly shows that the splenectomy patients were significantly younger than the patients without a splenectomy. Interpretation is thus difficult at least in part due to the natural bias for carrying out the procedure in patients who are young and in good shape. It also means that patients who are likely to come down with breast cancer would probably have had an early splenectomy vs. patients who had no splenectomy. The numbers are interesting but impossible to interpret definitely. Thus, what the authors have done is generate a hypothesis that needs some confirmation from other sources. Also, the chemotherapy may be another factor that received little attention in this analysis.

E. Glatstein, M.D.

Bladder Carcinoma and Other Second Malignancies After Radiotherapy for Prostate Carcinoma

Neugut AI, Ahsan H, Robinson E, et al (Columbia Univ, New York; Northern Israel Oncology Ctr, Haifa)

Cancer 79:1600–1604, 1997 20–6

Background.—Studies have shown that radiation therapy (RT) to the pelvis is associated with an increased risk of bladder cancer and other malignancies. To date, there have been no controlled studies of the risk of second malignancies after RT for prostate carcinoma.

TABLE 2.—Second Malignancies After Prostate Carcinoma

	6 mos < 5 yrs		5–8 yrs		> 8 yrs	
	O/E	RR (95% CI)	O/E	RR (95% CI)	O/E	RR (95% CI)
Bladder						
RT+	132/130.5	1.0 (0.8–1.2)	51/38.6	1.3 (1.0–1.7)	38/25.6	1.5 (1.1–2.0)
RT−	446/405.8	1.1 (1.0–1.2)	82/106.8	0.7 (0.6–0.9)	72/73.7	1.0 (0.7–1.2)
Rectal						
RT+	65/94.0	0.7 (0.5–0.9)	22/26.9	0.8 (0.5–1.2)	14/17.8	0.8 (0.4–1.3)
RT−	215/275.4	0.8 (0.7–0.9)	54/71.4	0.8 (0.6–1.0)	41/49.2	0.8 (0.6–1.1)
Acute nonlymphocytic leukemia						
RT+	20/13.3	1.5 (0.9–2.3)	5/4.2	1.2 (0.4–2.8)	1/2.8	0.4 (0.0–2.0)
RT−	30/41.95	0.7 (0.5–1.0)	9/11.6	0.8 (0.4–1.5)	9/7.9	1.1 (0.5–2.2)
Chronic lymphocyte leukemia						
RT+	7/22	0.3 (0.1–0.7)	3/6.5	0.5 (0.1–1.3)	6/4.5	1.3 (0.5–2.9)
RT−	38/72.3	0.5 (0.4–0.7)	27/19.3	1.4 (0.9–2.0)	8/13.9	0.6 (0.2–1.1)

Abbreviations: O/E, Observed/expected; *CI*, confidence interval; *RR*, relative risk.

(Courtesy of Neugut AI, Ahsan H, Robinson E, et al: Bladder carcinoma and other second malignancies after radiotherapy for prostate carcinoma. *Cancer* 79:1600–1604, 1997. Copyright © 1997 American Cancer Society. Reprinted by permission of Wiley-Liss, Inc., a subsidiary of John Wiley & Sons, Inc.)

Methods and Findings.—Data on a cohort of patients with prostate carcinoma were analyzed retrospectively. Radiation therapy had been performed in 34,889, and no RT had been performed in 106,872. The RT group had a relative risk of 1.5 for bladder carcinoma after 8 years. The risk in the no-RT group was 1.0. In addition, the RT group had a relative risk of 1.3 for bladder carcinoma. Neither group had an increased risk for rectal carcinoma, acute nonlymphocytic leukemia, or chronic lymphocytic leukemia (Table 2).

Conclusions.—Patients undergoing RT for prostate carcinoma had an increased risk of bladder carcinoma several years later, but the increase was not dramatic. These patients had no increased risk of rectal carcinoma or leukemia.

► When I look at the fields that are applied to prostatic cancer today, they seem bigger than the fields that I am used to treating. Typically, when I arced patients, I set the upper border of the field 1–1.5 cm above the top of the prostate, clipping the floor of the bladder. Today, I see fields in which the entire bladder is being treated in many instances, and obviously that is true when they decide to treat the whole pelvis to incorporate the lymph nodes, for which there is absolutely no evidence of benefit.

This article looks at almost 35,000 patients with carcinoma of the prostate who had undergone radiotherapy and more than 100,000 patients who had not. After 8 years of follow-up, the risk of bladder cancer had increased modestly in the radiotherapy group. That risk may be considerably more with time, but it is hard to tell. It is relevant to note that there was no increase in rectal carcinoma or leukemia during the same 8-year follow-up.

The data were collected from the Surveillance, Epidemiology, and End Results (SEER) program of the National Cancer Institute. This program began in 1973. For part of that time, there were no national figures; the national estimates were projected from the state of Connecticut and a 5-county area in California, where a diagnosis of cancer had to be reported by law. In 1973, the National Cancer Institute set up a program with roughly 10% of the hospitals in the United States in which the hospitals fed information into a computer system. The SEER system has worked surprisingly well, although it is not foolproof by any stretch of the imagination. I think it works quite well for incidence figures, although I am not sure that the survival data generated by SEER are as good as people assume. When events take place outside the hospital setting, it is not always easy for the hospital to find out about them, and it is the hospitals that are the source of the information for the SEER program, not individual offices. Also, events that take place outside the hospital setting may not get recorded in the hospital database for months, for years, or ever. It depends on the tenacity of the hospital and that of their tumor registrar. Unfortunately, tumor registrars have significant turnover in many of these institutions.

This article suggests that we should be careful about the volume that we are treating. I certainly agree with that, but I am concerned that our prostatic volumes are way too generous.

E. Glatstein, M.D.

Bilateral Diaphragmatic Weakness: A Late Complication of Radiotherapy

Brander PE, Järvinen V, Lohela P, et al (Kiljava Hosp, Finland; Helsinki Univ)

Thorax 52:829–831, 1997 20–7

Background.—Sometimes, many years after radiotherapy to the chest, brachial plexus neuropathy develops. Its development is related, among other factors, to the total dose of radiation, the duration of radiotherapy, and the patient's age. In this case report, the authors described a woman in whom not only brachial plexus neuropathy developed many years after radiotherapy, bilateral phrenic nerve weakness that caused bilateral weakness of the diaphragm also developed later.

Case Report.—Women, 67, had received 4 courses of radiotherapy for Hodgkin's disease from 1962 to 1964. The dose was 100 Gy delivered to the axillary and supraclavicular regions. After the fourth treatment, the Hodgkin's disease did not recur. A few years later, pain and muscular weakness began developing in the patient's arms, until electroneuromyography, in 1983, showed a severe bilateral brachial plexus injury. Surgery to break the brachial plexus adhesions and to cut the left scalenus anterior muscle relieved the pain but did not improve function.

Eleven years later, in 1994, the now 67-year-old woman was seen with severe orthopnea but no signs of heart failure or obstructive sleep apnea. Ventilatory function was impaired and was worse when she changed from a sitting to a supine position. She also had mild hypoxemia and a low maximal inspiratory mouth pressure. A high-resolution CT scan, done while the patient was standing, showed that the diaphragm moved about 3 cm during normal breathing. While the patient was supine, however, the diaphragm did not move at all during normal breathing. Electroneuromyography identified the previous brachial plexus injury from a decade earlier; it also indicated bilateral phrenic nerve weakness. Phrenic nerve stimulation of the diaphragm resulted in delayed latencies (12.5 msec; normal less than 9 msec). The patient was discharged with a bilevel positive airway pressure ventilator for use at night and was still using this device 2 years later.

Conclusion.—This patient was seen with the classic signs of bilateral diaphragmatic weakness. Although this condition is typically associated with generalized neuromuscular disease, this patient had no such history, nor any indications for other causes of the brachial plexus injury. The most likely cause was the radiation therapy some 30 years earlier, which led to brachial plexus injury and, eventually, the bilateral diaphragmatic weakness secondary to phrenic nerve injury.

► Most of us have seen brachial plexus neuropathy, usually after treatment for breast cancer. It is an uncommon phenomenon, but, at the same time, it does have a finite rate of occurrence. This paper is unusual in that it describes not brachial plexopathy, but phrenic plexopathy 30 years after radiotherapy for Hodgkin's disease and more than 10 years after the development of bilateral brachial plexus neuropathy. The patient was seen with bilateral diaphragmatic weakness secondary to phrenic nerve effects. Prior radiotherapy is thought to be the explanation.

Although I have certainly seen tumor injure phrenic nerves to an irreparable degree, I have only seen a therapeutic injury to the phrenic nerve on 1 occasion, when we treated an unresectable primary sarcoma of the esophagus to 7,200 rad with shrinking field technique and idoxuridine on a twice-a-day basis . We kept shrinking the field, in conjunction with the radiosensitizer IUdR, but 10 years after such treatment, a paralyzed phrenic nerve developed. The patient's other nerve remained stable and functional. This is the only time I have seen a phrenic nerve injury resulting from radiation therapy. In any event, this particular case report seemed to have some interest.

E. Glatstein, M.D.

21 Supportive Care

Impact of a Clinical Guidelines Program for Breast and Colon Cancer in a French Cancer Center

Ray-Coquard I, Philip T, Lehmann M, et al (Centre Léon Bérard, Lyon, France; Fédération Nationale des Centres de Lutte Contre le Cancer, Paris)

JAMA 278:1591–1595, 1997 21–1

Introduction.—Systematically developed statements to assist both practitioner and patient decisions about appropriate health care for specific clinical circumstances is the definition for clinical practice guidelines, which are being promoted to reduce unnecessary costs in health care services and to assist clinical decision making. A comprehensive cancer center in France implemented clinical practice guidelines by 1995 that were based on an analysis of the literature and the consensus of intra-institutional experts. The guidelines were created to help community-based oncologists in their decision making, to optimize health benefits, to ensure rational chemotherapy drug prescriptions, to minimize inappropriate variation in practice, and to provide leadership for cancer treatment. Institutional computerized records of patients with breast or colon cancer were reviewed to conduct a before-and-after study.

Methods.—There were 100 women with localized breast cancer and 158 patients with colon cancer whose records from 1993 and 1995 were reviewed. To assess compliance with clinical practice guidelines, investigators analyzed the medical decisions on these records. The scientific evidence for noncompliant decisions was determined via a systematic search of the literature.

Results.—Three hundred fifty of the 375 available medical decisions could be assessed. In 1995, the compliance rate with clinical practice guidelines for breast cancer was significantly higher than in 1993 (54% vs. 19%). In 1995, the compliance rate for colon cancer was significantly higher than in 1993 (70% vs. 50%). In 1995, 68% of medical decisions for breast cancer conformed with the clinical practice guidelines or were judged to be based on "scientific evidence," whereas 42% of medical decisions for breast cancer were based on clinical practice guidelines in 1993. In 1995, 81% of medical decisions for colon cancer were judged to be based on scientific evidence or conformed with the clinical practice guidelines, and in 1993, 71% of medical decisions for colon cancer were based on clinical practice guidelines.

Conclusion.—For both cancers, compliance rates were significantly higher. Significant changes in medical practice seem to result from the development and implementation of clinical practice guidelines; however, this study did not demonstrate a causal relationship between the guidelines and the changes.

► No one particularly likes having someone else tell them what to do. Nonetheless, for practical and economic reasons, a mandate for clinical practice guidelines has evolved in this country as well as in others. Are these guidelines effective in changing physician behavior? This report from a French comprehensive cancer center suggests an affirmative reply. The authors did demonstrate a significant difference in patient care offered by physicians in a 2-year period from 1993 to 1995. The authors believe that part of the reason for the success of the clinical practice guidelines is that the physicians participated in the development of the guidelines that were imposed and that these guidelines were also introduced as part of the continuing medical education curriculum. This seems like a very logical approach for changing behavior, even that of physicians.

P.J. Loehrer, Sr., M.D.

Efficacy of Pamidronate in Reducing Skeletal Complications in Patients With Breast Cancer and Lytic Bone Metastases

Hortobagyi GN, for the Protocol 19 Aredia Breast Cancer Study Group (Univ of Texas, Houston; Saint Thomas Hosp, Nashville, Tenn; Saint Vincent Med Ctr, Los Angeles; et al)

N Engl J Med 335:1785–1791, 1996 21–2

Introduction.—Most women with advanced breast cancer have bone metastases. Osteoclast-induced bone resorption causes the destruction of bone in these lesions, and cytotoxic chemotherapy or hormone therapy is the treatment most often preferred. However, this therapy causes progressive skeletal destruction, which leads to immobility and more pain. Potent inhibitors of osteoclastic bone resorption are biphosphonates, which are effective in treating cancer that has metastasized to bone. Skeletal complications may be reduced by pamidronate disodium, a second-generation bisphosphonate. A randomized, double-blind study was conducted to compare monthly infusions of pamidronate (90 mg) with a placebo to prevent skeletal complications.

Methods.—Placebo or pamidronate at 90 mg was given to 380 women with stage IV breast cancer as a 2-hour IV infusion monthly for 12 cycles. The women also were receiving cytotoxic chemotherapy and had at least one lytic bone lesion. Each month, an assessment was made to determine whether the patient had skeletal complications, including pathologic fractures, the need for radiation to bone or bone surgery, spinal cord compression, and hypercalcemia (a serum calcium concentration above 12 mg/dL [3.0 mmol/L] or elevated to any degree and requiring treatment).

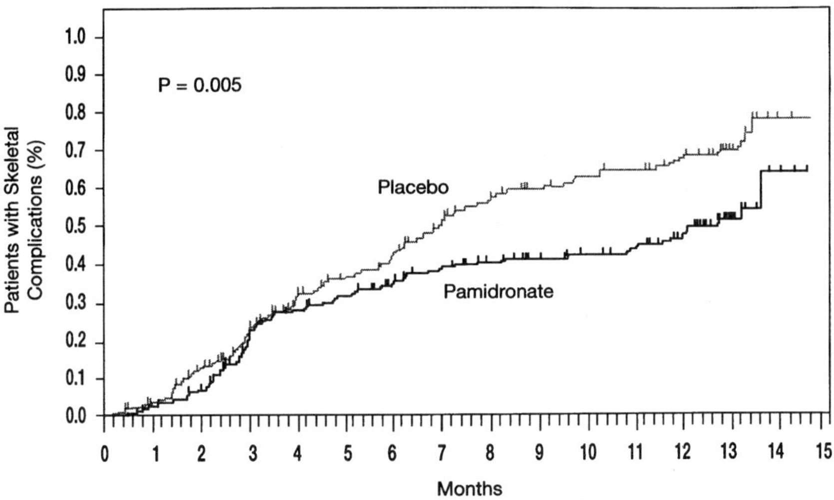

FIGURE 1.—Kaplan-Meier estimates of the time to the first skeletal complication. (Reprinted by permission of the New England Journal of Medicine, from Hortobagyi GN, for the Protocol 19 Aredia Breast Cancer Study Group: Efficacy of pamidronate in reducing skeletal complications in patients with breast cancer and lytic bone metastases. *N Engl J Med* 335:1785–1791, copyright 1996, Massachusetts Medical Society. All rights reserved.)

Evaluations were also done on bone pain, performance status, use of analgesic drugs and quality of life.

Results.—There was a greater length of time for the occurrence of the first skeletal complication among the women receiving the pamidronate (13.1 months) than in the group receiving placebo (7 months) (Fig 1). In the pamidronate group, 43% of women had skeletal complications compared to 56% of women in the placebo group. In the pamidronate group, there was significantly less increase in bone pain and deterioration of performance status than in the placebo group. The women tolerated the pamidronate well.

Conclusion.—Women with stage IV breast cancer who have osteolytic bone metastases are more protected against skeletal complications with monthly infusions of pamidronate as a supplement to chemotherapy.

► Symptomatic bone metastases are a major cause of morbidity from advanced breast cancer. Osteoclast-induced bone resorption causes destruction of bones leading to both pain and skeletal fractures. Bisphosphonates, by virtue of their inhibition of osteoclastic bone resorption, are effective in treating cancer-related hypercalcemia, which is often associated with widespread bony metastases. This study clearly demonstrates that pamidronate is also effective in reducing skeletal complications in patients with breast cancer and lytic bone metastases. Pamidronate can now be considered the standard of care to be used in conjunction with systemic chemotherapy or hormonal therapy to decrease skeletal complications in women with osteolytic bone metastases.

R.F. Ozols, M.D., Ph.D.

Ondansetron Versus Metoclopramide, Both Combined With Dexamethasone, in the Prevention of Cisplatin-induced Delayed Emesis

Roila F, and the Italian Group for Antiemetic Research (Policlinico Hosp, Italy)

J Clin Oncol 15:124–130, 1997 21–3

Background.—Delayed emesis 24 hours after cisplatin dosing is often treated with oral metoclopramide combined with dexamethasone. However, delayed emesis still occurs in about half of patients, and thus better methods to control this problem are needed. Suggested alternatives include the 5-HT_3 receptor antagonists, and the utility of ondansetron plus dexamethasone and that of metoclopramide plus dexamethasone in preventing cisplatin-induced delayed emesis were evaluated.

Methods.—In this randomized, double-blind, parallel groups study, 318 patients undergoing chemotherapy received dexamethasone (20 mg) and ondansetron (8 mg) immediately before cisplatin dosing (less than 50 mg/m^2) as prophylaxis for acute emesis. Then, after cisplatin administration, 160 patients received metoclopramide (20 mg every 6 hours on days 2–4) plus dexamethasone (8 mg twice a day on days 2 and 3, and 4 mg twice a day on day 4) and 158 received ondansetron (8 mg every 12 hours on days 2–4) plus dexamethasone (according to the same dosing schedule). Vomiting and nausea episodes were documented after cisplatin dosing at 2, 4, 6, and 8 hours and once a day for another 6 days.

Findings.—Patient compliance with both regimens was good. The 2 groups did not differ significantly in complete protection from nausea (62% vs 60%, ondansetron plus dexamethasone vs. metoclopramide plus dexamethasone) or vomiting (44% vs. 54%). However, a significant effect was observed when both treatments were regarded in concert. Treatment with either regimen gave complete protection from delayed vomiting in 73% of patients who did not vomit on day 1 and 19% of those who did; the corresponding numbers for those with complete protection from delayed nausea who did not or did vomit on day 1 were 45% and 9%, respectively. Within this analysis, patients with acute vomiting who received ondansetron plus dexamethasone had better protection from delayed vomiting (29% vs. 9%).

Conclusions.—Regardless of the antiemetic regimen used, preventing acute nausea and vomiting has the best effect on the delayed occurrence of these symptoms. Both regimens had similar effects on acute and delayed vomiting, except that ondansetron plus dexamethasone may be of more use in patients who experience acute vomiting. Because of its decreased cost and similar efficacy, metoclopramide plus dexamethasone is the recommended treatment for cisplatin-induced emesis.

▶ The 5-HT_3 receptor antagonists have proved to be very effective in the management of acute nausea and vomiting associated with cisplatin and other highly emetogenic chemotherapeutic agents. Before they were available, a widely used combination consisted of metoclopramide with dexamethasone. In this study, patients receiving cisplatin were randomly assigned in a double-blind manner to either ondansetron or metoclopramide, and both were combined with dexamethasone in patients receiving cisplatin chemotherapy. It was of interest that effective management of acute nausea and vomiting was associated with less delayed vomiting and nausea, which is frequently observed with cisplatin. Both combinations in the study were similarly effective in the prevention of delayed emesis induced by cisplatin. Ondansetron plus dexamethasone appears to be more effective in the management of acute vomiting. Consequently, ondansetron appears to be the preferable agent to use with cisplatin, although investigators in this study continue to recommend metoclopramide with dexamethasone, primarily because of decreased cost.

R.F. Ozols, M.D., Ph.D.

Randomized Study of Prophylactic Platelet Transfusion Threshold During Induction Therapy for Adult Acute Leukemia: 10,000/μL Versus 20,000/μL

Heckman KD, Weiner GJ, Davis CS, et al (Univ of Iowa, Iowa City)

J Clin Oncol 15:1143–1149, 1997 21–4

Background.—In patients undergoing chemotherapy for acute leukemia, prophylactic platelet transfusions can decrease the risk of hemorrhage. However, transfusions increase the risk of transmission of viral hepatitis, HIV, and other infectious agents, and they are expensive. This study evaluated whether total utilization of platelets might safely be decreased by making a platelet count of 10,000/μL the threshold for prophylactic administration.

Methods.—Over approximately 4.5 years, 82 adult patients receiving induction therapy for acute leukemia entered the study. Seventy-eight were found to be eligible and assessable. They were randomly assigned to receive prophylactic transfusions at a platelet count of 20,000/μL (41 patients) or 10,000/μL (37 patients).

Results.—As expected, patients in the 10,000/μL group required fewer prophylactic transfusions than those in the 20,000/μL group. They were found to require more therapeutic transfusions, but overall platelet utilization was still lower than in the 20,000/μL group. There was no statistically significant difference between the groups in morbidity from bleeding. No bleeding was fatal or required surgery or transfer to ICU. Neither age nor status of leukemia (newly diagnosed vs. relapsed) affected the number of bleeding episodes. In both the 10,000/μL and 20,000/μL groups, febrile patients required more platelets than nonfebrile patients, but the incidence of severe bleeding was minimal.

Conclusions.—In deciding how to administer prophylactic platelet transfusions to adults undergoing chemotherapy for acute leukemia, physicians should consider that a threshold platelet count of 10,000/µL seems to be safe and should result in cost savings. Patients with thrombocytopenia were not evaluated, but the authors see no scientific reason why the 10,000/µL threshold could not apply to them as well, as long as they have no coagulation or anatomic abnormalities that might predispose them to bleeding.

► The conventional threshold for platelets, in cases in which the potential for bleeding is sufficient to warrant a platelet transfusion, has been 20,000/µL. However, it has recently been suggested that this threshold may be lowered. This study is important because it represents the few prospective trials randomizing patients to a threshold of either 10,000/µL or 20,000/µL. Importantly, the lower threshold caused only a minimal adverse effect on bleeding, with no statistically significant effect on morbidity, but there was a meaningful decrease in the total utilization of platelets. This article suggests we may change the way we care for patients with acute leukemia.

M.S. Tallman, M.D.

Impact of Therapy With Epoetin Alfa on Clinical Outcomes in Patients With Nonmyeloid Malignancies During Cancer Chemotherapy in Community Oncology Practice

Glaspy J, Bukowski R, Steinberg D, et al (Univ of California, Los Angeles; Pacific Shores Med Group, Long Beach, Calif; Cleveland Clinic, Ohio; et al)
J Clin Oncol 15:1218–1234, 1997 21–5

Background.—Anemia is a common complication of chemotherapy in patients with cancer, resulting in reduced functional capacity and quality of life and necessitating red blood cell transfusion with its associated risks, inconvenience, and costs. The effect of epoetin alfa on quality of life, transfusion requirements, and hemoglobin in patients with cancer and anemia during chemotherapy was studied.

Methods.—A total of 2,342 patients in more than 500 community-based oncology practices were enrolled in the open-label study. All were being treated with cytotoxic chemotherapy for malignancies. Epoetin alfa, 150 U/kg 3 times a week, was administered for up to 4 months. The dose was doubled in patients with inadequate responses.

Findings.—One thousand forty-seven patients completed all 4 months of epoetin alfa treatment. Significant increases in mean self-rated scores for energy level, activity level, and overall quality of life were noted. These improvements were correlated with the magnitude of the hemoglobin increase and were independent of tumor response. Epoetin alfa treatment was also associated with a significant increase in mean hemoglobin and a significant reduction in the proportion of patients needing transfusions. The patients tolerated epoetin alfa well.

Conclusions.—Epoetin alfa improves the functional status and quality of life in anemic cancer patients receiving chemotherapy. It also increases hemoglobin levels and reduces transfusion requirements. Further research is needed to delineate optimal doses and schedules.

▶ It certainly is possible that clinicians have not fully appreciated the impact of cancer-associated anemia upon the quality of life of cancer patients undergoing chemotherapy. This study demonstrates that epoetin alfa is effective in increasing hemoglobin levels in anemic cancer patients. This improvement in hemoglobin and hematocrit is associated with improvement in functional status as well as in self-assessment and quality of life. Epoetin alfa was associated with little toxicity, and virtually all patients could complete 4 months of epoetin alfa therapy. Questions remain regarding the cost benefit associated with epoetin alfa compared with transfusions as well as what is the optimal dose and schedule for this cytokine.

R.F. Ozols, M.D., Ph.D.

Corticosteroids Significantly Delay the Onset of Docetaxel-induced Fluid Retention: Final Results of a Randomized Study of the European Organization for Research and Treatment of Cancer Investigational Drug Branch for Breast Cancer

Piccart MJ, Klijn J, Paridaens R, et al (Universitair Ziekenhuis Gasthuisberg, Leuven, Belgium; Academisch Ziekenhuis, Leiden, The Netherlands; Fondation Bergonié, Bordeaux, France; et al)

J Clin Oncol 15:3149–3155, 1997 21–6

Introduction.—Because of their novel mechanism of action and promising cytotoxic activity in a number of solid tumors, the taxoids, such as paclitaxel and docetaxel, have generated significant interest. In phase I trials, docetaxel was administered as a 1-hour intravenous infusion on days 1 and 8 every 3 weeks. For phase II trials, the recommended dosage of docetaxel was 50 mg/m^2 to be administered on days 1 and 8. Corticosteroids were also suggested to delay fluid retention, a frequent cause of premature discontinuation of docetaxel. The efficacy of docetaxel in women with breast cancer was determined, and the incidence of fluid retention and skin toxicity was compared when docetaxel was administered with and without prophylactic corticosteroids.

Methods.—There were 83 women who were pretreated with 1 chemotherapy regimen for metastatic breast cancer with bidimensionally measurable and progressive disease. On days 1 and 8 every 21 days, docetaxel with prophylactic oral antihistamine was administered at a dose of 50mg/m^2 as a 1-hour infusion. The patients were divided into 2 groups. One received methylprednisolone, 40 mg, on days −1, 0, 1, 7, 8, and 9 of each cycle, and the other group did not.

Results.—An objective response was achieved by 28 patients (34%). The median time to disease progression was 5 months, and the median

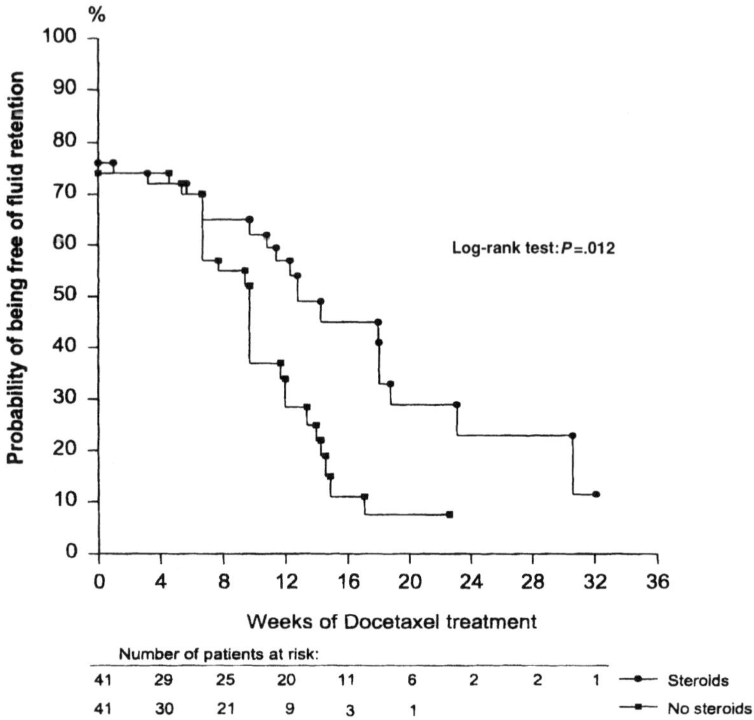

FIGURE 1.—Docetaxel-induced fluid retention: time to onset. (Courtesy of Piccart MJ, Klijn J, Paridaens R, et al: Corticosteroids significantly delay the onset of docetaxel-induced fluid retention: Final results of a randomized study of the European Organization for Research and Treatment of Cancer Investigational Drug Branch for Breast Cancer. *J Clin Oncol* 15:3149–3155, 1997.)

time to overall survival was 13.5 months. There were 415 cycles of docetaxel administered, and the most common toxicity was grade 3 or 4 neutropenia, which occurred in 79% of patients. Skin reactions and asthenia were clinically significant nonhematologic side effects. In an intent-to-treat analysis, patients who received methylprednisolone premedication had a delayed onset of fluid retention (Fig 1). They also received a higher cumulative dose of docetaxel before the onset of fluid retention (333 mg/m^2 vs. 215 mg/m^2).

Conclusions.—Docetaxel demonstrated definite antitumor activity in pretreated metastatic breast cancer patients at this dose and schedule. Corticosteroids were shown to have a favorable impact on docetaxel-induced fluid retention.

▶ The taxanes are highly active anticancer drugs for the treatment of breast, lung, ovary, and other cancers. Paclitaxel and docetaxel are taxanes with a similar spectrum of activity but with different toxicity profiles. Induced fluid retention and myelosuppression have been Docetaxel's dose-limiting toxicities. In this randomized study, corticosteroids were shown to delay the onset of fluid retention. Although there was a delay, as seen in Figure 1, fluid retention remains a concern at higher cumulative doses. In particular, corticosteroids did not appear to decrease the incidence of pleural effusions developing in this group of patients. In addition, 79% of the patients still encountered grade 3 or 4 neutropenia. Direct comparisons of paclitaxel and docetaxel in patients with metastatic breast cancer are in progress to determine the relative activity and toxicity profiles.

R.F. Ozols, M.D., Ph.D.

Thoracoscopic Talc Poudrage Pleurodesis for Malignant Effusions: A Review of 360 Cases

Viallat J-R, Rey F, Astoul P, et al (Paoli Calmettes Inst, Marseilles, France; La Conception Hosp, Marseilles, France)

Chest 110:1387–1393, 1996 21–7

Background.—A renewed interest in talc pleurodesis has been expressed recently in North America. The efficacy and safety of thoracoscopic talc poudrage for pleurodesis in patients with malignant effusions were reported.

Methods.—Thoracoscopy was performed for diagnosis and subsequent talc pleurodesis in 215 patients and for pleurodesis only in 145 patients. Two hundred seventy-two patients had pleural metastases and 88 had mesothelioma. Mean follow-up was 12 months.

Findings.—Thirty-three critically ill patients died in the first month and were not included in the final analysis. These patients had illnesses that should have contraindicated the procedure. Of the remaining patients, 90.2% had a successful pleurodesis at 1 month and 82.1% had a lifelong pleural symphysis. Adverse effects were fever in 9.8%, empyema in 2.5%, pulmonary infection in 0.8%, and malignant invasion of the scar in 1 patient. In addition, 1 patient died with end-stage disease 3 days after the procedure.

Conclusion.—Thoracoscopic talc poudrage is effective and safe for lifelong pleurodesis. It should be done early in the course of malignant effusions to avoid the risk of respiratory failure. The use of no more than 5 gm of talc for malignant effusions and 1–2 g for pneumothoraces is recommended.

► The study reviews the efficacy of thoracoscopic talc poudrage pleurodesis for the management of malignant effusions. This technique has been primarily used in Europe; in North America, the primary method of pleurodesis has been the installation of tetracycline, bleomycin, or talc via a chest tube. A prospective, randomized comparison of different techniques for pleurodesis is in progress in the United States. What is clear is that thoracoscopic talc poudrage pleurodesis is effective and safe. In addition, the efficacy of any method of pleurodesis is increased when it is administered early on in the management of chronic malignant pleural effusions. Repeat thoracentesis in dyspneic patients with malignant pleural effusions should be avoided because symptomatic relief is brief and there is resulting depletion in fluids, proteins, and electrolytes. Pleurodesis should, therefore, be considered early in the treatment of this common problem.

R.F. Ozols, M.D., Ph.D.

Sucralfate for Radiation Mucositis: Results of a Double-blind Randomized Trial

Meredith R, Salter M, Kim R, et al (Univ of Alabama, Birmingham)

Int J Radiat Oncol Biol Phys 37:275–279, 1997 21–8

Background.—Head, neck, and chest irradiation can cause mucositis that, if severe enough, may compromise therapy. The standard treatment to prevent or ameliorate radiation-induced mucositis is a suspension of antacids, diphenhydramine, and viscous lidocaine. These authors evaluated this regimen alone and with the addition of sucralfate to see whether the polysaccharide conferred any extra benefits.

Methods.—Patients undergoing radiation therapy to the oral cavity, pharynx, or esophagus who had not previously undergone radiation therapy were eligible for the study. Those with allergies to the medications, those who had received or were receiving chemotherapy, and those using other medications to treat mucositis were excluded. Radiation therapy consisted of once-daily irradiation with more than 40 Gy in 1.8 Gy fractions delivered 5 times a week. If mucositis developed, patients were randomized to receive a bedtime dose of either the standard suspension (150 mg diphenhydramine, 10 mL 2% viscous lidocaine plus antacids [225 mg aluminum hydroxide, and 200 mg magnesium hydroxide]; n = 31) or the sucralfate suspension (12 gm sucralfate plus the standard suspension; n = 34). Patients reported their degree of soreness (scale of 0 to 20), ability to eat various foods (scale of 0 to 5), and other symptoms as mucositis occurred. Tissue samples were collected to screen for candidiasis.

TABLE 2.—Comparison of Mucositis in Radiation Patients Receiving Sucralfate Solution or Standard Medication

Extent of mucositis	Sucralfate group No. of patients (%)	Standard medication No. of patients (%)
Absent	20 (59)	15 (48)
Erythema not requiring systemic analgesia	10 (29)	8 (26)
Patchy mucositis, <50%	4 (12)	6 (19)
>50% mucosa involved	0	2 (6)

(Reprinted by permission of the publisher from Meredith R, Salter M, Kim R, et al. Sucralfate for radiation mucositis: Results of a double-blind randomized trial. *Int J Radiat Oncol Biol Phys* 37:275–279, copyright 1997 by Elsevier Science Inc.)

Findings.—Although the result was not statistically significant, patients taking the sucralfate suspension had a lesser extent of mucositis and fewer involved patches (less than 50%) compared with patients taking the standard suspension (Table 2). The 2 treatment groups did not differ with respect to soreness or dietary changes to softer foods, and less than 10% in each group reported drug-related side effects (mainly a sore mouth).

Conclusion.—There was a trend toward better control of mucositis in the group taking the sucralfate suspension compared with the standard lidocaine-diphenhydramine-antacid suspension. The lack of a significant effect may be, in part, related to the action of sucralfate: This drug has an affinity for ulcer sites, and none of these patients had ulcers. Thus, results in patients with mouth ulcers may have been more substantial.

▶ These investigators carried out a study evaluating sucralfate in the management of radiation mucositis. They compared a standard regimen with the same regimen plus sucralfate. With 111 patients entered over 2 years; the authors saw a trend (that was not statistically significant) toward less severe radiation mucositis in the patients who were receiving sucralfate in addition to their standard combination of viscous lidocaine, diphenhydramine, and antacid. I think it is interesting to look at this paper, which is fairly well done. Those of us who see radiation mucositis are certainly looking for ways to improve it. I, for one, will be trying this in the future to see whether it represents an improvement.

E. Glatstein, M.D.

Subject Index

A

Abdomen
colectomy in hereditary nonpolyposis colorectal cancer, rectal cancer risk after, 161
Absidia
infection after allogeneic bone marrow transplantation, incidence and risk factors for, 279
Acetaminophen
ovarian cancer risk with, 7
Aclarubicin
plus cytosine arabinoside in acute myeloid leukemia, survival and secondary malignancies after, 205
Adenocarcinoma
colon, laparoscopic *vs.* open resection for, 141
gastric, laparoscopy in, 156
pancreas, pancreaticoduodenectomy for, and preoperative and postoperative chemoradiation strategies, 169
Adenomas
colon, 5 mm or less in diameter, importance of detection by sigmoidoscopy, 183
Adenopathy
in Sézary syndrome, 211
African-Americans
ovarian carcinoma in, epithelial, 6
Age
effect on outcome of autologous bone marrow transplantation for hematologic malignancies, 282
Altretamine
in ovarian carcinoma, relapsed, 95
5-Aminolevulinic acid
induced protoporphyrin IX, fluorescence imaging and spectroscopy for detection of neoplastic lesions in oral cavity, 55
Amphotericin B
in *Fusarium* infections in hematologic cancer patients, 335
Amsacrine
in leukemia, acute adult lymphoblastic, 203
Analgesics
over-the-counter, and risk of ovarian cancer, 7
Anaplastic
lymphoma, primary large-cell, in adults, 213
Androgen
suppression with goserelin after radiotherapy in prostate cancer, 108
Anemia
after topotecan in resistant ovarian cancer, 94
Angiogenesis
-related gene expression and progression of ovarian carcinoma (in mice), 27
Angiographic
response of locally advanced soft tissue sarcoma after hyperthermic isolated limb perfusion with tumor necrosis factor, 271
Anthracycline
-containing chemotherapy regimen in operable breast cancer, 71
Antigen
carcinoembryonic, monitoring, value in curative surgery for recurrent colorectal carcinoma, 174
Antineoplastic
agents, in vitro tumor cell killing by, telomerase activity decline as measure of, 13
Anus
carcinoma, National Cancer Data Base report on, 142
Apoptosis
p53-dependent, role of *bax* in (in mice), 53
Ara-C
plus aclarubicin or daunorubicin in acute myeloid leukemia, survival and secondary malignancies after, 205
Arthralgia
after stem cell transplantation, allogeneic blood, 284
Ascitic fluid
oncofetal fibronectin in, in advanced epithelial ovarian cancer, 58
Aspergillus
infection after allogeneic bone marrow transplantation, incidence and risk factors for, 279
Aspiration
cytology, fine-needle, in pancreatic cancer
resectable, 168
suspected, 162
Aspirin
dose in suppression of colorectal mucosal prostaglandins, 163
ovarian cancer risk with, 7

Ataxia
truncal, after TNP-470 in squamous cell cancer of cervix, 324
Attitudes
of clinicians toward clinical trials of cancer therapy, 322
Autopsy
series used to estimate disease "reservoir" for ductal carcinoma in situ of breast, 77
Axillary
lymph node
dissection in T1a breast cancer, 83
metastasis of breast carcinoma, detection with Tc-99m sestamibi scintimammography, 41
lymphadenectomy for breast cancer, overnight closed suction drainage after, 78

B

Basal cell
carcinoma of face, surgery *vs.* radiotherapy for, 258
bax
role in p53-dependent apoptosis (in mice), 53
B-cell
leukemia, de novo prolymphocytic, cladribine in, 199
lymphoma, marginal zone, of parotid glands, radiotherapy *vs.* combined therapy in, 209
Behavior
health risk, physician discussion of, relation to patient income, 2
Biology
cancer, 13
radiation
basic, 291
in brachytherapy, 291
Biopsy
aspiration, fine-needle, in pancreatic cancer
resectable, 168
suspected, 162
prostate, results after interstitial brachytherapy in early prostate cancer, 112
sentinel node, to avoid axillary dissection in breast cancer with clinically negative nodes, 75
skin, in Sézary syndrome, 211
Bladder
cancer
invasive, hypofractionated radiotherapy for, 299
muscle infiltrating, transurethral resection for, long-term follow-up, 120
after radiotherapy for prostate carcinoma, 339
carcinoma *(see* cancer *above)*
irritability after primary therapy for early prostate cancer, 103
Blastic
morphologic features in mantle cell lymphoma, 208
Bleomycin
/etoposide with cisplatin *vs.* carboplatin in good-prognosis metastatic nonseminomatous germ cell cancer, 125
in germ cell tumor, poor-prognosis metastatic nonseminomatous, 135
in Hodgkin's disease, 215
importance in combination chemotherapy for good-prognosis nonseminomatous testicular cancer, 130
Blood
disorders, fatal, after combined modality therapy in advanced Hodgkin's disease, 219
peripheral
involvement in mantle cell lymphoma, 208
progenitor cell mobilization and transplantation in non-Hodgkin's lymphoma, recombinant methionyl human stem cell factor and filgrastim for, 328
stem cell, transplantation (*see* Transplantation, stem cell)
Bone
cancer, primary, CT and MRI in local staging of, 263
marrow transplantation (*see* Transplantation, bone marrow)
metastases, lytic, and breast cancer, pamidronate in prevention of skeletal complications in, 346
BOP/VIP-B
intensive induction-sequential chemotherapy for poor-prognosis metastatic nonseminomatous germ cell tumor, 135
Bowel
irritability after primary therapy for early prostate cancer, 103
preparation, outpatient, for elective colon resection, 170
Brachytherapy
interstitial

of breast, ultrasound localization of lumpectomy cavity for, 79
in prostate cancer, early, biopsy results after, 112
intracavitary, in cervix cancer, dynamics of pear-shaped dimensions and volumes of, 292
radiation biology in, 291
radiotherapy combined with, external beam, in high-grade soft tissue sarcomas of extremity with positive microscopic margin, 296

Brain
tumors, 227
vertex field treatment of, dose estimation to critical organs from, 227

BRCA1
breast cancer patients, survival of, 8
mutations
in breast cancer, differences between *BRCA2* mutations and, 37
in breast cancer, prevalence and contribution of, 33
inherited predisposition to cancer and, recommendations for follow-up care of individuals with, 36
in ovarian cancer, 25
in ovarian cancer, prevalence and contribution of, 33
ovarian cancer patients, survival of, 8

BRCA2
mutations
in breast cancer, differences between *BRCA1* mutations and, 37
and inherited predisposition to cancer, recommendations for follow-up care of individuals with, 36

Breast
brachytherapy of, interstitial, ultrasound localization of lumpectomy cavity for, 79
cancer, 61
advanced, locally, breast conservation after induction chemotherapy for, 69
BRCA1, survival of patients with, 8
BRCA1 mutations in, prevalence and contribution of, 33
clinical guidelines program for, impact of, 345
cyclophosphamide and fluorouracil combined with mitoxantrone *vs.* doxorubicin for, 67
docetaxel in, fluid retention due to, corticosteroids delay onset of, 351
ductal in situ, 76
ductal in situ, autopsy series used to estimate disease "reservoir" for, 77
estrogen receptor-positive, tamoxifen in, response to, and HER-2 expression, 62
estrogen-receptor positive, node-negative, tamoxifen and chemotherapy for, 63
familial, pathology of, 37
incidence after mantle field radiation, 336
intraductal, lumpectomy and radiotherapy for, 80
lymphadenectomy in, axillary, overnight closed suction drainage after, 78
lymphadenectomy in, sentinel, 82
metastases, lytic bone, pamidronate in prevention of skeletal complications in, 346
metastasis of, axillary node, detection with Tc-99m scintimammography, 41
node-negative, sentinel node biopsy to avoid axillary dissection in, 75
node-positive, in premenopausal women, radiotherapy and chemotherapy for, 72
node-positive, postmenopausal, chemotherapy/tamoxifen in, 64
operable, primary chemotherapy in, 70
primary, doxorubicin/cyclophosphamide regimen in, increased intensification and total dose of cyclophosphamide in, 68
regional, surgical treatment for, stress and immune responses after, 74
risk after radiotherapy for Hodgkin's disease in splenectomized patients, 337
screening in public hospital emergency room, costs and effects of, 32
sentinel lymph node hypothesis for, histopathologic validation of, 39
T1a, axillary lymph node dissection in, 83
carcinoma (*see* Breast, cancer *above*)
conservation after induction chemotherapy for locally advanced breast cancer, 69
masses in women treated for childhood cancer, incidence and screening guidelines, 61

Bronchial
  epithelium of smokers, molecular damage in, 3
Busulfan
  levels, plasma, effect on outcome after marrow transplantation for chronic myeloid leukemia, 281
L-*S,R*-Buthionine sulfoximine
  continuous infusion, with IV melphalan, phase I study of, 325

C

CA 125
  levels
    raised serum, risk of ovarian cancer diagnosis after, 24
    response to altretamine in relapsed ovarian carcinoma by, 95
Cancer
  biology, 13
  bladder (*see* Bladder, cancer)
  bone, primary, CT and MRI in local staging of, 263
  breast (*see* Breast, cancer)
  cervix (*see* Cervix, cancer)
  chemotherapy modulation by green tea (in mice), 321
  childhood, breast masses in women treated for, incidence and screening guidelines, 61
  colon (*see* Colon, cancer)
  colorectal (*see* Colorectal, cancer)
  diagnosis, 13
  endometrium, relationship of local and distant failure from, 87
  epidemiology, 1
  etiology, 1
  gastric (*see* Gastric, cancer)
  gastrointestinal, 139
  genitourinary, 115
  germ cell, metastatic
    good-prognosis nonseminomatous, bleomycin/etoposide/cisplatin *vs.* bleomycin/etoposide/carboplatin in, 125
    prognostic factor-based staging system for, 115
  gynecologic, 85
  head and neck, 243
  lung (*see* Lung, cancer)
  markers, 13
  noncolorectal, nonneuroendocrine, hepatic resection for metastases from, 152
  nonmyeloid, chemotherapy in, effect of epoetin alfa on clinical outcomes, 350
  ovaries (*see* Ovaries, cancer)
  pancreas (*see* Pancreas, cancer)
  predisposition to, inherited, recommendations for follow-up care of individuals with, 36
  prostate (*see* Prostate, cancer)
  rectum (*see* Rectum, cancer)
  second, risk among long-term survivors of testicular cancer, 121
  secondary, after aclarubicin or daunorubicin plus cytosine arabinoside in acute myeloid leukemia, 205
  skin, 255
  testes (*see* Testes, cancer)
  therapy, clinicians' attitudes to clinical trials of, 322
  undefeated, 1
  urothelium, metastatic, previously untreated, gemcitabine in, 128
Candida
  infection after allogeneic bone marrow transplantation, incidence and risk factors for, 279
Candidiasis
  hepatosplenic, and acute leukemia, 200
Carboplatin
  in chemotherapy regimen, subsequent, in platinum pretreated ovarian cancer, predictors of response to, 99
  in ovarian cancer
    dose-effect study of, 314
    persistent/relapsed, with autologous transplantation, 286
  /paclitaxel
    in ovarian cancer, stage III and IV, 316
    in urothelial carcinoma, advanced, 127
Carboxyamidotriazole
  oral, phase I clinical and pharmacokinetic study of, 326
Carboxylesterase
  rabbit liver, overexpression sensitizes human tumor cells to CPT-11, 311
Carcinoembryonic
  antigen monitoring, value in curative surgery for recurrent colorectal carcinoma, 174
Carcinoid
  pleural, surgically treated, adjuvant photodynamic therapy in, 331
Carcinoma
  adenocarcinoma (*see* Adenocarcinoma)
  anus, National Cancer Data Base report on, 142

basal cell, of face, surgery *vs.* radiotherapy for, 258
bladder (*see* Bladder, cancer)
breast (*see* Breast, cancer)
cervix (*see* Cervix, cancer)
colon (*see* Colon, cancer)
colorectal (*see* Colorectal, cancer)
extrapulmonary small cell, 231
gastric (*see* Gastric, cancer)
larynx, glottic, T3 squamous cell, definitive radiotherapy for, 250
lung (*see* Lung, cancer)
nasopharynx
pterygopalatine fossa and maxillary nerve infiltration in, 245
radiotherapy alone in, 248
ovaries (*see* Ovaries, cancer)
pancreas (*see* Pancreas, cancer)
prostate (*see* Prostate, cancer)
rectum (*see* Rectum, cancer)
testis (*see* Testes, cancer)
urothelium, advanced, paclitaxel/carboplatin in, 127
Care
follow-up, recommendations for individuals with inherited predisposition to cancer, 36
support, best, alone or with chemotherapy in advanced gastric cancer, 177
supportive, 345
for women with ovarian cancer, patterns of, in U.S., 85
CEA
monitoring, value in curative surgery for recurrent colorectal carcinoma, 174
Cell(s)
basal cell carcinoma of face, surgery *vs.* radiotherapy for, 258
B-cell
leukemia, de novo prolymphocytic, cladribine in, 199
lymphoma, marginal zone, of parotid glands, radiotherapy *vs.* combined therapy in, 209
germ (*see* Germ cell)
granulosa cell tumors, ovarian, serum inhibin and disease status in, 23
killer, natural, responses after surgical treatment for regional breast cancer, effect of stress on, 74
lung cancer, small, activated raf-1 causes growth arrest in, 47
mantle cell lymphoma, clinicopathologic study of, 208
ovarian carcinoma, growth inhibitory effects of sodium phenylacetate on, in vitro, 313
progenitor, peripheral blood, mobilization and transplantation in non-Hodgkin's lymphoma, recombinant methionyl human stem cell factor and filgrastim for, 328
Reed-Sternberg, of Hodgkin's disease, fascin as marker for, 16
squamous cell carcinoma (*see* Squamous cell carcinoma)
stem (*see* Stem cell)
T-, circulating atypical, with cerebriform nuclei, in Sézary syndrome, 211
tumor
killing by antineoplastic agents in vitro, telomerase activity decline as measure of, 13
sensitivity to CPT-11, effect of overexpression of rabbit liver carboxylesterase on, 311
Central nervous system
toxicity after cisplatin/ifosfamide in advanced squamous carcinoma of cervix, 89
Cerebellar
neurotoxicity after oral carboxyamidotriazole, 326
Cerebriform
nuclei, circulating atypical T-cells with, in Sézary syndrome, 211
Cervix
cancer
brachytherapy in, intracavitary, dynamics of pear-shaped dimensions and volume of, 292
invasive, papillomavirus infection as risk factor for, 10
screening in public hospital emergency room, costs and effects of, 32
squamous cell, advanced, cisplatin alone *vs.* cisplatin/mitolactol *vs.* cisplatin/ifosfamide in, 89
squamous cell, advanced, TNP-470 in, 324
stage Ib-IIa, radical surgery *vs.* radiotherapy for, 100
carcinoma *(see* cancer *above)*
Chemoradiation
adjuvant, with pelvic exenteration for locally advanced rectal carcinoma, 139
of anal carcinoma, 143
in breast cancer in premenopausal women, 72

node-positive, 72
in Hodgkin's disease, stage I to IIA, *vs.* subtotal lymphoid irradiation, 215
in lymphoma, marginal zone B-cell, 211
strategies, pre- and postoperative, in patients treated with pancreaticoduodenectomy for pancreas adenocarcinoma, 169
Chemotherapy
adjuvant, for localized resectable soft tissue sarcoma, 266
agents, selective resistance to, p53-dependent regulation of *MDR1* gene expression causing (in rodent), 54
in anal carcinoma, 143
cancer, modulation by green tea (in mice), 321
combination, importance of bleomycin in, for good-prognosis nonseminomatous testicular cancer, 130
in extrapulmonary small cell carcinoma, 232
fluorouracil-modulated, combined with pelvic radiotherapy for rectal cancer, 164
in gastric cancer, advanced, plus best supportive care, 177
high-dose
with autologous transplantation for persistent/relapsed ovarian cancer, 286
stem cell transplantation and, autologous, for relapsing Hodgkin's disease, prognostic factors for survival after, 288
induction
for breast cancer, locally advanced, breast conservation after, 69
for leukemia, adult acute, prophylactic platelet transfusion during, 349
induction-sequential, intensive, for poor-prognosis metastatic nonseminomatous germ cell tumor, 135
in leukemia, acute
lymphoblastic, adult, intensive postremission chemo without maintenance therapy, 202
myeloid, intensive consolidation chemo after aclarubicin or daunorubicin plus ara-C, survival and secondary malignancies after, 205
in lymphoma, non-Hodgkin's, intermediate- and high-grade, CHOP regimen, in patients over 70, 207
in nonmyeloid malignancies, effect of epoetin alfa on clinical outcomes during, 350
in ovarian cancer, stage III and IV, combination paclitaxel and carboplatin as first-line chemo, 316
primary, in operable breast cancer, 70
/radiotherapy (*see* Chemoradiation)
salvage, with vinblastine, ifosfamide, and cisplatin in recurrent seminoma, 129
in seminoma
metastatic, radiotherapy after, 132
residual mass after, 133
stage II, 122
subsequent, in platinum pretreated ovarian cancer, predictors of response to, 99
/tamoxifen in breast cancer
node-negative estrogen-receptor positive, 63
node-positive postmenopausal, 64
in testicular cancer, metastatic, residual masses after, 134
Children
cancer in, treatment, breast masses in women after, incidence and screening guidelines, 61
cryptorchidism in, and risk of testicular cancer, 118
medulloblastoma in, potential role of proton therapy in, 225
neuro-ectodermal tumors in, primitive, potential role of proton therapy in, 225
solid tumors in, 225
Chills
after stem cell transplantation, allogeneic blood, 284
2-Chlorodeoxyadenosine
in leukemia, de novo B-cell prolymphocytic, 199
Cholangiopancreatography
endoscopic retrograde, in diagnostic workup for suspected pancreatic carcinoma, 162
CHOP
regimen in lymphoma, intermediate- and high-grade non-Hodgkin's, in patients over 70, 207
Chromosome
Philadelphia chromosome-positive chronic myelogenous leukemia, all-trans retinoic acid in, 201

Cigarette
smokers, molecular damage in bronchial epithelium of, 3
smoking causing mitochondrial genome damage, 35
Cisplatin
alone or with mitolactol or ifosfamide in advanced squamous carcinoma of cervix, 89
-based chemotherapy
induction, for metastatic testicular cancer, residual masses after, 134
of seminoma, residual mass after, 133
/bleomycin/etoposide *vs.* carboplatin/bleomycin/etoposide in good-prognosis metastatic nonseminomatous germ cell cancer, 125
/docetaxel in advanced solid tumors, phase I and pharmacologic study of, 312
in germ cell tumor, poor-prognosis metastatic nonseminomatous, 135
-induced delayed emesis, ondansetron/dexamethasone *vs.* metoclopramide/dexamethasone in prevention of, 348
/paclitaxel in advanced ovarian cancer, cost-effectiveness of, 90
in seminoma, recurrent, 129
with stem cell transplantation, tandem autologous, for multiple myeloma, 285
Cladribine
in leukemia, de novo B-cell prolymphocytic, 199
Clinical
guidelines program for breast and colon cancer, impact of, 345
trials of cancer therapy, clinicians' attitudes toward, 322
Clinicians
attitudes to clinical trials of cancer therapy, 322
Clinicopathologic
study of mantle cell lymphoma, 208
Coagulopathy
disseminated intravascular, after suramin/leuprolide/flutamide in previously untreated metastatic prostate cancer, 107
Cognitive
impairment after TNP-470 in squamous cell cancer of cervix, 324
Colectomy
abdominal, in hereditary nonpolyposis colorectal cancer, rectal cancer risk after, 161
Collagenase
type IV expression and progression of ovarian carcinoma (in mice), 27
Colon
adenocarcinoma, laparoscopic *vs.* open resection for, 141
adenomas 5 mm or less in diameter, importance of detection by sigmoidoscopy, 183
cancer
(*See also* Colorectal, cancer)
clinical guidelines program for, impact of, 345
hemicolectomy for, open *vs.* laparoscopic right, cost of, 149
node-negative, vessel counts and expression of vascular endothelial growth factor as prognostic factors in, 157
nonpolyposis, hereditary, follow-up care of individuals with inherited predisposition to, 190
survival in, mutated p53 gene as independent adverse predictor of, 194
carcinoma *(see* cancer *above)*
resection, elective, outpatient bowel preparation for, 170
Colony-stimulating factor
granulocyte
in *Fusarium* infections in hematologic cancer patients, 335
with paclitaxel/topotecan in ovarian epithelial malignancies, 327
stem cell factor and, recombinant methionyl human, for peripheral blood progenitor cell mobilization and transplantation in non-Hodgkin's lymphoma, 328
in stem cell transplantation, allogeneic blood, for hematologic malignancies, hematopoietic recovery after, 283
granulocyte-macrophage, with tandem autologous transplantation for multiple myeloma, 284–285
Colorectal
cancer
(*See also* Colon, cancer; Rectum, cancer)
K-*ras* DNA mutation detected in plasma or serum of patients with, 21
liver metastases from, resection of, significance of lymph node involvement at hepatic hilum in, 147

locally advanced, extended resection for, 151
metastases from, hepatic, cryosurgical ablation of, 159
metastases from, hepatic, recurrent, survival after repeat hepatic resection for, 146
nonpolyposis, hereditary, abdominal colectomy in, rectal cancer risk after, 161
recurrent, value of carcinoembryonic antigen monitoring in curative surgery for, 174
resection for, follow-up after, 150
stage B, identifying patients at high risk of tumor recurrence and death, 158
surgery for, radical, follow-up after, 184
surgery for, radioimmunoguided, 329
carcinoma *(see* cancer *above)*
mucosal prostaglandins, suppression of, 163
Complications of therapy, 333
Computed tomography (*see* Tomography, computed)
Corticosteroids
delay onset of docetaxel-induced fluid retention, 351
Cost(s)
of bowel preparation for elective colon resection, 170
of cervical and breast cancer screening in public hospital emergency room, 32
-effectiveness
of extending screening mammography guidelines to include women 40 to 49 years of age, 34
of paclitaxel in combination therapy for advanced ovarian cancer, 90
of hemicolectomy for cancer, open *vs.* laparoscopic right, 149
of soft tissue reconstruction of posterior oral cavity and oropharynx, free *vs.* pedicled, 243
Counseling
telephone, to enhance adherence after abnormal Pap smears among low-income minority women, 86
CPT-11
human tumor cell sensitivity to, effect of overexpression of rabbit liver carboxylesterase on, 311
Cryosurgical
ablation of hepatic metastases from colorectal carcinoma, 159
Cryptorchidism
risk of testicular cancer in boys with, 118
CT (*see* Tomography, computed)
Cutaneous (*see* Skin)
Cyclophosphamide
in breast cancer
node-positive, in premenopausal women, with radiotherapy, 72
operable, 71
radiotherapy with, in premenopausal women, 73
in chemotherapy regimen plus tamoxifen in breast cancer
node-negative estrogen-receptor positive, 63
node-positive postmenopausal, 66
/doxorubicin regimen in primary breast cancer, increased intensification and total dose of cyclophosphamide in, 68
/fluorouracil combined with mitoxantrone *vs.* doxorubicin for breast cancer, 67
in induction chemotherapy for locally advanced breast cancer, breast conservation after, 69
in lymphoma, intermediate- and high-grade non-Hodgkin's, in patients over 70, 207
in lymphoma, marginal zone B-cell, 211
in ovarian cancer, persistent/relapsed, with autologous transplantation, 286
with stem cell transplantation, tandem autologous, for multiple myeloma, 284
Cyclosporine
in ovarian cancer, persistent/relapsed, with autologous transplantation, 286
in stem cell transplantation, allogeneic blood, for hematologic malignancies, hematopoietic recovery after, 283
Cyst
ovaries, telomerase activity in, 30
Cystadenoma
ovarian, telomerase activity in, 29
Cytarabine
in leukemia, acute adult lymphoblastic, 202
with stem cell transplantation, tandem autologous, for multiple myeloma, 285

Cytokines
hematopoietic, to accelerate recovery of immune system after irradiation (in mice), 19
Cytology
fine-needle aspiration, in pancreatic cancer
resectable, 168
suspected, 162
Cytoreductive
surgery, secondary, at second-look laparotomy in advanced ovarian cancer, 97
Cytosine arabinoside
plus aclarubicin or daunorubicin in acute myeloid leukemia, survival and secondary malignancies after, 205

D

Daunorubicin
plus cytosine arabinoside in acute myeloid leukemia, survival and secondary malignancies after, 205
Dental
extraction timing in management of oral cavity and oropharyngeal malignancies, 247
Deoxyribonucleic acid
K-*ras,* mutant, detection in plasma or serum of colorectal cancer patients, 21
Dexamethasone
/ondansetron *vs.* dexamethasone/metoclopramide in prevention of cisplatin-induced delayed emesis, 348
with stem cell transplantation, tandem autologous, for multiple myeloma, 284
Diagnosis
cancer, 13
Diaphragmatic
weakness, bilateral, as late complication of radiotherapy, 342
Diarrhea
after TNP-470 in squamous cell cancer of cervix, 324
after topotecan, oral, in solid tumors in adults, 310
Difluorodeoxycytidine
in chemotherapy regimen, subsequent, in platinum pretreated ovarian carcinoma, predictors of response to, 99
in urothelium cancer, previously untreated metastatic, 128
Diplopia
after TNP-470 in squamous cell cancer of cervix, 324
Disseminated intravascular coagulopathy
after suramin/leuprolide/flutamide in previously untreated metastatic prostate cancer, 107
DNA
K-*ras,* mutant, detection in plasma or serum of colorectal cancer patients, 21
Docetaxel
in chemotherapy regimen, subsequent, in platinum pretreated ovarian cancer, predictors of response to, 99
/cisplatin in advanced solid tumors, phase I and pharmacologic study of, 312
-induced fluid retention, corticosteroids delay onset of, 351
Dose
estimation to critical organs from vertex field treatment of brain tumors, 227
Doxorubicin
-based adjuvant chemotherapy for localized resectable soft tissue sarcoma, 266
in breast cancer, operable, 71
combined with cyclophosphamide/fluorouracil for breast cancer, 67
/cyclophosphamide regimen in primary breast cancer, increased intensification and total dose of cyclophosphamide in, 68
effect of green tea on (in mice), 321
in induction chemotherapy for locally advanced breast cancer, breast conservation after, 69
liposomal, in refractory ovarian cancer, 96
in lymphoma, intermediate- and high-grade non-Hodgkin's, in patients over 70, 207
with stem cell transplantation, tandem autologous, for multiple myeloma, 284
Drainage
suction, overnight closed, after axillary lymphadenectomy for breast cancer, 78
Drug(s)
antineoplastic, in vitro tumor cell killing by, telomerase activity decline as measure of, 13

chemotherapy, selective resistance to, p53-dependent regulation of *MDR1* gene expression causing (in rodent), 54
resistance
multiple, circumvention by sphinxolides, 307
promoted by *bax*-deficiency, and p53-dependent apoptosis (in mice), 53
synergistic, plus sulfonamide for nocardiosis after bone marrow transplantation, 335
Dysmetria
after TNP-470 in squamous cell cancer of cervix, 324

E

Edentulation
timing in management of oral cavity and oropharyngeal malignancies, 247
Elderly
gastric cancer in, advanced, chemotherapy plus best supportive care *vs.* supportive care alone in, 177
incontinence in, urinary, after primary therapy for early prostate cancer, 103
lymphoma in, non-Hodgkin's, intermediate- and high-grade, CHOP regimen in, 207
ovarian cancer in, 86
advanced, secondary cytoreductive surgery at second-look laparotomy in, 97
prostate cancer in, metastatic, previously untreated, suramin, leuprolide, and flutamide in, 107
Electrolyte
-polyethylene glycol lavage solution in outpatient bowel preparation for elective colon resection, 170
Emergency
room, public hospital, costs and effects of cervical and breast cancer screening in, 32
Emesis
after altretamine in relapsed ovarian carcinoma, 95
after carboxyamidotriazole, oral, 326
cisplatin-induced delayed, ondansetron/dexamethasone *vs.* metoclopramide/dexamethasone in prevention of, 348
Endometrium
cancer, relationship of local and distant failure from, 87
Endoscopic
retrograde cholangiopancreatography in diagnostic workup for suspected pancreatic carcinoma, 162
Endothelial
growth factor, vascular (*see* Growth, factor, vascular endothelial)
Environmental
tobacco smoke, and lung cancer, 5
Epidemiology
of cancer, 1
Epirubicin
in chemotherapy regimen, subsequent, in platinum pretreated ovarian cancer, predictors of response to, 99
Epithelial
ovarian cancer (*see* Ovaries, cancer, epithelial)
ovarian tumors, benign, telomerase activity in, 29
Epithelium
bronchial, of smokers, molecular damage in, 3
Epoetin
alfa, effect on clinical outcomes of nonmyeloid malignancies during cancer chemotherapy, 350
Erythroderma
in Sézary syndrome, 211
Estrogen
receptor-positive breast cancer
node-negative, tamoxifen and chemotherapy for, 63
tamoxifen in, response to, and HER-2 expression, 62
Etiology
of cancer, 1
Etoposide
/bleomycin with cisplatin *vs.* carboplatin in good-prognosis metastatic nonseminomatous germ cell cancer, 125
in chemotherapy plus supportive care in advanced gastric cancer, 177
in germ cell tumor, poor-prognosis metastatic nonseminomatous, 135
in leukemia, acute adult lymphoblastic, 203
with stem cell transplantation, tandem autologous, for multiple myeloma, 285
topotecan and, effect on topoisomerase IIα levels (in mice), 309

Extraction
  timing in management of oral cavity and oropharyngeal malignancies, 247
Extramedullary
  leukemia, adverse effect on hematologic complete remission rate and survival in patients with t(8;21)(q22;q22), 203
Extrapulmonary
  small cell carcinoma, 231
Extremity
  sarcoma, soft tissue (*see* Sarcoma, soft tissue, extremity)

F

Face
  carcinoma, basal cell, surgery *vs.* radiotherapy for, 258
Fascin
  as marker for Reed-Sternberg cells of Hodgkin's disease, 16
Fatigue
  after altretamine in relapsed ovarian carcinoma, 95
  after carboxyamidotriazole, oral, 326
FDG
  PET in lymph node staging in non-small cell lung cancer, 48
    vs. CT, 50
Fever
  after stem cell transplantation, allogeneic blood, 284
Fibroblast
  growth factor, basic, expression, and progression of ovarian carcinoma (in mice), 27
Filgrastim (*see* Colony-stimulating factor, granulocyte)
Flaps
  free *vs.* pedicled pectoralis major myocutaneous, in reconstruction of posterior oral cavity and oropharynx, 243
Fluid
  retention, docetaxel-induced, corticosteroids delay onset of, 351
Fluorescence
  imaging and spectroscopy of 5-aminolevulinic acid induced protoporphyrin IX for detection of neoplastic lesions in oral cavity, 55
Fluoro-1-deoxy-D-glucose
  PET in lymph node staging in non-small cell lung cancer, 48
    vs. CT, 50
Fluorouracil
  -based chemotherapy plus supportive care in advanced gastric cancer, 177
  in breast cancer
    node-positive, in premenopausal women, with radiotherapy, 72
    operable, 71
    radiotherapy with, in premenopausal women, 73
  in chemotherapy regimen plus tamoxifen in breast cancer
    node-negative estrogen-receptor positive, 63
    node-positive postmenopausal, 66
  /cyclophosphamide combined with mitoxantrone *vs.* doxorubicin for breast cancer, 67
  in induction chemotherapy for locally advanced breast cancer, breast conservation after, 69
  -modulated chemotherapy combined with pelvic radiation therapy for rectal cancer, 164
  in rectal carcinoma, locally advanced, with preoperative and intraoperative radiotherapy, 144
Flutamide
  /suramin/leuprolide in prostate cancer, previously untreated metastatic, 107
Follicular
  lymphoma, incidence, predictive factors, and outcome of lymphoma transformation in, 214
Foot
  hand-foot syndrome after liposomal doxorubicin in ovarian cancer, 97
Fossa
  pterygopalatine, infiltration in nasopharyngeal carcinoma, 245
Fungal
  infections, invasive, incidence and risk factors after allogeneic bone marrow transplantation, 279
Fusarium
  infection
    after bone marrow transplantation, allogeneic, incidence and risk factors for, 279
    hematologic malignancy and, 334

G

Gastric
  adenocarcinoma, laparoscopy in, 156
  cancer

advanced, chemotherapy plus best supportive care *vs.* best supportive care alone in, 177
lymph node dissection in, effect on survival, 186
proximal, survival benefit of extended D1 resection for, 187
carcinoma *(see* cancer *above)*
Gastrointestinal
cancer, 139
toxicity of TNP-470 in squamous cell cancer of cervix, 324
Gemcitabine
in chemotherapy regimen, subsequent, in platinum pretreated ovarian cancer, predictors of response to, 99
in urothelium cancer, previously untreated metastatic, 128
Gene(s)
angiogenesis-related, expression, and progression of ovarian carcinoma (in mice), 27
BRCA1 (see BRCA1)
BRCA2
mutations, and inherited predisposition to cancer, recommendations for follow-up care of individuals with, 36
mutations in breast cancer, differences between *BRCA1* mutations and, 37
MDR1, expression, p53-dependent regulation of, and selective resistance to chemotherapy agents (in rodent), 54
p53, mutation as independent adverse predictor of survival in colon carcinoma, 194
Wilms' tumor, mRNA levels, in acute myeloid leukemia, and long-term outcome, 18
Genitourinary
cancer, 115
Genome
mitochondrial, damage associated with smoking, 35
Germ cell
cancer, metastatic
good-prognosis nonseminomatous, bleomycin/etoposide/cisplatin *vs.* bleomycin/etoposide/carboplatin in, 125
staging system for, prognostic factor-based, 115
tumor, metastatic, poor-prognosis nonseminomatous, intensive induction-sequential chemotherapy for, 135
Glottic
larynx, T3 squamous cell carcinoma of, definitive radiotherapy for, 250
Goserelin
in prostate cancer after radiotherapy, 108
Graft
-*vs.*-host disease as risk factor for invasive fungal infections after allogeneic bone marrow transplantation, 279
xenografts of non-small cell lung carcinoma, advantage of residualizing iodine radiolabel for radioimmunotherapy of, 52
Granulocyte
colony-stimulating factor (*see* Colony-stimulating factor, granulocyte)
-macrophage colony-stimulating factor with tandem autologous transplantation for multiple myeloma, 284–285
transfusions in *Fusarium* infections in hematologic cancer patients, 335
Granulocytopenia
after docetaxel/cisplatin in advanced solid tumors, 312
Granulosa
cell tumors, ovarian, serum inhibin and disease status in, 23
Green tea
modulation of cancer chemotherapy by (in mice), 321
Growth
factor
basic fibroblast, expression, and progression of ovarian carcinoma (in mice), 27
vascular endothelial, content in prostatic tissue, regulation by androgens, 44
vascular endothelial, expression, and progression of ovarian carcinoma (in mice), 27
vascular endothelial, expression as prognostic factor in node-negative colon cancer, 157
Guidelines
clinical guidelines program for breast and colon cancer, impact of, 345
mammography, screening, cost-effectiveness of extending to include women 40 to 49 years of age, 34
Gynecologic
cancer, 85

H

Hand
 -foot syndrome after liposomal doxorubicin in ovarian cancer, 97
Head and neck
 cancer, 243
Headache
 after stem cell transplantation, allogeneic blood, 284
Health
 risk behaviors, physician discussion of, relation to patient income, 2
Hematologic
 complete remission rate in patients with t(8;21) (q22;q22), extramedullary leukemia adversely affects hematologic complete remission rate and overall survival in patients with, 203
 malignancies
  bone marrow transplantation for, autologous, effect of age on outcome after, 282
  Fusarium infection and, 334
  stem cell transplantation in, autologous blood, *vs.* allogeneic bone marrow transplantation, hematopoietic recovery after, 283
 toxicity
  after paclitaxel/topotecan in ovarian epithelial malignancies, 327
  after topotecan in resistant ovarian cancer, 94
Hematopoietic
 cytokines to accelerate recovery of immune system after irradiation (in mice), 19
 recovery after allogeneic blood stem cell transplantation *vs.* allogeneic bone marrow transplantation in hematologic malignancies, 283
Hemicolectomy
 right, open *vs.* laparoscopic, for cancer, cost of, 149
Hepatic (*see* Liver)
Hepatosplenic
 candidiasis and acute leukemia, 200
HER-2
 expression and response to tamoxifen in estrogen-receptor positive breast cancer, 62
Hilum
 hepatic, lymph node involvement at, significance in resection of colorectal liver metastases, 147
Histology
 retroperitoneal and pulmonary, and residual masses after chemotherapy for metastatic testicular cancer, 134
Histopathologic
 assessment for identification of stage A nonseminomatous testis cancer patients at extremely low risk for metastatic disease, 42
 validation of sentinel lymph node hypothesis for breast carcinoma, 39
Histopathology
 cutaneous, of Sézary syndrome, 211
HLA
 class II matching, effect on unrelated donor marrow transplantation for chronic myeloid leukemia, 280
Hodgkin's disease
 advanced, is combined modality therapy necessary for? 217
 bone marrow transplantation for, autologous, effect of age on outcome of, 282
 radiotherapy for
  diaphragmatic weakness as late complication of, bilateral, 342
  mantle field, breast cancer incidence after, 336
  in splenectomized patients, breast cancer risk after, 337
 Reed-Sternberg cells of, fascin as marker for, 16
 relapsing, prognostic factors for survival after high-dose therapy and autologous stem cell transplantation for, 288
 stage I, treatment, long-term outcome of, 222
 stage I to IIA, chemotherapy plus regional irradiation *vs.* subtotal lymphoid irradiation in, 215
Hormone
 treatment, immediate *vs.* deferred, for advanced prostate cancer, 106
Hospital
 emergency room, public, costs and effects of cervical and breast cancer screening in, 32
 volume influences outcome of pancreatic resection for cancer, 140
Hybridization
 in situ, of messenger RNA for angiogenesis-related genes in ovarian carcinoma (in mice), 27
Hydrocortisone
 /suramin/leuprolide/flutamide in previously untreated metastatic prostate cancer, 107

Hyperthermic
isolated limb perfusion with tumor necrosis factor, angiographic response of locally advanced soft tissue sarcoma after, 271
Hysterectomy
radiotherapy after, for endometrial cancer, relationship of local and distant failure after, 87

I

Ibuprofen
ovarian cancer risk with, 7
Ifosfamide
/cisplatin in advanced squamous carcinoma of cervix, 89
in germ cell tumor, poor-prognosis metastatic nonseminomatous, 135
in seminoma, recurrent, 129
Imaging
fluorescence, of 5-aminolevulinic acid induced protoporphyrin IX for detection of neoplastic lesions in oral cavity, 55
magnetic resonance
in local staging of primary malignant musculoskeletal neoplasms, 263
of pterygopalatine fossa and maxillary nerve infiltration in nasopharyngeal carcinoma, 245
Immune
responses after surgical treatment for regional breast cancer, and stress, 74
system recovery after irradiation, acceleration by hematopoietic cytokines (in mice), 19
Immunohistochemical
analysis for angiogenesis-related genes in ovarian carcinoma (in mice), 27
assessment for identification of stage A nonseminomatous testis cancer patients at extremely low risk for metastatic disease, 42
Immunophenotype
in lymphoma, primary anaplastic large-cell, 213
Impotence
patient-reported, after nerve-sparing radical prostatectomy, 104
Income
low-income minority women, enhancing adherence after abnormal Pap smears among, 86
patient, related to physician discussion of health risk behaviors, 2
Incontinence
urinary
after primary therapy for early prostate cancer, in elderly, 103
after prostatectomy, nerve-sparing radical, 104
Infection
fungal, invasive, incidence and risk factors after allogeneic bone marrow transplantation, 279
after suramin/leuprolide/flutamide in previously untreated metastatic prostate cancer, 107
Infertile
couples, prevalence of carcinoma in situ of testis in oligozoospermic men from, 137
Inhibin
serum, and disease status in ovarian granulosa cell tumors, 23
Interferon
-gamma in hyperthermic isolated limb perfusion, angiographic response of locally advanced soft tissue sarcoma after, 271–272
Interleukin
-3 combined with IL-11 to accelerate recovery of immune system after irradiation (in mice), 19
-8 expression and progression of ovarian carcinoma (in mice), 27
International Prognostic Scoring System
for myelodysplastic syndromes, 198
Intravascular
coagulation, disseminated, after suramin/leuprolide/flutamide in previously untreated metastatic prostate cancer, 107
Iodine
radiolabel for radioimmunotherapy of xenografts of non-small cell lung carcinoma, advantage of residualizing, 52
Iodine-125
radiation, interstitial, in localized prostate cancer, 110
Irinotecan
in chemotherapy regimen, subsequent, in platinum pretreated ovarian cancer, predictors of response to, 99
Irradiation (*see* Radiation)

K

Keratopathy
  vortex, after suramin/leuprolide/flutamide in previously untreated metastatic prostate cancer, 107
Killer cell
  natural, responses after surgical treatment for regional breast cancer, effect of stress on, 74
K-*ras*
  DNA, mutant, detection in plasma or serum of colorectal cancer patients, 21

L

Laparoscopy
  colonic resection by, *vs.* open, for adenocarcinoma, 141
  in diagnostic workup for suspected pancreatic carcinoma, 162
  hemicolectomy by, *vs.* open procedure for cancer, cost of, 149
  management of gastric adenocarcinoma by, 156
Laparotomy
  second-look, in advanced ovarian cancer, secondary cytoreductive surgery at, 97
Larynx
  glottic, T3 squamous cell carcinoma of, definitive radiotherapy for, 250
Lavage
  solution, polyethylene glycol-electrolyte, in outpatient bowel preparation for elective colon resection, 170
Leucovorin
  added to fluorouracil-modulated chemotherapy combined with pelvic radiation therapy for rectal cancer, 164
  in chemotherapy plus supportive care in advanced gastric cancer, 177
Leukemia
  acute
    adult, prophylactic platelet transfusion during induction therapy for, 349
    candidiasis and, hepatosplenic, 200
  adult, 197
  extramedullary, adverse effect on hematologic complete remission rate and survival in patients with t(8;21) (q22;q22), 203
  lymphoblastic, acute adult, intensive postremission chemotherapy without maintenance therapy in, 202
  lymphocytic, chronic, splenectomy in, 197
  myelogenous
    acute, bone marrow transplantation for, autologous, effect of age on outcome of, 282
    Philadelphia chromosome-positive, all-trans retinoic acid in, 201
  myeloid
    acute, aclarubicin or daunorubicin plus cytosine arabinoside in, survival and secondary malignancies after, 205
    acute, Wilms' tumor gene mRNA levels in, and long-term outcome, 18
    acute, with t(8;21) translocation, effect of extramedullary leukemia on hematologic remission and survival in, 203
    chronic, bone marrow transplantation for, effect of plasma busulfan levels on outcome, 281
    chronic, bone marrow transplantation for, matched unrelated donor, effect of HLA class II matching on, 280
  prolymphocytic, de novo B-cell, cladribine in, 199
Leukocytopenia
  after docetaxel/cisplatin in advanced solid tumors, 312
Leukopenia
  after cisplatin/ifosfamide in advanced squamous carcinoma of cervix, 89
Leuprolide
  /suramin/flutamide in prostate cancer, previously untreated metastatic, 107
Levamisole
  added to fluorouracil-modulated chemotherapy combined with pelvic radiation therapy for rectal cancer, 164
Limb
  perfusion, hyperthermic isolated, with tumor necrosis factor, angiographic response of locally advanced soft tissue sarcoma after, 271
Liposarcoma
  outcome and prognostic factors after conservation surgery and radiation therapy, 276

Liposomal
doxorubicin in refractory ovarian cancer, 96
Liver
carboxylesterase, rabbit, overexpression sensitizes human tumor cells to CPT-11, 311
hilum, lymph node involvement at, significance in resection of colorectal liver metastases, 147
metastases (*see* Metastases, liver)
resection
for metastases, noncolorectal, nonneuroendocrine, 152
for metastatic colorectal cancer results in cure for some patients, 155
repeat, for recurrent colorectal hepatic metastases, survival after, 146
veno-occlusive disease after busulfan in marrow transplantation for chronic myeloid leukemia, 281–282
Lobectomy
vs. wedge resection for stage I non-small cell lung cancer, 237
Lumpectomy
in breast carcinoma, ductal in situ, radiotherapy after, 76
cavity for interstitial brachytherapy of breast, ultrasound localization of, 79
/radiotherapy for intraductal breast cancer, 80
Lung
cancer, 231
non-small cell, lymph node staging in, 48
non-small cell, lymph node staging in, FDG-PET *vs.* CT for, 50
non-small cell, radioimmunotherapy of xenografts of, advantage of residualizing iodine radiolabel for, 52
non-small cell, radiotherapy of, conformal, dose escalation, 298
non-small cell, stage I, wedge resection *vs.* lobectomy for, 237
non-small cell, with ipsilateral mediastinal node involvement, surgical adjuvant thoracic radiation therapy in, 234
small cell, activated raf-1 causes growth arrest in cells of, 47
small cell, utility of screening procedures for detecting recurrence of disease after complete response in, 233
tobacco smoke and, environmental, 5
carcinoma *(see* cancer *above)*
metastasectomy, factors influencing long-term survival after, 239
resection, wedge, *vs.* lobectomy for stage I non-small cell lung cancer, 237
Lymph node
axillary
dissection in T1a breast cancer, 83
metastasis of breast carcinoma, detection with Tc-99m sestamibi scintimammography, 41
dissection in gastric cancer, effect on survival, 186
involvement at hepatic hilum in resection of colorectal liver metastases, 147
mediastinal, ipsilateral involvement in non-small cell lung cancer, surgical adjuvant thoracic radiation therapy in, 234
sentinel
biopsy, to avoid axillary dissection in breast cancer with clinically negative nodes, 75
dissection, optimal selective, in primary melanoma, 255
hypothesis for breast carcinoma, histopathologic validation of, 39
staging in non-small cell lung cancer, 48
FDG-PET *vs.* CT for, 50
Lymphadenectomy
axillary, for breast cancer, overnight closed suction drainage after, 78
sentinel, in breast cancer, 82
Lymphatic
irradiation, comprehensive, in low-grade non-Hodgkin's lymphoma, 220
Lymphoblastic
leukemia, acute adult, intensive postremission chemotherapy without maintenance therapy in, 202
Lymphocytic
leukemia, chronic, splenectomy in, 197
Lymphoid
irradiation, subtotal, in clinical stage I to IIA Hodgkin's disease, 215
Lymphoma
adult, 207
B-cell, marginal zone, of parotid glands, radiotherapy *vs.* combined therapy in, 209
follicular, incidence, predictive factors, and outcome of lymphoma transformation in, 214

large-cell, primary anaplastic, in adults, 213
mantle cell, clinicopathologic study of, 208
non-Hodgkin's
bone marrow transplantation for, autologous, effect of age on outcome of, 282
intermediate- and high-grade, CHOP regimen in, in patients over 70, 207
low-grade, comprehensive lymphatic irradiation in, 220
progenitor cell mobilization and transplantation in, peripheral blood, recombinant methionyl human stem cell factor and filgrastim for, 328
Lytic
bone metastases and breast cancer, pamidronate in prevention of skeletal complications in, 346

M

Macrophage
-granulocyte colony-stimulating factor with tandem autologous transplantation for multiple myeloma, 284–285
Magnetic resonance imaging
in local staging of primary malignant musculoskeletal neoplasms, 263
of pterygopalatine fossa and maxillary nerve infiltration in nasopharyngeal carcinoma, 245
Malignancies
hematologic (*see* Hematologic, malignancies)
oral cavity and oropharyngeal, timing of edentulation and extraction in, 247
pleural, surgically treated, adjuvant photodynamic therapy in, 330
second, after radiotherapy for prostate carcinoma, 339
Mammography
scintimammography, technetium-99m sestamibi, detection of axillary node metastasis of breast carcinoma with, 41
screening
benefit, role of numeracy in understanding, 35
guidelines, cost-effectiveness of extending to include women 40 to 49 years of age, 34
Mandible
osteoradionecrosis, resection and immediate microvascular reconstruction for, 244
Mantle
cell lymphoma, clinicopathologic study of, 208
Markers
cancer, 13
Marrow
transplantation (*see* Transplantation, bone marrow)
Maxillary
nerve infiltration in nasopharyngeal carcinoma, 245
MDR1
gene expression, p53-dependent regulation of, and selective resistance to chemotherapy agents (in rodent), 54
Mediastinal
lymph node involvement, ipsilateral, in non-small cell lung cancer, surgical adjuvant thoracic radiation therapy in, 234
Medulloblastoma
pediatric, potential role of proton therapy in, 225
Melanoma
primary, optimal selective lymph node dissection in, 255
stage III, computed tomography in evaluation of, 257
thin, ambulatory narrow excision for, 256
Melphalan
in hyperthermic isolated limb perfusion, angiographic response of locally advanced soft tissue sarcoma after, 271
IV, with L-*S*,*R*-buthionine sulfoximine, phase I study of, 325
in ovarian cancer, persistent/relapsed, with autologous transplantation, 286
with stem cell transplantation, tandem autologous, for multiple myeloma, 285
Meningioma
ordinary, poor outcome predicted by telomerase activity, 14
Mesothelioma
malignant pleural, surgically treated, adjuvant photodynamic therapy in, 331
Metastasectomy
lung, factors influencing long-term survival after, 239

Metastases
bone, lytic, and breast cancer, pamidronate in prevention of skeletal complications in, 346
distant metachronous, from rectal cancer, effect of surgery on, 173
germ cell cancer
good-prognosis nonseminomatous, bleomycin/etoposide/cisplatin *vs.* bleomycin/etoposide/carboplatin in, 125
staging system for, prognostic factor-based, 115
germ cell tumor, poor-prognosis nonseminomatous, intensive induction-sequential chemotherapy for, 135
liver
from colorectal cancer, cryosurgical ablation of, 159
from colorectal cancer, resection of, significance of lymph node involvement at hepatic hilum in, 147
from colorectal cancer, resection results in cure for some patients, 155
noncolorectal, nonneuroendocrine, resection for, 152
recurrent, from colorectal cancer, survival after repeat hepatic resection for, 146
lymph node, axillary, of breast carcinoma, detection with Tc-99m sestamibi scintimammography, 41
prostate cancer, previously untreated, suramin, leuprolide, and flutamide in, 107
seminoma, radiotherapy after chemotherapy for, 132
testis cancer patients at extremely low risk for, stage A nonseminomatous, identification of, 42
urothelium cancer, previously untreated, gemcitabine in, 128
Methionyl
human stem cell factor, recombinant, with filgrastim for peripheral blood progenitor cell mobilization and transplantation in non-Hodgkin's lymphoma, 328
Methotrexate
in breast cancer
node-positive, in premenopausal women, with radiotherapy, 72
operable, 71
radiotherapy with, in premenopausal women, 73
in chemotherapy regimen plus tamoxifen in breast cancer
node-negative estrogen-receptor positive, 63
node-positive postmenopausal, 66
in Hodgkin's disease, 215
in leukemia, acute adult lymphoblastic, 203
Methylprednisolone
delays onset of docetaxel-induced fluid retention, 351
Metoclopramide
/dexamethasone *vs.* ondansetron/dexamethasone in prevention of cisplatin-induced delayed emesis, 348
Microfilament
depletion and circumvention of multiple drug resistance by sphinxolides, 307
Microvascular
reconstruction, immediate, after resection for osteoradionecrosis of mandible, 244
Minority women
low-income, enhancing adherence after abnormal Pap smears among, 86
Mitochondrial
genome damage associated with smoking, 35
Mitolactol
/cisplatin in advanced squamous carcinoma of cervix, 89
Mitotic
activity increase in mantle cell lymphoma, 208
Mitoxantrone
combined with cyclophosphamide/fluorouracil for breast cancer, 67
-containing chemotherapy regimen in operable breast cancer, 71
in leukemia, acute adult lymphoblastic, 203
in ovarian cancer, persistent/relapsed, with autologous transplantation, 286
Molecular
damage in bronchial epithelium of smokers, 3
Monitoring
carcinoembryonic antigen, value in curative surgery for recurrent colorectal carcinoma, 174

Morbidity
after preoperative radiation therapy, resection, and intraoperative radiation therapy for locally advanced rectal carcinoma, 144
Mortality
of bone marrow transplantation for hematologic malignancies, effect of age on, 282
cancer, 1
MRI
in local staging of primary malignant musculoskeletal neoplasms, 263
of pterygopalatine fossa and maxillary nerve infiltration in nasopharyngeal carcinoma, 245
Mucosa
colorectal, suppression of prostaglandins in, 163
Mucositis
after busulfan in marrow transplantation for chronic myeloid leukemia, 281
radiation, sucralfate for, trial results, 354
Muscle
infiltrating bladder carcinoma, transurethral resection for, long-term follow-up, 120
Musculoskeletal
neoplasms, primary malignant, CT and MRI in local staging of, 263
Myalgia
after stem cell transplantation, allogeneic blood, 284
Myelodysplastic
syndromes, international scoring system for evaluating prognosis in, 198
Myelogenous
leukemia
acute, bone marrow transplantation for, autologous, effect of age on outcome of, 282
Philadelphia chromosome-positive, all-trans retinoic acid in, 201
Myeloid
leukemia (*see* Leukemia, myeloid)
Myeloma
multiple
bone marrow transplantation for, autologous, effect of age on outcome of, 282
previously untreated, superiority of tandem autologous transplantation over standard therapy for, 284
Myelosuppression
after paclitaxel/topotecan in ovarian epithelial malignancies, 327
after topotecan in resistant ovarian cancer, 94
Myocutaneous
flaps, pedicled pectoralis major, *vs.* free flaps, in reconstruction of posterior oral cavity and oropharynx, 243

N

Nasopharynx
carcinoma
pterygopalatine fossa and maxillary nerve infiltration in, 245
radiotherapy alone in, 248
Natural killer cell
responses after surgical treatment for regional breast cancer, effect of stress on, 74
Nausea
after altretamine in relapsed ovarian carcinoma, 95
after carboxyamidotriazole, oral, 326
after TNP-470 in squamous cell cancer of cervix, 324
Neck
cancer, 243
Neoplastic
lesions in oral cavity, fluorescence imaging and spectroscopy of 5-aminolevulinic acid induced protoporphyrin for detection of, 55
Nephrotoxicity
after cisplatin/ifosfamide in advanced squamous carcinoma of cervix, 89
Nerve
maxillary, infiltration in nasopharyngeal carcinoma, 245
phrenic, injury, after radiotherapy causing bilateral diaphragmatic weakness, 342
-sparing radical prostatectomy, patient-reported impotence and incontinence after, 104
Nervous system
central, toxicity, after cisplatin/ifosfamide in advanced squamous carcinoma of cervix, 89
Neuro-ectodermal
tumors, primitive, potential role of proton therapy in, 225
Neurologic
toxicity (*see* Neurotoxicity)
Neurotoxicity
cerebellar, after oral carboxyamidotriazole, 326
peripheral, after cisplatin/ifosfamide in advanced squamous carcinoma of cervix, 89

of TNP-470 in squamous cell cancer of cervix, 324
Neutropenia
after paclitaxel/carboplatin in ovarian cancer, 317
after paclitaxel/topotecan in ovarian epithelial malignancies, 327
after suramin/leuprolide/flutamide in previously untreated metastatic prostate cancer, 107
after topotecan in ovarian cancer, 92
resistant, 94
Nocardiosis
after bone marrow transplantation, 335
Node (*see* Lymph node)
Northern blot
analysis for angiogenesis-related genes in ovarian carcinoma (in mice), 27
Novel therapy, 321
NSC 3039
growth inhibitory effects on ovarian carcinoma cells, in vitro, 313
Numeracy
role in understanding benefit of screening mammography, 35
Nystagmus
after TNP-470 in squamous cell cancer of cervix, 324

O

Oligozoospermic
men from infertile couples, prevalence of carcinoma in situ of testis in, 137
Oncofetal
fibronectin in advanced epithelial ovarian cancer, 58
Oncogenic
transformation promoted by *bax*-deficiency, and p53-dependent apoptosis (in mice), 53
Oncologists' attitudes
to clinical trials of cancer therapy, 322
Ondansetron
/dexamethasone *vs.* metoclopramide/dexamethasone in prevention of cisplatin-induced delayed emesis, 348
Oral
cavity
lesions, neoplastic, fluorescence imaging and spectroscopy of 5-aminolevulinic acid induced protoporphyrin for detection of, 55
malignancies, timing of edentulation and extraction in, 247
posterior, reconstruction of, comparison of cost and function in, 243
Orchiectomy
for prostate cancer, osteoporosis after, 333
in seminoma, reproductive function after, 119
Organs
critical, dose estimation from vertex field treatment of brain tumors to, 227
visceral and solid, prevention of radiation damage to, during radiation therapy of trunk, 302
Oropharynx
malignancies, timing of edentulation and extraction in, 247
reconstruction of, comparison of cost and function in, 243
Osteoporosis
after orchiectomy for prostate cancer, 333
Osteoradionecrosis
mandible, resection and immediate microvascular reconstruction for, 244
Ovaries
cancer
advanced, paclitaxel in combination therapy for, cost-effectiveness of, 90
advanced, secondary cytoreductive surgery at second-look laparotomy in, 97
BRCA1, survival of patients with, 8
BRCA1 mutations in, 25
BRCA1 mutations in, prevalence and contribution of, 33
carboplatin in, dose-effect study of, 314
cells, growth inhibitory effects of sodium phenylacetate on, in vitro, 313
diagnosis, and serum CA 125 level, 24
epithelial, advanced, oncofetal fibronectin in, 58
epithelial, in African-Americans, 6
epithelial, p53 overexpression in, mutant, relation to lifetime ovulatory cycles, 22
epithelial, recurrent, topotecan *vs.* paclitaxel for, 91
epithelial, telomerase activity in, 29
paclitaxel sensitivity in, no effect of p53 status on, 318
paclitaxel-resistant, topotecan in, 93

patterns of care for women with, in U.S., 85
persistent/relapsed, high-dose chemotherapy with autologous transplantation for, 286
platinum pretreated, predictors of response to subsequent chemotherapy in, 99
platinum-resistant, topotecan in, 93
progression of, and expression of angiogenesis-related genes (in mice), 27
refractory, liposomal doxorubicin in, 96
relapsed, altretamine in, 95
relapsed, weekly paclitaxel in, phase I and pharmacologic study of, 319
risk, and over-the-counter analgesics, 7
stage III and IV, combination paclitaxel and carboplatin as first-line chemotherapy in, 316
telomerase activity in, 30
carcinoma *(see* cancer *above)*
lesions, malignant, premalignant, and benign, telomerase activity in, 30
tumors
epithelial, benign, telomerase activity in, 29
granulosa cell, serum inhibin and disease status in, 23
Over-the-counter
analgesics and risk of ovarian cancer, 7
Ovulatory
cycles, lifetime, relation to overexpression of mutant p53 in epithelial ovarian cancer, 22

P

p53
-dependent apoptosis, role of *bax* in (in mice), 53
-dependent regulation of *MDR1* gene expression causes selective resistance to chemotherapy agents (in rodent), 54
mutation as independent adverse predictor of survival in colon carcinoma, 194
overexpression, mutant, in epithelial ovarian cancer, relation to lifetime ovulatory cycles, 22
status, no effect on paclitaxel sensitivity in ovarian cancer, 318
Paclitaxel
/carboplatin
in ovarian cancer, stage III and IV, 316
in urothelial carcinoma, advanced, 127
in chemotherapy regimen, subsequent, in platinum pretreated ovarian cancer, predictors of response to, 99
in combination therapy for advanced ovarian cancer, cost-effectiveness of, 90
in ovarian cancer, persistent/relapsed, with autologous transplantation, 286
-resistant ovarian cancer, topotecan in, 93
sensitivity in ovarian cancer, no effect of p53 status on, 318
/topotecan in ovarian epithelial malignancies, phase I and pharmacologic trial of, 327
vs. topotecan for recurrent epithelial ovarian cancer, 91
weekly, in relapsed ovarian cancer, phase I and pharmacologic study of, 319
Pain
after suramin/leuprolide/flutamide in previously untreated metastatic prostate cancer, 107
Pamidronate
in prevention of skeletal complications in patients with breast cancer and lytic bone metastases, 346
Pancreas
adenocarcinoma, pancreaticoduodenectomy for, and preoperative and postoperative chemoradiation strategies, 169
cancer
resectable, fine-needle aspiration in, 168
resection for, hospital volume influences outcome of, 140
suspected, diagnostic workup for, 162
carcinoma *(see* cancer *above)*
Pancreaticoduodenectomy
for pancreas adenocarcinoma, and preoperative and postoperative chemoradiation strategies, 169
Pap smears
abnormal, among low-income minority women, enhancing adherence after, 86
Papillomavirus
infection as risk factor for invasive cervical cancer, 10

Paracetamol
  ovarian cancer risk with, 7
Parotid
  glands, marginal zone B-cell lymphoma of, radiotherapy *vs.* combined therapy in, 209
Pathology
  of breast cancer, familial, 37
Patient
  income related to physician discussion of health risk behaviors, 2
PCR
  for Kl-*ras* DNA mutation in plasma or serum of colorectal cancer patients, 21
Pediatric (*see* Children)
Pelvic
  control after preoperative radiation therapy, resection, and intraoperative radiation therapy for locally advanced rectal carcinoma, 144
  exenteration for locally advanced rectal carcinoma, 139
  radiotherapy with fluorouracil-modulated chemotherapy for rectal cancer, 164
Perfusion
  limb, hyperthermic isolated, with tumor necrosis factor, angiographic response of locally advanced soft tissue sarcoma after, 271
PET
  FDG, in lymph node staging in non-small cell lung cancer, 48
    vs. CT, 50
Pharmacokinetic
  study of oral carboxyamidotriazole, 326
Pharmacologic
  study
    of docetaxel and cisplatin in advanced solid tumors, 312
    of paclitaxel, weekly, in relapsed ovarian cancer, 319
    of paclitaxel/carboplatin combination as first-line chemotherapy in stage III and IV ovarian cancer, 316
    of topotecan, oral, for solid tumors in adults, 310
  trial of paclitaxel/topotecan in ovarian epithelial malignancies, 327
Pharmacology, 307
Philadelphia chromosome
  -positive chronic myelogenous leukemia, all-trans retinoic acid in, 201
Photodynamic therapy
  adjuvant, in surgically treated pleural malignancies, 330
Phrenic
  nerve injury causing bilateral diaphragmatic weakness after radiotherapy, 342
Physician
  discussion of health risk behaviors related to patient income, 2
Platelet
  transfusion, prophylactic, during induction therapy for adult acute leukemia, 349
Platinum
  -based chemotherapy of extrapulmonary small cell carcinoma, 232
  pretreated ovarian cancer, predictors of response to subsequent chemotherapy in, 99
  -resistant ovarian cancer, topotecan in, 93
Pleural
  effusions, malignant, thoracoscopic talc poudrage pleurodesis for, 353
  malignancies, surgically treated, adjuvant photodynamic therapy in, 330
Pleurodesis
  thoracoscopic talc poudrage, for malignant effusions, 353
Polyethylene
  glycol-electrolyte lavage solution in outpatient bowel preparation for elective colon resection, 170
Polymerase chain reaction
  for K-*ras* DNA mutation in plasma or serum of colorectal cancer patients, 21
Positron emission tomography
  FDG, in lymph node staging in non-small cell lung cancer, 48
    vs. CT, 50
Postmenopausal women
  breast cancer in, node-positive, chemotherapy/tamoxifen in, 64
Poudrage
  thoracoscopic talc, for pleurodesis for malignant effusions, 353
Prednisone
  in lymphoma
    B-cell, marginal zone, 211
    non-Hodgkin's, intermediate- and high-grade, in patients over 70, 207
Premalignant
  ovarian lesions, telomerase activity in, 30
Premenopausal
  women, breast cancer in
    node-positive, radiotherapy and chemotherapy for, 72

radiotherapy/chemotherapy in, 72
Progenitor cell
peripheral blood, mobilization and transplantation in non-Hodgkin's lymphoma, recombinant methionyl human stem cell factor and filgrastim for, 328
Prolymphocytic
leukemia, de novo B-cell, cladribine in, 199
Prostaglandins
colorectal mucosal, suppression of, 163
Prostate
biopsy results after interstitial brachytherapy in early prostate cancer, 112
cancer, 103
advanced, treatment for, immediate *vs.* deferred, 106
early, brachytherapy in, interstitial, biopsy results after, 112
early, patient-reported symptoms after primary therapy for, 103
localized, interstitial iodine-125 radiation in, 110
metastatic, previously untreated, suramin, leuprolide, and flutamide in, 107
orchiectomy for, osteoporosis after, 333
prostatectomy in, radical, nerve-sparing, patient-reported impotence and incontinence after, 104
radiotherapy for, bladder carcinoma and other second malignancies after, 339
radiotherapy in, goserelin after, 108
carcinoma *(see* cancer *above)*
tissue, vascular endothelial growth factor content in, regulation by androgens, 44
Prostatectomy
radical, in prostate cancer
early, patient-reported symptoms after, 103
nerve-sparing, patient-reported impotence and incontinence after, 104
Proton
therapy, potential role in pediatric medulloblastoma/primitive neuro-ectodermal tumors, 225
Protoporphyrin
IX, 5-aminolevulinic acid induced, fluorescence imaging and spectroscopy for detection of neoplastic lesions in oral cavity, 55
Pruritus
in Sézary syndrome, 211
Pterygopalatine
fossa infiltration in nasopharyngeal carcinoma, 245
Pulmonary
histology and residual masses after chemotherapy for metastatic testicular cancer, 134
toxicity of bleomycin-based combination chemotherapy in testicular cancer, 131

R

Radiation
biology
basic, 291
in brachytherapy, 291
damage to visceral and solid organs during radiation therapy of trunk, prevention of, 302
immune system recovery after, acceleration by hematopoietic cytokines (in mice), 19
iodine-125 interstitial, in localized prostate cancer, 110
mucositis, sucralfate for, trial results, 354
therapeutic (*see* Radiotherapy)
Radiochemotherapy (*see* Chemoradiation)
Radioimmunoguided
surgery for colorectal cancer, 329
Radioimmunotherapy
of xenografts of non-small cell lung carcinoma, advantage of residualizing iodine radiolabel for, 52
Radiolabel
iodine, for radioimmunotherapy of xenografts of non-small cell lung carcinoma, advantage of residualizing, 52
Radiologic
assessment for identification of stage A nonseminomatous testis cancer patients at extremely low risk for metastatic disease, 42
Radiotherapy
adjuvant, of sarcoma, extremity soft tissue, 267
of anal carcinoma, 143
basic, 291
of brain tumors, dose estimation to critical organs from vertex field in, 227
/chemotherapy (*see* Chemoradiation)

definitive, for T3 squamous cell carcinoma of glottic larynx, 250
diaphragmatic weakness as late complication of, bilateral, 342
dose escalation for non-small cell lung cancer, 298
external beam, combined with brachytherapy in high-grade soft tissue sarcomas of extremity with positive microscopic margin, 296
of extrapulmonary small cell carcinoma, 232
of face carcinoma, basal cell, 258
of Hodgkin's disease
in splenectomized patients, breast cancer risk after, 337
stage I, long-term outcome of, 222
hypofractionated, for invasive bladder cancer, 299
after hysterectomy for endometrial cancer, relationship of local and distant failure after, 87
intraoperative, with preoperative radiotherapy and resection for locally advanced rectal carcinoma, pelvic control and morbidity after, 144
of liposarcoma, outcome and prognostic factors after, 276
/lumpectomy for intraductal breast cancer, 80
after lumpectomy in ductal in situ breast carcinoma, 76
lymphatic, comprehensive, in low-grade non-Hodgkin's lymphoma, 220
lymphoid, subtotal, in clinical stage I to IIA Hodgkin's disease, 215
of lymphoma, marginal zone B-cell, 209
mantle field, breast cancer incidence after, 336
of nasopharyngeal carcinoma, 248
pelvic, with fluorouracil-modulated chemotherapy for rectal cancer, 164
postoperative, of rectal cancer
combined with radical surgery, 175
mobile, 172
preoperative, of rectal cancer
locally advanced, with resection and intraoperative radiotherapy, pelvic control and morbidity after, 144
with radical surgery, 304
resectable, 180
T3 and T4, long-term results of, 191
of prostate cancer
bladder carcinoma and other second malignancies after, 339
early, patient-reported symptoms after, 103
goserelin after, 108
repeat, palliative, for recurrent rectal cancer, 178
of rhabdomyosarcoma, 269
of seminoma
metastatic, after chemotherapy, 132
reproductive function after, 119
stage II, 122
thoracic
for childhood cancer, breast masses in women after, 61
surgical adjuvant, in non-small cell lung carcinoma with ipsilateral mediastinal node involvement, 234
of trunk, prevention of radiation damage to visceral and solid organs during, 302
vs. surgery, radical, for stage Ib-IIa cervical cancer, 100
Raf-1
activated, causes growth arrest in small cell lung cancer cells, 47
Reconstruction
microvascular, immediate, after resection for osteoradionecrosis of mandible, 244
of posterior oral cavity and oropharynx, comparison of cost and function in, 243
Rectum
cancer
(*See also* Colorectal, cancer)
locally advanced, pelvic control and morbidity after preoperative radiation therapy, resection, and intraoperative radiation therapy, 144
locally advanced, pelvic exenteration for, 139
mobile, surgery alone *vs.* surgery followed by radiotherapy for, 172
radiotherapy in, pelvic, fluorouracil-modulated chemotherapy combined with, 164
radiotherapy in addition to radical surgery in, 304
recurrent, aggressive surgical management of, is it worthwhile? 166
recurrent, reirradiation for, palliative, 178
resectable, preoperative radiotherapy in, 180
risk after abdominal colectomy in hereditary nonpolyposis colorectal cancer, 161

stage T3 and T4, long-term results of preoperative radiation therapy for, 191
surgery, effect on metachronous distant metastases and survival, 173
surgery, radical, combined with postoperative radiotherapy, 175
carcinoma *(see* Rectum, cancer *above)*
Reed-Sternberg cells
of Hodgkin's disease, fascin as marker for, 16
Reirradiation
palliative, for recurrent rectal cancer, 178
Renal
failure, acute, after suramin/leuprolide/flutamide in previously untreated metastatic prostate cancer, 107
toxicity after cisplatin/ifosfamide in advanced squamous carcinoma of cervix, 89
Reproductive
function after radiotherapy and orchidectomy in seminoma, 119
Retinoic acid
all-trans, in Philadelphia chromosome-positive chronic myelogenous leukemia, 201
Retroperitoneal
histology and residual masses after chemotherapy for metastatic testicular cancer, 134
sarcoma, prognostic factors associated with long-term survival for, 273
Rhabdomyosarcoma
radiotherapy for, 269
mRNA
hybridization of, in situ, for angiogenesis-related genes in ovarian carcinoma (in mice), 27
levels, Wilms' tumor gene, in acute myeloid leukemia, and long-term outcome, 18

S

Sarcoma, 261
retroperitoneal, prognostic factors associated with long-term survival for, 273
soft tissue
extremity, high-grade, with positive microscopic margin, effect of combined external beam radiotherapy and brachytherapy on, 296
extremity, local recurrence associated with subsequent survival in, 261
extremity, local recurrence in patients treated by initial unplanned resection for, impact of residual disease on, 262
extremity, radiation therapy in, adjuvant, 267
locally advanced, angiographic response after hyperthermic isolated limb perfusion with tumor necrosis factor, 271
resectable, localized, adjuvant chemotherapy for, 266
Scintimammography
technetium-99m sestamibi, detection of axillary node metastasis of breast carcinoma with, 41
Seminoma
chemotherapy of, residual mass after, 133
metastatic, radiotherapy after chemotherapy for, 132
radiotherapy and orchidectomy in, reproductive function after, 119
recurrent, salvage chemotherapy with vinblastine, ifosfamide, and cisplatin in, 129
stage II, management of, 122
Sentinel
lymph node (*see* Lymph node, sentinel)
lymphadenectomy in breast cancer, 82
Seroepidemiologic
study of papillomavirus infection as risk factor for invasive breast cancer, 10
Sestamibi
scintimammography, Tc-99m, detection of axillary node metastasis with, 41
Sexual
dysfunction
after primary therapy for early prostate cancer, 103
after prostatectomy, nerve-sparing radical, 104
Sézary syndrome
cutaneous histopathology of, 211
Sigmoidoscopy
importance of adenomas 5mm or less in diameter detected by, 183
Skeletal
complications prevented by pamidronate in patients with breast cancer and lytic bone metastases, 346
Skin
biopsy in Sézary syndrome, 211
cancer, 255
histopathology of Sézary syndrome, 211

Smears
Pap, abnormal, among low-income minority women, enhancing adherence after, 86
Smoke
tobacco, environmental, and lung cancer, 5
Smokers
bronchial epithelium of, molecular damage in, 3
Smoking
mitochondrial genome damage due to, 35
Sodium
phenylacetate, growth inhibitory effects on ovarian carcinoma cells, in vitro, 313
Soft tissue
sarcoma (*see* Sarcoma, soft tissue)
transfer, free *vs.* pedicled, in reconstruction of posterior oral cavity and oropharynx, 243
tumors, primary, CT and MRI in local staging of, 263
Solid organs
prevention of radiation damage to, during radiation therapy of trunk, 302
Solid tumor (*see* Tumor, solid)
Spectroscopy
fluorescence, of 5-aminolevulinic acid induced protoporphyrin IX for detection of neoplastic lesions in oral cavity, 55
Sphinxolides
microfilament depletion and circumvention of multiple drug resistance by, 307
Splenectomy
in leukemia, chronic lymphocytic, 197
patients undergoing radiation therapy for Hodgkin's disease, breast cancer risk after, 337
Squamous cell carcinoma
cervix, advanced
cisplatin alone *vs.* cisplatin/mitolactol *vs.* cisplatin/ifosfamide in, 89
TNP-470 in, 324
larynx, glottic, T3, definitive radiotherapy for, 250
Stem cell
factor, recombinant-methionyl human, with filgrastim for peripheral blood progenitor cell mobilization and transplantation in non-Hodgkin's lymphoma, 328
support, 279
transplantation (*see* Transplantation, stem cell)
Stomatitis
after doxorubicin, liposomal, in ovarian cancer, 97
after TNP-470 in squamous cell cancer of cervix, 324
Stress
immune responses after surgical treatment for regional breast cancer and, 74
Sucralfate
for radiation mucositis, trial results, 354
Suction
drainage, overnight closed, after axillary lymphadenectomy for breast cancer, 78
Sulfonamide
plus synergistic agents for nocardiosis after bone marrow transplantation, 335
Supportive care, 345
best, alone or with chemotherapy in advanced gastric cancer, 177
Suramin
/leuprolide/flutamide in prostate cancer, previously untreated metastatic, 107
Synergistic
agents plus sulfonamide for nocardiosis after bone marrow transplantation, 335

T

t(8;21) (q22;q22)
extramedullary leukemia adversely affects hematologic complete remission rate and survival in patients with, 203
Talc
poudrage pleurodesis, thoracoscopic, for malignant effusions, 353
Tamoxifen
in breast cancer, estrogen receptor-positive, response to, and HER-2 expression, 62
/chemotherapy in breast cancer
estrogen-receptor positive
node-negative, 63
node-positive postmenopausal, 64
T-cell(s)
circulating atypical, with cerebriform nuclei, in Sézary syndrome, 211
responses after surgical treatment for regional breast cancer, effect of stress on, 74

Tea
green, modulation of cancer chemotherapy by (in mice), 321
Technetium-99m
sestamibi scintimammography, detection of axillary node metastasis of breast carcinoma with, 41
Telephone
counseling to enhance adherence after abnormal Pap smears among low-income minority women, 86
Telomerase
activity
decline as measure of tumor cell killing by antineoplastic agents in vitro, 13
in ordinary meningiomas predicts poor outcome, 14
in ovarian lesions, malignant, premalignant, and benign, 30
in ovarian tumors, benign and malignant, 29
Testes
cancer
familial, prevalence of, 117
in situ, prevalence in oligozoospermic men from infertile couples, 137
metastatic, chemotherapy of, residual masses after, 134
nonseminomatous, good-prognosis, importance of bleomycin in combination chemotherapy for, 130
nonseminomatous, stage I, identification of patients at extremely low risk for metastasis from, 42
risk in boys with cryptorchidism, 118
survivors, long-term, risk of second malignancy among, 121
carcinoma *(see* cancer *above)*
seminoma (*see* Seminoma)
Therapy
complications of, 333
novel, 321
Thoracic
radiation therapy, surgical adjuvant, in non-small cell lung carcinoma with ipsilateral mediastinal node involvement, 234
radiotherapy for childhood cancer, breast masses in women after, 61
Thoracoscopic
talc poudrage pleurodesis for malignant effusions, 353
Thrombocytopenia
after paclitaxel/carboplatin in ovarian cancer, 317
after paclitaxel/topotecan in ovarian epithelial malignancies, 327
after suramin/leuprolide/flutamide in previously untreated metastatic prostate cancer, 107
after topotecan in resistant ovarian cancer, 94
Tissue
prostatic, vascular endothelial growth factor content in, regulation by androgens, 44
soft (*see* Soft tissue)
TNP-470
in cervix cancer, advanced squamous cell, 324
Tobacco
smoke, environmental, and lung cancer, 5
Tomography
computed
in diagnostic workup for suspected pancreatic carcinoma, 162
in local staging of primary malignant musculoskeletal neoplasms, 263
in lymph node staging in non-small cell lung cancer, 50
in melanoma evaluation, stage III, 257
positron emission, FDG, in lymph node staging in non-small cell lung cancer, 48
vs. CT, 50
Topoisomerase IIα
levels, effect of topotecan and etoposide on (in mice), 309
Topotecan
increases topoisomerase IIα levels and sensitivity to treatment with etoposide in schedule-dependent process (in mice), 309
oral, for solid tumors in adults, phase I and pharmacologic study of, 310
in ovarian cancer, platinum- and paclitaxel-resistant, 93
/palictaxel in ovarian epithelial malignancies, phase I and pharmacologic trial of, 327
vs. paclitaxel for recurrent epithelial ovarian cancer, 91
Toxicity
CNS, after cisplatin/ifosfamide in advanced squamous carcinoma of cervix, 89
of docetaxel/cisplatin in advanced solid tumors, 312
hematologic
after paclitaxel/topotecan in ovarian epithelial malignancies, 327

after topotecan in resistant ovarian cancer, 94
neurotoxicity, cerebellar, after oral carboxyamidotriazole, 326
pulmonary, of bleomycin-based combination chemotherapy in testicular cancer, 131
renal, after cisplatin/ifosfamide in advanced squamous carcinoma of cervix, 89
of TNP-470 in squamous cell cancer of cervix, 324
Transaminases
elevated, after suramin/leuprolide/flutamide in previously untreated metastatic prostate cancer, 107
Transfusion
granulocyte, in *Fusarium* infections in hematologic cancer patients, 335
platelet, prophylactic, during induction therapy for adult acute leukemia, 349
Transplantation
bone marrow, 279
allogeneic, for leukemia, chronic myeloid, effect of plasma busulfan levels on outcome, 281
allogeneic, fungal infections after, invasive, incidence and risk factors for, 279
allogeneic, *vs.* allogeneic blood stem cell transplantation in hematologic malignancies, hematopoietic recovery after, 283
autologous, for hematologic malignancies, effect of age on outcome after, 282
nocardiosis after, 335
unrelated donor, matched, for chronic myeloid leukemia, effect of HLA class II matching on, 280
progenitor cell, peripheral blood, in non-Hodgkin's lymphoma, recombinant methionyl human stem cell factor and filgrastim for peripheral blood cell mobilization in, 328
stem cell
allogeneic, *vs.* allogeneic bone marrow transplantation in hematologic malignancies, hematopoietic recovery after, 283
autologous, for ovarian cancer, persistent/relapsed, with high-dose chemotherapy, 286
autologous, in Hodgkin's disease, relapsing, prognostic factors for survival after, 288
autologous, tandem, superiority over standard therapy for previously untreated multiple myeloma, 284
Transurethral
resection of bladder for muscle infiltrating carcinoma of bladder, long-term follow-up, 120
Trials
clinical, of cancer therapy, clinicians' attitudes toward, 322
Truncal
ataxia after TNP-470 in squamous cell cancer of cervix, 324
Trunk
radiation therapy of, prevention of radiation damage to visceral and solid organs during, 302
Tumor(s)
brain, 227
vertex field treatment of, dose estimation to critical organs from, 227
cell(s)
killing by antineoplastic agents in vitro, telomerase activity decline as measure of, 13
sensitivity to CPT-11, effect of overexpression of rabbit liver carboxylesterase on, 311
germ cell, metastatic, poor-prognosis nonseminomatous, intensive induction-sequential chemotherapy for, 135
musculoskeletal, primary malignant, CT and MRI in local staging of, 263
necrosis factor, hyperthermic isolated limb perfusion with, angiographic response of locally advanced soft tissue sarcoma after, 271
neuro-ectodermal, primitive, potential role of proton therapy in, 225
ovaries
epithelial, benign, telomerase activity in, 29
granulosa cell, serum inhibin and disease status in, 23
solid
adult, oral topotecan in, phase I and pharmacologic study of, 310
advanced, docetaxel and cisplatin in, phase I and pharmacologic study of, 312
pediatric, 225

Wilms' tumor gene mRNA levels in acute myeloid leukemia, and long-term outcome, 18

U

Ultrasound
localization of lumpectomy cavity for interstitial brachytherapy of breast, 79
Urinary
genitourinary cancer, 115
incontinence
after primary therapy for early prostate cancer, in elderly, 103
after prostatectomy, nerve-sparing radical, 104
Urothelium
cancer, metastatic, previously untreated, gemcitabine in, 128
carcinoma, advanced, paclitaxel/carboplatin in, 127

V

Vascular
endothelial growth factor (*see* Growth, factor, vascular endothelial)
intravascular coagulation, disseminated, after suramin/leuprolide/flutamide in previously untreated metastatic prostate cancer, 107
permeability factor expression and progression of ovarian carcinoma (in mice), 27
Veno-occlusive
disease of liver after busulfan in marrow transplantation for chronic myeloid leukemia, 281–282
Vertex
field treatment of brain tumors, dose estimation to critical organs from, 227
Vertigo
after TNP-470 in squamous cell cancer of cervix, 324
Vessel
counts as prognostic factor in node-negative colon cancer, 157
Video
-assisted wedge resection *vs.* lobectomy for stage I non-small cell lung cancer, 237
Vinblastine
in Hodgkin's disease, 215
in seminoma, recurrent, 129
Vincristine
in germ cell tumor, poor-prognosis metastatic nonseminomatous, 135
in lymphoma
B-cell, marginal zone, 211
non-Hodgkin's, intermediate- and high-grade, in patients over 70, 207
with stem cell transplantation, tandem autologous, for multiple myeloma, 284
Virus
papillomavirus infection as risk factor for invasive cervical cancer, 10
Visceral
organs, prevention of radiation damage to, during radiation therapy of trunk, 302
Vomiting (*see* Emesis)
Vortex
keratopathy after suramin/leuprolide/flutamide in previously untreated metastatic prostate cancer, 107

W

Weakness
after TNP-470 in squamous cell cancer of cervix, 324
Weight
loss after suramin/leuprolide/flutamide in previously untreated metastatic prostate cancer, 107
Wilms' tumor
gene mRNA levels in acute myeloid leukemia, and long-term outcome, 18
Women
minority, low-income, enhancing adherence after abnormal Pap smears among, 86
postmenopausal, chemotherapy/tamoxifen in node-positive breast cancer in, 64
premenopausal, breast cancer in
node-positive, radiotherapy and chemotherapy for, 72
radiotherapy/chemotherapy in, 72

Wound
complications
in soft tissue sarcomas of extremity with positive microscopic margin, high-grade, effect of combined external beam radiotherapy and brachytherapy on, 296
wt1
mRNA levels in acute myeloid leukemia, and long-term outcome, 18

X

Xenografts
of lung carcinoma, non-small cell, advantage of residualizing iodine radiolabel for radioimmunotherapy of, 52

Author Index

A

Abbruzzese JL, 169
Adams JF, 337
Aghajanian C, 319
Ahmad NR, 178, 191
Ahsan H, 339
Alekhteyar KM, 296
Allemann F, 50
Altendorf-Hofmann A, 173
Ambrogi V, 239
Anaissie EJ, 334
Andersen BL, 74
Andersen JE, 314
Anderson S, 68
Anttila V-J, 200
Arbitrio M, 19
Argatoff LH, 208
Arikian S, 90
Arimori K, 54
Arnaud JP, 175
Arnott SJ, 172
Arthur DC, 203
Astoul P, 353
Auperin A, 258
Avilés A, 209
Avril M-F, 258

B

Baas P, 330
Bailar JC III, 1
Bailey HH, 325
Baker AR, 267
Baker SD, 327
Ballinger SW, 45
Balshem AM, 168
Barlogie B, 284
Bartoli C, 256
Bastion Y, 214
Bastos E, 22
Bayer R, 286
Beard CJ, 144
Beckurts KTE, 147
Behrens C, 3
Benko FA, 21
Bennett CJ, 217
Berchuck A, 22
Berger F, 214
Bergmann L, 18
Berlin J, 326
Bertelsen K, 314
Bilker WB, 58
Bines SD, 146
Birnbaum EH, 166
Bishop MR, 283
Björge T, 10
Black WC, 35, 77
Blasko JC, 110
Blessing JA, 89
Bogart JA, 337
Boggess JF, 23
Bokey EL, 149
Bonadonna G, 70
Bonner JA, 234
Bono A, 256
Borg A, 8
Bosset JF, 175
Bouabdallah R, 288
Bouder TG, 45
Boutati EI, 334
Brambilla C, 70
Brander PE, 342
Brennan M, 82
Brennan MF, 152, 296
Brenner DJ, 291
Brice P, 288
Brunetto VL, 97
Buckner CD, 281
Bukowski R, 350
Burke EC, 156
Burke W, 36, 190
Butterly LF, 183
Byhardt RW, 108
Byrd JC, 203

C

Caplan R, 108
Caranto JF, 292
Carmichael J, 91
Castiglione-Gertsch M, 64
Chang AE, 267
Cheng C-W, 227
Chong VFH, 245
Chontos AJ, 83
Chung CT, 337
Ciocca D, 62
Clark JA, 103
Clemente C, 256
Clift RA, 281
Coit DG, 257
Collins CD, 299
Colombo A, 100
Conlon KC, 156
Connor TMF, 53
Connors JM, 208
Cooper MR, 107
Cordeiro PG, 244
Corn BW, 87
Cortes J, 201
Cox C, 198
Cramer DW, 7
Crawford M, 95
Creemers GJ, 310
Crispens MA, 27
Curtis RE, 121
Cusack JD, 197

D

D'Agostino R Jr, 87
Daniell HW, 333
Danks MK, 311
Das IJ, 227
Davies AP, 24
Davis AM, 262
Davis CS, 349
Davis GS, 45
Dawson NA, 107
Debernardis D, 318
DeBiose DA, 79
De Feudis P, 318
Dekker AW, 202
Deleyiannis F W-B, 243
Delgado S, 209
De Los Santos JF, 220
Denmeade SR, 44
de Nully Brown P, 205
Desyatnikova SS, 243
Devergie A, 280
de Wit R, 130
Dieckmann K-P, 117
Dignam J, 63, 80
Dillner J, 10
Doerr TD, 247
Donohue JH, 155
Doolas A, 146
Driscoll DL, 187
Duchesne GM, 132
Duggan BD, 29

E

Eckardt JR, 310
Eisenhauer EA, 99
Ekström K, 177
Elledge RM, 62
Elonen E, 200
Errante D, 207
Evans WK, 67

F

Fallowfield L, 322
Fan Y-F, 245

Faraoni I, 13
Farrar WB, 74
Fein DA, 227
Fenger C, 184
Fennelly D, 319
Ferrandina G, 313
Figg WD, 107
Finkelstein SD, 194
Fisher B, 63, 68, 80
Fleming GF, 327
Fonseca R, 76
Fortunato L, 159
Fossa S, 135
Fosså SD, 125
Foster RS, 42
Frasca D, 19
Freeman H, 32
Friend WG, 329
Frost DB, 151
Frytak S, 231
Fuller LM, 222

G

Galanis E, 231
Galimberti V, 75
Garden AS, 248
Gathright JB Jr, 170
Gatsonis C, 263
Gayther SA, 25
Geara FB, 248
Gelb Safran D, 2
Gerrits CJH, 310
Giacco GG, 139
Giuliano AE, 82
Giwercman A, 137
Glasgow RE, 140
Glaspy J, 350
Glimelius B, 177, 304
Gloor B, 162
Goff BA, 23
Goldenberg DM, 52
Golden-Kreutz D, 74
Gong G, 33
Gonin R, 129
Gordon MS, 328
Gordon NH, 309
Gordon W JR, 119
Gore M, 91
Gornik HL, 1
Gospodarowicz M, 122
Goswitz MS, 276
Gould PM, 234
Green S, 62
Greenberg P, 198
Grimm PD, 110, 112
Guhlmann A, 48
Guidi F, 19

H

Habib FA, 255
Hackman RC, 335
Hackshaw AK, 5
Hagemeister FB, 222
Hainsworth JD, 96
Hanfelt JJ, 269
Hansen K, 194
Harlan LC, 85
Harlow BL, 7
Harrison LE, 152
Hart MJ, 329
Hartmann LC, 76
Hauser M, 50
Hazuka MB, 298
Heckman KD, 349
Hertz J, 137
Heslin M, 261
Heslin MJ, 273
Hicks ML, 6
Hidalgo DA, 244
Higgins CD, 118
Hirota S, 321
Hoak DC, 112
Hoekstra HJ, 271
Hoffman JP, 159
Hoffman K, 177
Hölscher AH, 147
Hoppe RT, 215
Horning SJ, 215
Hortobagyi GN, 346
Horwich A, 125, 133
Horwitz EM, 79
Huang S, 151
Hudson MM, 61
Huerta-Guzmán J, 209
Huizing MT, 316
Hutson P, 326

I

Iborra I, 120
Isacsson U, 304
Itnyre J, 33

J

Jackson SM, 72
Jacobs IJ, 24
Jagannath S, 284
Jakobsen A, 314
Jamison RL, 155
Jantunen E, 279
Järvinen V, 342
Jeffers S, 96
Jenkins L, 146
Jessup JM, 144
Jóhansson OT, 8
Johnson DE, 168
Jones DJ, 61
Jones RC, 82
Joseph IBJK, 44
Jung B, 304

K

Kandel RA, 262
Kantarjian H, 201
Karnell LH, 142
Karpeh MS Jr, 156
Kaste SC, 61
Kaye SB, 130, 135
Kennedy BJ, 186
Kerger C, 286
Kerlikowske K, 34
Khalkhali I, 41
Kim HK, 144
Kim R, 354
Kim RY, 292
Kirk D, 106
Kitadai Y, 157
Kjeldsen BJ, 184
Klasa RJ, 208
Klein EE, 336
Klijn J, 351
Kling KM, 69
Knudson CM, 53
Köckerling F, 173
Köln, 147
Kopecky KK, 42
Kopreski MS, 21
Kotzerke J, 48
Krasne DL, 39
Krishnan K, 163
Kronborg O, 184
Kudelka AP, 324
Kuniyasu H, 27
Kurtz C, 257
Kusnierz-Glaz CR, 282
Kuvshinoff BW, 257
Kuzel T, 128
Kwee C, 21
Kyo S, 30

L

Lam S, 3
Lanciano RM, 87
Landoni F, 100
Landreneau RJ, 237
Langford LA, 14
Langhoff E, 16

Law MR, 5
Le N, 72
Le TH, 170
LeBeau MM, 198
Lee CG, 302
Lee JE, 169
Lee T, 199
Leer J-WH, 299
Lehmann M, 345
Lehtinen M, 10
Leibovitch I, 42
Leong SPL, 255
Lerner SA, 197
Leung D, 261
Leung DH, 296
Leunig A, 55
Levy T, 324
Lewis JJ, 261, 273
Li W-Z, 29
Lingareddy V, 178
Liu CD, 78
Lloyd RV, 231
Loehrer PJ, 129
Loercher A, 313
Lohela P, 342
Lomax A, 225
Loprinzi CL, 233
Loret de Mola JR, 58
Lucha PA Jr, 174
Lynch JW Jr, 217, 220

M

Mack MJ, 237
Maher DP, 83
Malkowicz SB, 127
Manayan RC, 329
Mancuso AA, 250
Mandelblatt J, 32
Maneo A, 100
Margulis A, 258
Martinez AA, 79
Marunick MT, 247
Masci G, 13
Mason J, 215
Maurer U, 18
McCurrach ME, 53
McFadden DW, 78
McGuire W, 90
McKenna K, 166
McLeod RS, 150
McMahon M, 47
Mead GM, 115, 135
Melichar B, 313
Menck HR, 142
Mendenhall NP, 217, 220
Mendenhall WM, 250
Menzin AW, 58
Meredith R, 354
Mermillod B, 239
Meterissian SH, 139
Miething C, 18
Miller KD, 129
Miller SM, 86
Miloro SM, 187
Minale L, 307
Miralbell R, 225
Mohiuddin M, 178
Moller P, 141
Moore JWE, 149
Moreau P, 288
Morton CL, 311
Moskowitz CH, 328
Muggia FM, 96
Mulcahy HE, 158
Mulvhill SJ, 140
Muñoz KA, 85
Murrer L, 330
Mutch DG, 93
Myerson RJ, 142

N

Nadeem SQ, 335
Nadler E, 273
Nagle D, 191
Nagorney DM, 155
Nelson JB, 44
Nelstrop AE, 95
Neugut AI, 339
Neugut AL, 90
Newman E, 152
Niskanen L, 279
Nordling S, 200
Nordlinger B, 175
Norman A, 133

O

O'Brien S, 201
O'Connell MJ, 164
Ogunbiyi OA, 166
Olenwine JA, 174
Olieman AFT, 271
Ollila DW, 39
Omura GA, 89
Orchard GE, 211
O'Reilly S, 327
Ostrzega N, 69
Overgaard M, 72

P

Paganelli G, 75
Påhlman L, 180
Paluchowska B, 133
Panicek DM, 263
Panzarella T, 122
Pareek PN, 292
Parham G, 6
Paridaens R, 351
Parsons JT, 250
Patchett SE, 158
Pavletic ZS, 283
Pawlik CA, 311
Pendurthi TK, 168
Perez EA, 233
Petersen IA, 76
Petroni GR, 164
Philip T, 345
Philipson BM, 149
Phillips JL, 6
Phillips K, 34
Piatyszek MA, 14
Piccart MJ, 351
Pichlmeier U, 117
Pike MC, 118
Pilepich MV, 108
Pinkus GS, 16
Pinkus JL, 16
Planting AST, 312
Pollack A, 276
Prestidge BR, 112
Pricolo VE, 194
Pronk LC, 312
Propert KJ, 104

R

Rader JS, 93
Ragaz J, 72
Ragde H, 110
Ranstam J, 8
Ratcliffe D, 322
Ratzer ER, 83
Ravi RK, 47
Ray-Coquard I, 345
Read JD, 183
Read TE, 183
Reber HA, 162
Rey F, 353
Reymond MA, 173
Ricós JV, 120
Richard CS, 150
Rick K, 55
Ricós JV, 120
Rieker P, 103, 104
Ripple G, 325

Ritter EF, 302
Robert JH, 239
Robertson JM, 298
Robinson E, 339
Rock CL, 163
Rodríguez-Bigas MA, 161
Roila F, 348
Rosen L, 174
Rosenthal DI, 263
Rosing H, 316
Roth B, 128
Rowe VL, 151
Ruffin MT IV, 163
Ruishu XU, 14
Russell P, 25
Russo M, 225
Rustin GJS, 95
Ruutu P, 279

S

Sadzuka Y, 321
Salter M, 354
Salzmann P, 34
Sanguineti G, 248
Saven A, 199
Sawyer TE, 234
Schellens JHM, 312
Schildkraut JM, 22
Schlegel PG, 282
Schlutz M, 199
Schmit P, 69
Scholten AN, 299
Schroeder CM, 86
Schulze S, 141
Schwartz LM, 35
Sebban C, 214
Seto TB, 2
Seymour JF, 197
Shaha AR, 244
Shapiro F, 319
Shepherd FA, 67
Siegmund K, 119
Siejak KK, 86
Siré EG, 318
Skates S, 24
Skibber JM, 139
Slattery JT, 281
Sleijfer DT, 125
Sloan JA, 233
Solsona E, 120
Souhami R, 322
Soules MR, 23
Spitz FR, 169
Stadler WM, 128
Stage JG, 141
Stanisic TH, 119
Stein R, 52
Steinberg D, 350
Steinert HC, 50
Steinmetz I, 255
Stepp H, 55
Stewart DJ, 67
Steyerberg EW, 134
Stiff P, 328
Stiff PJ, 286
Storck M, 48
Storm H, 121
Stoter G, 130
Stratton JF, 25
Stratton MR, 37
Sugarbaker DJ, 237
Sugiyama T, 321
Swerdlow AJ, 118
Swisher EM, 93

T

Taira DA, 2
Takahashi Y, 157
Takakura M, 30
Talcott JA, 103, 104
Tanaka M, 30
Tarantolo SR, 283
Tefft MC, 269
ten Bokkel Huinink W, 91
Ten Haken RK, 298
Tepper JE, 164
Thomsen JK, 137
Thorban ST, 147
Thorpe SR, 52
Thottassery JV, 54
Tierney JF, 266
Tilly H, 213
Timmcke AE, 170
Tinger A, 336
Tirelli U, 207
Titus-Ernstoff L, 7
Todd KE, 162
Tolmos J, 41
Toner M, 158
Travis LB, 121
Trimble EL, 85
Trotter MJ, 211
Tsue TT, 243
Tucker SL, 157
Turner RR, 39
Turriziani M, 13
Tutsch KD, 325, 326
Tyler D, 302

V

Vaccarello L, 89
Valagussa P, 70
van Burik J-A, 335
van Ginkel RJ, 271
van Glabbecke M, 99
Van Glabbeke M, 207
van Warmerdam LJC, 316
Vargas H, 41
Vaughn DJ, 127
Vermorken JB, 99
Veronesi U, 75
Verschraegen CF, 324
Vesole DH, 284
Viallat J-R, 353
Vlachaki MT, 222
Volpe CM, 187

W

Wald NJ, 5
Wan M, 29
Wanebo HJ, 186
Warde P, 122
Wasserman TH, 336
Weber E, 47
Weiner GJ, 349
Weiss RB, 203
Welch HG, 77
Wharam MD, 269
Whitacre CM, 309
Whittaker SJ, 211
Whittemore AS, 33
Wickerham DL, 68
Williams L, 97
Winchester DP, 186
Winczewski D, 32
Wistuba II, 3
Wolmark N, 63, 80
Woloshin S, 35
Wong RM, 282
Wunder JS, 262

Y

Yang JC, 267
Yeh KA, 159
Yoneda J, 27
Yordan E, 97

Z

Zagars GK, 276
Zambetti GP, 54
Zampella A, 307
Zborowska E, 309
Zhang X, 307
Zoetmulder FAN, 330
Zoltick B, 127